STATISTICAL AND PROCESS MODELS
FOR
COGNITIVE NEUROSCIENCE AND AGING

The Notre Dame Series
on Quantitative Methodology

Building on the strength of Notre Dame as a center for training in quantitative psychology, the Notre Dame Series on Quantitative Methodology (NDSQM) offers advanced training in quantitative methods for social and behavioral research. Leading experts in data analytic techniques provide instruction in state–of–the–art methods designed to enhance quantitative skills in a selected substantive domain.

Each volume evolved from an annual conference that brings together expert methodologists and a workshop audience of substantive researchers. The substantive researchers are challenged with innovative techniques and the methodologists are challenged by innovative applications. The goal of each conference is to stimulate an emergent substantive and methodological synthesis, enabling the solution of existing problems and bringing forth the realization of new questions that need to be asked. The resulting volumes are targeted towards researchers in a specific substantive area, but also contain innovative techniques of interest to pure methodologists.

The books in the series are:

- *Methodological issues in aging research*, co-edited by Cindy S. Bergeman and Steven M. Boker (2006)

- *Statistical and process models for cognitive neuroscience and aging*, co-edited by Michael J. Wenger and Christof Schuster (2006)

STATISTICAL AND PROCESS MODELS
FOR
COGNITIVE NEUROSCIENCE AND AGING

Edited by

Michael J. Wenger
The Pennsylvania State University

Christof Schuster
Justus-Liebig-Universität Giessen, Germany

LAWRENCE ERLBAUM ASSOCIATES, PUBLISHERS
2007   Mahwah, New Jersey   London

Camera ready copy for this book was provided by the editors.

Lawrence Erlbaum Associates, Inc., Publishers
10 Industrial Avenue
Mahwah, New Jersey 07430
www.erlbaum.com

Cover design by Kathryn Houghtaling Lacey

For cip information for this volume please contact the Library of Congress

ISBN 978-0-8058-5413-8 — 0-8058-5413-4 (cloth)
ISBN 978-0-8058-5414-5 — 0-8058-5414-2 (pbk.)
ISBN 978-1-4106-1401-8 — 1-4106-1401-8 (e book)

Books published by Lawrence Erlbaum Associates are printed on acid-free paper, and their bindings are chosen for strength and durability.

Printed in the United States of America
10 9 8 7 6 5 4 3 2 1

Contents

Preface

Michael J. Wenger
The Pennsylvania State University

Christof Schuster
Justus-Liebig-Universität Giessen

Age-related changes in cognitive abilities have gained increased attention in recent years, reflecting the concerns of a population that is living longer than was the case even a few decades ago. Although questions regarding age-related changes in cognitive function are being pursued from a variety of complementary perspectives—specifically, cognitive neuroscience, computational and mathematical modeling, and traditional biobehavioral assessment—the majority of the research being performed is conducted within disciplinary boundaries.

Over the past several decades, three significant changes relevant to quantitative scientists have taken place in areas related to the study of cognitive processes and cognitive aging. First, traditional behavioral and physiological methods have been augmented by the methods of cognitive neuroscience, particularly those related to brain imaging, and these methods have revealed a set of important challenges for statistical analysis and modeling. Second, the theoretical languages for discussing age-related changes in cognition have been augmented by the inclusion of formal (mathematical, algorithmic, and computational) models of the cognitive processes under study (e.g., memory, categorization, etc.), with one important class being neural network models. Third, it has become critically important to consider both the complexity and flexibility of formal models and the inherent complexity of the patterns predicted or accounted for by those models in evaluating the link between formal models and the types of data that are obtained in the newer experimental methods. This confluence of changes presents significant challenges to both quantitative professionals and subject-matter experts.

The present volume is a second in a series of volumes, all originating in a set of intensive workshops and seminars held at the University of Notre Dame, intended to bring together significant contributions from a range of disciplines, with all relevant to the goal of furthering research in cognitive aging. The scope of this volume is, by design, quite broad. Our intent in bringing together the contributions contained in this volume was to expose researchers working on a range of issues associated with cognitive aging to approaches, accomplishments, and technologies of which they might not otherwise be aware, thereby helping to cross disciplinary boundaries. Thus, each of the contributors faced the somewhat daunting task of crafting presentations and (ultimately) chapters describing sophisticated and complex work that could be read by working scientists from outside their field of expertise. We believe that readers of the chapters in this volume will find that all of the contributors produced both exceptional and accessible works.

The book is intended for scientists and advanced students in any of the areas associated with cognitive and behavioral neuroscience. The methods presented here are, in the best tradition of psychonomic and psychometric modeling, intended to illustrate general principles and approaches. Consequently, we believe the chapters will have interest to behavioral neuroscientists, gerontologists, and developmental and cognitive psychologists, as well as to computational neuroscientists, psychometricians, and computational and mathematical modelers.

The volume begins with Edland and Petersen's overview (Chapter 1) of work on cognitive aging, mild cognitive impairment, and Alzheimer's disease. This chapter provides a summary of clinical research in these areas and emphasizes the critical role that psychometrics, in a range of applications, has played in advancing this particular field. This chapter provides a context for all the work that follows, in that the research challenges (and accomplishments) it describes offer important targets for application of the methods and models that are described in the remaining chapters.

Ashby and Valentin (Chapter 2) follow with a chapter that begins a series of looks at formal and computational modeling of *mechanisms* in cognitive neuroscience at a variety of levels of analysis. Ashby and Valentin outline an algorithm for the process of developing computational models that are grounded in the biophysics and structure of the nervous system. They illustrate this algorithm with a set of applications drawn from the extensive body of work produced in their laboratory. Hasselmo, McGaughy, and Linster (Chapter 3) follow with a chapter detailing their innovative and important investigations of acetylcholine and hippocampal theta rhythm in tasks that are critically dependent on memory. Along with presenting a number of critical insights, this chapter nicely illustrates how formal modeling allows numerous levels of analysis to be integrated in pursuit of a research question. Similarly, Murre, Meeter, and Chessa (Chapter 3) brings together multiple levels of analysis, with the focus being their long-term project of modeling a variety of memory deficits. They present work aimed at understanding the mechanisms of a set of important memory phenomena, including Alzheimer's, semantic, and Korsakoff's dementia. Rounding out the set of chapters on formal and computational models is the contribution from Keinan, Kaufman, Hilgetag, Meilijson, and Ruppin (Chapter 5). This work gives an overview of a novel application of fundamental concepts from game theory to the question of understanding how the components of biological neural networks function together in the support of cognitive behavior.

Quantitative work in cognitive neuroscience is not limited to models of mechanisms. As such, Cichocki (Chapter 6) begins the series of contributions focusing on models for *data*. He presents a careful, detailed tutorial on the blind source signal separation and generalized component analysis, and he illustrates the use of these methods in the context of early detection of Alzheimer's disease. Ferree, Kramer, McGonigle, and Hwa (Chapter 7) follow with a chapter on the scaling properties of EEG and MEG signals, as continuous time series. This chapter includes a discussion of the important role of detrended fluctuation analysis with these types of biophysical data. The volume closes with Jung and Lee's (Chapter 8) discussion of the use of independent components analysis with EEG data, placing this work in the broader context of applications of signal decomposition methods.

This volume documents what was an exceptional opportunity to bring together an internationally-recognized group of scholars for tutorial presentations and discussions. Our contributors came from North America, Japan, Europe, and Israel, and represent what we believe is some of the finest and most sophisticated work being done in this broad and important field. The volume would, of course, not have been possible without their involvement, and we as editors wish to offer our sincere thanks for all of their efforts.

The workshop was funded in part by a grant from the National Institute on Aging (1 R13 AG023103-01) and from an internal grant from the Graduate School and the Institute for Scholarship in the Liberal Arts at the University of Notre Dame. Special thanks are due to Rebecca Bickelhaupt, who provided an exceptional level of assistance to our visitors. We are also appreciative of all of the assistance provided by Connie Dosmann at the University of Notre Dame's Center for Continuing Education, the site of the workshop. Finally, we wish to thank our colleagues in the Quantitative Area of the Psychology Department at Notre Dame—Cindy Bergeman, Steve Boker, Scott Maxwell, and Ke-Hai Yuan—for their support in pulling this effort together.

1

Longitudinal Study in Cognition and Aging

Steven D. Edland and Ronald C. Petersen
Alzheimer's Disease Research Center, Mayo Clinic College of Medicine

Neuropsychometric data are integral to research in cognitive aging and Alzheimer's disease. Neuropsychometric data are required for a research diagnosis of Alzheimer's disease, are obtained as a matter of course in longitudinal studies of aging and dementia, and have been an integral component of thousands of publications on cognitive aging and Alzheimer's disease. This chapter provides some background on research in cognitive aging and Alzheimer's disease that may be relevant to quantitative psychology. The initial section provides a review of current clinical research activities in Alzheimer's disease, focusing on investigations of mildly cognitively impaired patients. The second section provides a historic overview of uses of neuropsychometric data in Alzheimer's disease research and explores possible areas for new research. It is hoped that this review stimulates interest among quantitative psychologists in Alzheimer's disease research.

1.1 CLINICAL CHARACTERIZATION

The study of aging and dementia can be approached from two perspectives: a clinical or patient oriented research approach and a basic science approach. The clinical approach proposes to study the diagnostic features of a variety of clinical conditions and characterize them longitudinally.

In current research on aging and dementia, increasing attention is being paid to identifying individuals at the earliest stage of cognitive impairment. As such, much of our work at Mayo Clinic College of

1

Medicine has focused on the condition known as mild cognitive impairment (MCI) as a means of moving the diagnostic threshold for Alzheimer's disease back to an earlier point in the disease process. We also do a great deal of neuroimaging research on these individuals.

On the basic science side of the research program, investigators are studying genetic predispositions and biomarkers and developing drugs for intervention at an early stage in the disease process. Ultimately, we hope to be able to bring these two lines of research together to enable us to identify the earliest features of the disease and intervene with effective therapeutics.

We tend to view MCI as an intermediate stage between the cognitive changes of normal aging and what constitutes the cognitive features of very early Alzheimer's disease. This transitional state is characterized by the following criteria:

1. Cognitive complaint, usually confirmed by an informant;

2. Cognitive impairment, usually memory impairment, for age;

3. General preservation of cognition in other non-memory domains;

4. Largely preserved activities of daily living; and

5. Does not meet criteria for dementia or Alzheimer's disease.

These criteria have been used to study many aspects of the aging continuum.

As mentioned, much of our work has focused on structural neuroimaging. In particular, we have demonstrated that subjects with MCI have volumetric appearances of the entorhinal cortex, hippocampal formation, whole brain and ventricular volumes which are intermediate between normal aging and mild Alzheimer's disease. These structures have been characterized both cross-sectionally and longitudinally and have been shown to be useful in predicting which subjects will progress to Alzheimer's disease most rapidly (Jack, Petersen, O'Brien, Smith & Ivnik, 2000).

We have also studied a large group of normal community-dwelling individuals who have been followed for up to 15 years. Most of these subjects have remained normal and have exhibited slight changes in cognition over the years. However, a subset has declined over this time frame and has transitioned into diagnoses of MCI or Alzheimer's disease. One subset of these individuals was a group of 874 normal subjects who were enrolled and evaluated on at least one additional occasion to allow them to have the opportunity to convert to MCI or Alzheimer's disease. The mean age of these subjects was 78.6 years, and they had a mean of 13.2 years of education. The median follow-up for this group was 4.8 years, and the mean Mini-Mental State Exam (MMSE) score at enrollment was 28.1. Over this time frame, 122 of these subjects progressed to dementia or MCI.

Using these data we have investigated whether there are variables that predict progression to MCI or Alzheimer's disease. We entered a large number of variables into a multivariate prediction equation and assessed the relative contribution of each of these predictors. Many of the measures of cognition, including primarily memory measures, were significant predictors of conversion in univariate analyses. When all of the positive univariate measures were put into a multivariate Cox model to predict MCI or Alzheimer's disease, five factors remained statistically significant predictors: age, apolipoprotein E (apoE) genotype, the Short Test of Mental Status, the Auditory Verbal Learning Test, measure of delayed recall, and the Free and Cued Selective Reminding Test, a measure of the effectiveness of cues. When the same approach was used to predict conversion to MCI or any form of dementia, the results were somewhat similar with the following measures remaining in the model: age, apoE genotype, Mini-Mental State Exam, Global Deterioration Scale, Auditory Verbal Learning Test-Delayed Recall, and Free and Cued Selective Reminding Test-Learning Measure. These are essentially the same parameters in the previous model, with the addition of the Global Deterioration Scale, indicating that the additional factor here concerns the subject's awareness of a subjective memory problem. That is, those individuals who reported a memory problem tended to convert more rapidly than those who did not.

From this work, we concluded that despite the fact that these individuals are normal at the time of enrollment in the study, certain demographic and cognitive measures do predict who is going to progress to MCI or Alzheimer's disease. These measures included age, a genetic factor (apoE), a measure of general cognition (the Short Test of Mental Status), and two measures of memory function—one for learning and one for delayed recall. As such, these measures can be used to predict who will be evolving to MCI and Alzheimer's disease and may be useful for guiding intervention decisions.

Ultimately, this research is designed to develop a profile of individuals who are at risk for developing MCI or Alzheimer's disease in the future. Hopefully, our colleagues in the basic science laboratories will be able to develop biomarkers to mirror this research process and ultimately to develop interventions that prevent Alzheimer's disease before it begins.

1.2 NEUROPSYCHOMETRIC DATA IN ALZHEIMER'S RESEARCH

1.2.1 Natural history of Alzheimer's disease described neuropsychometrically

The progression from normal cognitive function to MCI, and ultimately clinical dementia, can be tracked using neuropsychometric instruments. For example, the CERAD battery of neuropsychometric instruments (Welsh, Butters, Moh, Beekly, Edland & Fillenbaum, 1994) has been used to follow the progression of Alzheimer's disease longitudinally in a number of studies. The CERAD battery includes a global cognitive function test (the Mini-Mental State Exam, MMSE; Folstein, Folstein & McHugh, 1975), and instruments targeted to specific cognitive domains, including memory impairment, disorientation, expressive and receptive language, and dyspraxia (Welsh et al., 1994).

The CERAD battery is calibrated to measure cognitive function through the stages of mild, moderate, and severe Alzheimer's disease. Cognitively normal subjects tend to score near the ceiling on most CERAD instruments. Severely demented subjects, in contrast, are untestable, so most neuropsychometric instruments experience a floor effect if applied to subjects approaching the terminal stages of a dementing process. During intermediate stages of disease, a steady decline in scores on neuropsychometic instruments is typically observed. Ceiling and floor effects contribute to the s-shaped (Morris et al., 1993) or trilinear (Brooks, Kraemer, Tanke & Yesavage, 1993) pattern of progression typically seen when an Alzheimer patient's

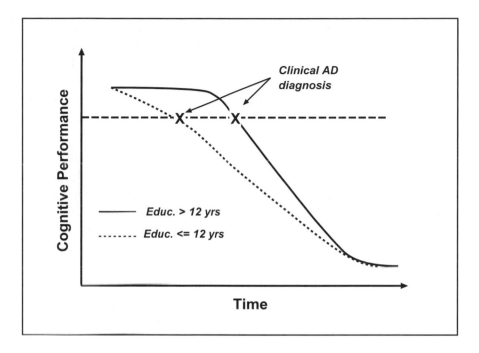

Fig. 1.1: Hypothetical progression of neuropsychometric performance in subjects with and without education-associated "cognitive reserve" against clinical manifestations of the Alzheimer's disease (AD) neurodegenerative process. The abscissa (Time) is time since the onset of the AD neurodegenerative process.

scores on a psychometric instrument are charted longitudinally.

Longitudinal neuropsychometric data have been used to describe the natural history of disease and to explore clinical heterogeneity within Alzheimer's disease. For example, education was found to predict faster decline in cognitive function within Alzheimer's disease in multiple studies (Koss et al., 1996). Based on longitudinal neuropsychometric data, it was hypothesized (Teri et al., 1995) that patients with higher educational attainment are diagnosed at a later stage of the Alzheimer neurodegenerative process, at which point progression on psychometric measures is accelerated (see Figure 1.1). Under this hypothesis, we expect higher education to be associated with a delay in onset of clinically diagnosable Alzheimer's disease, as has now been consistently observed in cohort studies following clinically normal subjects to incident dementia (Cobb et al., 1995; Kukull et al., 2002). This hypothesis also predicts that more highly educated subjects have more underlying neuropathology at a given clinical stage of disease than their less educated counterparts. This has been demonstrated by positron emission tomography (PET) studies of glucose metabolism within subjects with clinical dementia (Scarmeas et al., 2003).

The characterization of the relationship between education and Alzheimer's disease diagnosis and symptoms is an example of neuropsychometric data contributing to our understanding of Alzheimer's disease. A number of explanations for the different pattern of disease presentation in individuals at differing levels of education has been proposed. Educational training and associated factors may predict enhanced cognitive coping skills and thereby induce greater cognitive reserve against the effects of the Alzheimer neurodegenerative process. Education is also a crude surrogate of intelligence, participation in mentally engaging activities throughout life, and presumably neuronal synaptic density, which may further contribute to cognitive reserve against a clinical diagnosis of dementia.

Other findings from the neuropsychometric rate of decline literature include the observation that Alzheimer's disease cases with earlier onset disease decline more rapidly on neuropsychometric measures (Jacobs et al., 1994; Koss et al., 1996; Teri et al., 1995), consistent with the hypothesis that severity defined by age at onset is related to severity as defined by rate of decline once the disease is diagnosed. Different patterns of presentation by age at onset have also been described (Koss et al., 1996).

Another candidate predictor of faster decline is apoE genotype. Persons with one or two apoE ε4 alleles have a greater risk of disease (Farrer et al., 1997). Moreover, in prevalent case series (Farrer et al., 1997) and in population-based incidence studies (Miech et al., 2002), cases with an ε4 allele have an earlier onset age than cases without the ε4 allele. Subjects with an ε4 allele have an on average faster rate of decline on neuropsychometric measures in many, but not all, studies that have investigated this (reviewed in Craft et al., 1998). Inconsistencies in these studies may be explained in part by differences in analysis and interpretation of data (Craft et al., 1998). For example, controlling for the age effect on rate of decline tends to "wash out" any $\varepsilon 4$ effect. A conclusion consistent with most data is that subjects with an $\varepsilon 4$ allele have a faster rate of decline by virtue of their earlier age at onset, but that, given age, no or only a modest additional increase in average rate of decline is predicted by apoE genotype.

1.2.2 Neuropsychometric-neuropathologic correlations

Alzheimer's neuropathology progresses in a generally predictable, but not entirely deterministic, pattern. The two histopathological hallmarks of disease are intraneuronal tangles made of paired helical filament τ and extracellular plaques composed of amyloid β. The typical pattern of pathology on autopsy at various stages of clinical disease has been described by neuropathologists (Braak & Braak, 1991). Typically, lesions are present in the earliest stages of disease in the entorhinal region, are more dense in this region in more advanced disease, and are observed in increasing density in the neocortex in advanced cases. Accompanying the plaque and tangle pathology is neuronal loss and brain atrophy visible on brain magnetic resonance imaging (MRI). Advanced Alzheimer's disease cases have visibly smaller total brain volume, larger ventricles, and significantly atrophied or vacant hippocampal structures (Jack et al., 2004).

There is person-to-person variability in the typical pattern of disease progression. For example, right and left hippocampal structures may be differentially affected during each stage of disease in some persons. Because Alzheimer cases are still testable during early and intermediate stages of the disease, this phenomenon may provide an opportunity for quantitative psychologists to test various models of brain networking and function (see, e.g., Chapter 5 in this volume).

We have performed preliminary investigations in this regard by exploring the correlation between hippocampal volume and performance on various neuropsychometric instruments within Alzheimer's disease (Nair et al., 2004). Subjects were 76 Alzheimer's disease cases with mean age 83 years. Hippocampal volumes were estimated by manual tracing of successive (1.5 mm) cross-sectional MRI views along the long axis of the hippocampus. In regression analyses controlling for age, gender, total intracranial volume, and contralateral hippocampal volume, we found that left hippocampal volume pre-

Table 1.1: Regression coefficients (r) for right and left hippocampal volume ($mm^3 \times 10^{-3}$) in linear regression models predicting scores on various neuropsychological measurements within AD. Age, gender, and total intracranial volume were controlled for in all models.

Neuropsychological Measure	Hippocampal Volume	r	p-value
Delayed recall	Right	-0.30	.560
	Left	+1.00	.020
Visual reproduction	Right	+4.00	.020
	Left	-1.00	.480
Boston naming	Right	-17.00	.010
	Left	+20.00	.004

dicted better performance on a delayed recall test, and right hippocampal volume predicted better performance on a visual reproduction test (see Table 1.1). Interestingly, for performance on the Boston Naming test (Goodglass & Kaplan, 2001), which involves both visual recognition of line drawings and verbal recall of names, both the left and right hippocampal structure volumes were statistically significantly associated with performance (see Table 1.1).

1.2.3   Neuropsychological measurements in clinical trials

A final important application of neuropsychological measurements in Alzheimer's disease research is as outcome measures in clinical trials. Treatment trials are designed to test the ability of agents to slow the progression of Alzheimer's disease and typically use decline on a global cognitive scale as the endpoint for their primary analysis. For example, the cognitive component of the Alzheimer's Disease Assessment Scale (Mohs, Rosen & Davis, 1983) is the primary endpoint in many National Institute on Aging (NIA)-funded treatment trials performed by the Alzheimer's Disease Cooperative Study (e.g., Aisen et al., 2003). Global cognitive measures have also been successfully employed in studies of successful cognitive aging (Grodstein et al., 2003; Shadlen et al., 2005), and in primary prevention trials (Espeland et al., 2004; Raap et al., 2003). Neuropsychological measurements have the advantage of being measures of performance directly relevant to persons with disease.

A described limitation of neuropsychometric instruments for this application is that they are noisy instruments (Jack et al., 2004). In regard to clinical trials, their measurement variability is large relative to their annual rate of decline. This translates to large sample size requirements for clinical trials. An alternative measurement with less variability is rate of decline on volumetric measurements from serial MRIs (Jack et al., 2004). Volumetric MRI measurements, because of their smaller measurement error, may potentially dramatically reduce sample size requirements for clinical trials (see Table 1.2). The power calculations reported in Table 1.2 are for an analytic method that does not optimally utilize longitudinal psychometric data. Nonetheless, these sample size estimates give an indication of the potential magnitude of reduction in sample size that can be achieved by using instruments with less measurement error. A potential area of future research is refining or developing neuropsychometric instruments optimizing signal-to-noise properties for the purpose of clinical trials. Likewise, future investigation is required to compare and contrast the relative performance and utility of imaging versus neuropsychometric data as outcome measures for clinical trials.

1.3 CONCLUSIONS

Neuropsychometric measures have been and will continue to be a tool for understanding cognitive aging and Alzheimer's disease. Extensive neuropsychometric exams are routinely obtained in the course of most clinical research studies. Longitudinal data gathered by NIA funded Alzheimer's Disease Research Centers are maintained by the National Alzheimer's Coordinating Center at the University of Washington (Koepsell, Kukull, Beekly, van Belle, Higdon & Fitzpatrick, 2004), and are available to qualified researchers (application directions at www.alz.washington.edu). Quantitative psychologists may provide new perspectives on the interpretation and analysis of these data. As such, quantitative psychologists are well positioned to contribute to

Table 1.2: Estimated sample size for a treatment trial designed to detect a 25% reduction in rate of decline on various imaging and clinical measures of disease progression (assuming 1-5 years follow-up and 90% power).

Change Measurement		Sample Size
Volumetric	Hippocampus	102
	Entorhinal cortex	91
	Whole brain	130
	Ventricle	69
Psychometric	CDR	1,277
	MMSE	2,628

our understanding of Alzheimer's disease.

ACKNOWLEDGMENTS

This work supported in part by National Institute on Aging grants P50 AG005131, P50 AG16574, and U01 AG06786.

References

Aisen, P. S., Schafer, K. A., Grundman, M., Pfeiffer, E., Sano, M. & Davis, K. L. (2003). Effects of rofecoxib or naproxen vs. placebo on Alzheimer disease progression: A randomized controlled trial. *Jama-Journal Of The American Medical Association*, *289(21)*, 2819–2826.

Braak, H. & Braak, E. (1991). Neuropathological staging of Alzheimer related changes. *Acta Neuropathologica*, *82(4)*, 239–259.

Brooks, J. O., Kraemer, H. C., Tanke, E. D. & Yesavage, J. A. (1993). The methodology of studying decline in Alzheimer's disease. *Journal of the American Geriatrics Society*, *41(6)*, 623–628.

Cobb, J. L., Wolf, P. A., Au, R., White, R. & Dagostino, R. B. (1995). The effect of education on the incidence of dementia and

Alzheimer's disease in the Framingham Study. *Neurology, 45(9)*, 1707–1712.

Craft, S., Teri, L., Edland, S. D., Kukull, W. A., Schellenberg, G. & McCormick, W. C. (1998). Accelerated decline in apolipoprotein E-epsilon 4 homozygotes with Alzheimer's disease. *Neurology, 51(1)*, 149–153.

Espeland, M. A., Raap, S. R., Shumaker, S. A., Brunner, R., Manson, J. E. & Sherwin, B. B. (2004). Conjugated equine estrogens and global cognitive function in postmenopausal women: Women's Health Initiative Memory Study. *Jama-Journal Of The American Medical Association, 291(24)*, 2959–2968.

Farrer, L. A., Cupples, L. A., Haines, J. L., Hyman, B., Kukull, W. A. & Mayeux, R. (1997). Effects of age, sex, and ethnicity on the association between apolipoprotein E genotype and Alzheimer disease: A meta-analysis. *Jama Journal Of The American Medical Association, 278(16)*, 1349–1356.

Folstein, M. F., Folstein, S. E. & McHugh, P. R. (1975). Mini-mental state: A practical method for grading the cognitive state of patients for the clinician. *Journal Of Psychiatric Research, 12(3)*, 189–198.

Goodglass, H. & Kaplan, E. (2001). *Boston Naming Test (2nd ed.)*. Baltimore, MD: Lippincott Williams & Wilkins.

Grodstein, F., Chen, J. & Willett, W. C. (2003). High-dose antioxidant supplements and cognitive function in community-dwelling elderly women. *American Journal of Clinical Nutrition, 77(4)*, 975–984.

Jack, C. R., Petersen, R. C., O'Brien, P. C., Smith, G. E. & Ivnik, R. J. (2000). Rates of hippocampal atrophy correlate with change in clinical status in aging and AD. *Neurology, 55(4)*, 484–489.

Jack, C. R., Shiung, M. M., Gunter, J. L., O'Brien, P. C., Weigand, S. D. & Knopman, D. S. (2004). Comparison of different MRI brain atrophy rate measures with clinical disease progression in AD. *Neurology, 62(4)*, 591–600.

Jacobs, D., Sano, M., Marder, K., Bell, K., Bylsma, F. & Lafleche, G. (1994). Age at onset of Alzheimer's disease: Relation to pattern of cognitive dysfunction and rate of decline. *Neurology, 44(7)*, 1215–1220.

Koepsell, T. D., Kukull, W. A., Beekly, D., van Belle, G., Higdon, R. & Fitzpatrick, A. (2004). Public-use data from NACC. *Neurobiology Of Aging, 25*, S386–S386.

Koss, E., Edland, S., Fillenbaum, G., Mohs, R., Clark, C. & Galasko, D. (1996). Clinical and neuropsychological differences between patients with earlier and later onset of Alzheimer's disease: A CERAD analysis, Part XII. *Neurology, 46(1)*, 136–141.

Kukull, W. A., Higdon, R., Bowen, J. D., McCormick, W. C., Teri, L. & Schellenberg, G. D. (2002). Dementia and Alzheimer disease incidence: A prospective cohort study. *Archives Of Neurology, 59(11)*, 1737–1746.

Miech, R. A., Breitner, J. C. S., Zandi, P. P., Khachaturian, A. S., Anthony, J. C. & Mayer, L. (2002). Incidence of AD may decline in the early 90s for men, later for women: The Cache County study. *Neurology, 58(2)*, 209–218.

Mohs, R. C., Rosen, W. G. & Davis, K. L. (1983). The Alzheimer's Disease Assessment Scale: An instrument for assessing treatment efficacy. *Psychopharmacology Bulletin, 19(3)*, 448–450.

Morris, J. C., Edland, S., Clark, C., Galasko, D., Koss, E. & Mohs, R. (1993). The Consortium to Establish a Registry for Alzheimer's Disease (CERAD). Part IV. Rates of cognitive change in the longitudinal assessment of probable Alzheimer's disease. *Neurology, 43(23)*, 2457–2465.

Nair, A. K., Boeve, B. F., Edland, S. D., Jack, C. R., Slusser, T. C. & Knopman, D. S. (2004). Hippocampal asymmetry predicts neuropsychological performance in Alzheimer's disease. *Neurology, 62(S5)*, A238.

Raap, S. R., Espeland, M. A., Shumaker, S. A., Henderson, V. W., Brunner, R. L. & Manson, J. E. (2003). Effect of estrogen plus progestin on global cognitive function in postmenopausal women: The Women's Health Initiative Memory Study: A randomized controlled trial. *Jama-Journal Of The American Medical Association, 289(20)*, 2663–2672.

Scarmeas, N., Zarahan, E., Anderson, K. E., Harbeck, C. G., Hilton, J. & Flynn, J. (2003). Association of life activities with cerebral blood flow in Alzheimer disease: Implications for the cognitive reserve hypothesis. *Archives Of Neurology, 60(3)*, 359–365.

Shadlen, M. F., Larson, E. B., Wang, L., Phelan, E. A., McCormick, W. C. & Jolley, L. (2005). Education modifies the effect of apolipoprotein epsilon 4 on cognitive decline. *Neurobiology Of Aging, 26(1)*, 17–24.

Teri, L., McCurry, S. M., Edland, S. D., Kukull, W. A. & Larson, E. B. (1995). Cognitive decline in Alzheimer's disease: A longitudinal investigation of risk factors for accelerated decline. *Journals Of Gerontology Series A: Biological Sciences And Medical Sciences, 50(1)*, M49–M55.

Welsh, K. A., Butters, N., Moh, R. C., Beekly, D., Edland, S. & Fillenbaum, G. (1994). The Consortium to Establish a Registry for Alzheimer's Disease (CERAD). Part V. A normative study of the neuropsychological battery. *Neurology, 44(4)*, 609–614.

2

Computational Cognitive Neuroscience: Building and Testing Biologically Plausible Computational Models of Neuroscience, Neuroimaging, and Behavioral Data

F. Gregory Ashby and Vivian V. Valentin
University of California, Santa Barbara

The cognitive neuroscience revolution has profoundly altered the nature of theories in cognitive psychology. For many years, the only charge of these theories was to account for purely behavioral data from cognitive experiments that typically were performed on healthy young adults. Now, however, the validity of a cognitive theory may also be challenged by data from a wide variety of other sources— including functional magnetic resonance imaging (fMRI), neuropsychological patient studies, recordings of event-related potentials (ERPs), transcranial magnetic stimulation studies, and single-unit recordings. Clearly the converging evidence provided by these many methods adds tremendous new constraints to the underlying theories, and thereby almost guarantees faster progress in our understanding of the behaviors of interest. But the huge variety of data sources that a successful theory must resolve also greatly increases the difficulty of theory construction. In fact, a new type of theory is required, and along with it, new methods for constructing those theories.

This chapter describes a method we have developed over the past 5 or 6 years for constructing neurobiologically plausible computational models of behavior. The method is quite general and can be applied to a wide variety of behavioral phenomena. The components in the models that are constructed with this method are units that correspond to groups of similar cells in specific brain regions (e.g., cortical columns or hypercolumns). The resulting models are also quite flexible with respect to the types of data they can be tested against. For example, we describe detailed methods for fitting the models to single-cell recording data, fMRI data, and human behavioral data.

The method we describe is algorithmic in the sense that it consists of a discrete set of problems that must be solved. In this chapter, we define five specific problems, and we present detailed methods for solving all but one of these problems. These methods are all straightforward and easy to implement. The result is that, after working through this chapter, an interested reader who has an hypothesis about which brain regions may be mediating some behavior should be able to construct a computational version of that model and test its predictions against single-cell recordings, fMRI data, and behavioral data.

Of the five well-defined steps to be solved, the first and most difficult problem is to identify the brain areas that mediate performance in the behavior to be modeled. A necessary part of this process is to specify the interconnections among these areas and whether each projection is excitatory or inhibitory. The second problem is to write a set of differential equations that describe the neural activation in each of these brain regions. A related problem is to solve these (simultaneous nonlinear) differential equations. Solving these two problems results in a computational model that predicts dynamic changes in neural activation in each brain region specified by the model. To model real data, however, some interface needs to be added that describes how the dependent variable of interest is related to the neural activations that are the core currency of the model. The final three problems are directed at constructing these interfaces. Problem 3 is to find an interface to fit single-cell recording data—here we must convert the continuous neural activations obtained from solving the differential equations of Problem 2 into spike trains. The goal of Problem 4 is to fit fMRI data, which requires adding an interface that models the transformation from neural activation to the fMRI Blood Oxygen-Level Dependent (BOLD) signal. Finally, to fit behavioral data, Problem 5 seeks to add assumptions that relate neural activation in a particular brain region to behavior and then derive predictions for the relevant dependent variable (e.g., accuracy or response time). This chapter is organized around these five problems, with a major section devoted to each. After this we close with some general comments.

2.1   PROBLEM 1: IDENTIFYING RELEVANT BRAIN STRUCTURES

The first step in designing a computational neural network is to identify the brain structures that are hypothesized to mediate the performance in the behavior to be modeled. This task includes specifying the interconnections among these areas and whether each projection is excitatory or inhibitory. In most cases, this network is incomplete, in the sense that there generally are certain perceptual or cognitive processes omitted by the network that nonetheless are necessary for the expression of the behavior of interest. For example, a working memory model may specify the neural structures that mediate the maintenance of the memory, but say nothing about the neural networks that mediate the perception of the stimulus or the selection and execution of a motor response.

In general, there are two ways to deal with such omissions depending on whether the omitted processes are upstream from (i.e., precede) or downstream from (i.e., follow) the specified network. In the working memory example, perceptual processes should be upstream from the memory maintenance network and response execution processes downstream. Upstream processes must be directly modeled, in at least a rudimentary fashion, because they provide input to the specified network. Our approach has been to grossly oversimplify such upstream processes and simply model their input to the specified network as either on or off. Several examples of this technique appear throughout this chapter. Downstream processes can generally be ignored except when fitting the model to behavioral data that depend on these processes. In such cases, our approach has been to add a simple cognitive model of the downstream processes as an interface between the specified network and the observed behavior. Examples of such behavioral interfaces are given in the penultimate section of this chapter.

The problem of identifying even a partial neural network is, by far, the most difficult of the five problems that we discuss in this chap-

ter. It is also the only problem of the five that is not computational;
partly because of this qualitative difference, it is the only problem for
which we do not provide an algorithm for solving. Because the task
of identifying relevant brain areas is difficult and without set rules
to follow, our only recourse in the limited space we have here is to
provide some general guidelines and suggestions. These will surely
prove insufficient, so a realistic goal of this chapter is to provide algorithmic methods for building a computational model of an *existing*
neural network and for fitting that model to single-cell recording,
fMRI, and behavioral data.

Perhaps the most important advice we can give is not to expect
any simple solution to this problem. For example, it is highly unlikely
that a plausible neural network will be identified by studying only a
single type of data. Instead, solving this problem requires a thorough review and reconciliation of disconnected areas of the literature
in the brain sciences. When proposing a set of neural structures and
their interconnections, it is vital to consider evidence from converging methods that include many different levels of analysis, such as
neuroimaging, neuropsychology, behavioral neuroscience, neurophysiology, neuroanatomy, and neuropharmacology.

In trying to decide which structures are relevant for the model, a
useful approach is to establish which specific lesions impair the behavior of interest. A double dissociation is strong evidence that two
behaviors are mediated by two functionally separate brain systems
(Ashby & Ell, 2002). A wealth of such data comes from neuropsychological studies of human patients with specific brain lesions caused by
various kinds of injury or neurodegenerative disease, such as Huntington's, Parkinson's, or Alzheimer's disease. Temporary disabling
of a brain region that is required for a specific function can also be
achieved with experimental techniques such as transcranial magnetic
stimulation, Wada testing (disrupting activity in one hemisphere),
and electrical stimulation or cortical cooling during neurosurgery.
However, it is always important to confirm any double dissociation
observed in humans with similar dissociations from well-controlled
animal lesion studies (Ashby & Ell, 2002).

The techniques that investigate the loss of a given function due
to the disruption of a brain region are complemented with techniques
that measure brain activity associated with this function. These

methods include electroencephalography (EEG), ERPs, magnetoencephalography, fMRI, positron emission tomography, near-infrared spectroscopy, and single-cell recording. Due to its invasive nature, this latter technique is mostly used in animals. Pharmacological studies can also provide insights into both disruption and enhancement of specific neurotransmitter systems involved in certain behaviors. These kinds of experiments can provide powerful evidence, especially the animal studies that allow for more rigorous and flexible designs. For example, agonistic (or antagonistic) drugs that facilitate (or impair) a behavioral response can be injected into defined brain areas at various specific times within a behavioral paradigm.

The animal literature is highly relevant to understanding the neural basis of human behavior. The goal is to integrate the animal literature, human lesion findings, and results from functional neuroimaging studies. This goal often requires establishing the homology between the animal and human brain. The behavioral tasks given to animals and humans may also differ, even when both investigate the same psychological construct. Therefore, it is possible that some discrepancy in the brain-behavior relation may result from some behavioral or methodological differences. Still, to get the most comprehensive picture, both animal and human literatures should be consulted.

Interconnections among brain areas should be specified according to whether each of the projections is excitatory, inhibitory, or modulatory. The spontaneous basal firing rates can differ between structures as well and are usually associated with their inputs (e.g., structures with high basal firing rates often receive inhibitory inputs). A sophisticated dynamic model may also take into account the length and conducting speeds of axons and/or the number of synapses that occur between two functionally connected areas. The anatomical organization of projections is mapped out in studies using anterograde and retrograde tracing techniques. These findings can be complemented with those from a relatively new technique called functional connectivity analysis (using fMRI), which is useful in identifying functionally related brain areas and distributed networks by means of their synchronous fluctuations in signal intensity.

Completing this laborious chore of literature search to build the most plausible neural network is not only advantageous for increasing the chances of realistic and valid predictions that may result from the model, but it also provides a great service to the brain sciences community. Separate fields do not communicate enough to gain a more comprehensive picture of the current state of knowledge, although we all know that each technique is weak in isolation, but convergent findings from multiple techniques can be convincing. Therefore, using the most appropriate brain areas and projections to build the architecture of the model is an important step for distilling and clarifying a vast, disconnected literature. In addition, if a neural network is biologically accurate, it can confirm the neuroscience studies when it is tested with specific lesions, and it can also provide an artificial environment for testing various lesions that are impossible or too costly to attain in humans and other animals.

2.2   PROBLEM 2: WRITING THE DIFFERENTIAL EQUATIONS

After the relevant brain areas have been identified and their interconnections specified, the next step is to write a set of equations that describe the neural activation in these regions. The main challenge here is to select an appropriate level at which to direct the equations. If too global a level is chosen, the resulting model will lack biological plausibility, and, as a result, it will be unable to account for neuroscience data. If the model is too detailed, it may account spectacularly for single-cell phenomena, but it is likely to be too complex to account for human behavioral data.

Historically, two separate traditions have constructed computational models of neurons and neural networks. Within psychology, connectionist models have a long and successful history, and they have been used to account for a wide variety of behaviors (Rumelhart & McClelland, 1986). However, the units in connectionist models bear only superficial similarity to real neurons, and there is almost never an attempt to associate units with specific brain areas. Thus, although connectionist models provide powerful descriptions of human behavior, they are not able to account for single-cell recording data or other types of neuroscience data.

A separate discipline called *computational neuroscience* builds biologically realistic models that attempt to model biophysical properties of single neurons (e.g., Amini, Clark & Canavier, 1999; Brunel & Wang, 2001; Canavier & Wilson, 1999; Durstewitz, Kelc & Gunturkun, 1999; Durstewitz, Seamans & Sejnowski, 2000). Such models, which are often multicompartmental and include Hodgkin-Huxley-like dynamics, are applied to single-cell data, and typically no efforts are made to model behavior. Computational neuroscience models are often highly complex, and in some cases as many as hundreds of differential equations are used to model a single cell. Clearly, even with modern computing methods, this complexity is too high if one's goal is to model human behavior.

Thus, there is a pressing need for models that lie between the two extremes of the complex yet biophysically realistic models and the connectionist models that are computationally simple but lack neurobiological realism. For this reason, to accomplish our goals, we need to develop a new method of building neural network models that imbues the resulting models with more biological plausibility than is typically found in connectionist networks, but that also results in simpler models than are typically found in computational neuroscience.

The first step is to identify the key functional properties of the neural network that was hypothesized to mediate the behavior of interest (i.e., the network identified in the solution of Problem 1). For example, consider the network illustrated in Figure 2.1. Here the hypothesis is that whatever behavior we are modeling is mediated by a simple circuit consisting of two neural regions. Region A is assumed to receive an excitatory input from some lower-level sensory area and to send an excitatory projection to region B, whereas region B receives an excitatory projection from A and sends an inhibitory projection back to A. The model assumes that the behavior is mediated by these functional interconnections, so these interconnections must be captured in the mathematical equations that model the network. Any other features included in the equations must necessarily increase their complexity and thereby make the task of modeling behavior more difficult.

However, the simplest model of the interconnections shown in Figure 2.1 would have little biological plausibility, and hence could not be used to model neuroscience data. So some extra complexity is necessary. The key is to add the minimum amount of complexity needed

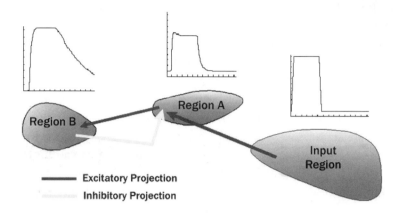

Fig. 2.1: A simple neural network model consisting of two neural regions and an input region. Also shown are the neural activations predicted by the computational model that describes processing in this network.

to model the most important biophysical properties of neurons. Our approach has been to model two key biophysical properties that are shared by all neurons: (a) saturation—every neuron has a maximum firing rate; and (b) decay—if all inputs to a neuron cease, then the activation in that cell will decay to some baseline firing level. In our applications, these biophysical properties, together with the hypothesized interconnections, have been sufficient for modeling single-cell recording data, neuroimaging data, and human behavioral data. Yet as the modeling efforts focus more heavily on neuroscience data, it may be necessary to increase the complexity of the models by trying to model other, more subtle biophysical properties.

We illustrate the approach by writing differential equations that describe the neural activation in regions A and B in the Figure 2.1 network. All of the equations have identical structure, and there is a straightforward algorithm for constructing these equations. In fact, the algorithm is so simple that no special mathematical expertise is required. We begin with region A. The left side of each equation is the derivative of the activation in the region we are modeling. For region A, we can denote the activation at time t as $A(t)$, in which case the left side becomes

$$\frac{dA(t)}{dt} = \tag{2.1}$$

An intuitive description of this derivative is that it equals the firing rate of the cells in neural region A. Any excitatory input to region A will increase this firing rate and hence will appear on the right side as a positive term, and any inhibitory input to region A will decrease the firing rate and therefore appear as a negative term on the right side.

We begin with the excitatory input $I(t)$ from the input region. We model this as a simple square wave that has the value $I(t) = 1$ if the stimulus is present and $I(t) = 0$ if the stimulus is absent. More detailed models of the input region could be used, but of course this would complicate the analysis. For example, if the task is primarily cognitive and regions A and B are somewhere in the frontal cortex, it is quite plausible that the neural dynamics in the visual cortex may not have significant effects either on the observable behavior or the neural dynamics in regions A and B. Because the projection from this input area is assumed to be excitatory, $I(t)$ appears on the right side as a positive term.

$$\frac{dA(t)}{dt} = \alpha_A I(t) \tag{2.2}$$

The constant α_A is a measure of the strength of the synapse between the input area and region A. In most applications, α_A is unknown and must be determined from some data source. Our approach has been to estimate constants such as α_A from single-cell recording data and then leave these constants fixed in all other applications.

The problem with the model so far is that a continual input will cause activation in region A to increase to infinity. As mentioned earlier, one of our goals was to build saturation into our models. This is accomplished in a straightforward fashion by adding a multiplier to the input term

$$\frac{dA(t)}{dt} = \alpha_A I(t)[1 - A(t)] \tag{2.3}$$

As the activation $A(t)$ increases from 0, the multiplier $1 - A(t)$ decreases, which reduces the excitatory effects of the input. As $A(t)$

approaches 1, $1 - A(t)$ approaches 0 and the effect of the constant
input is further reduced. Eventually the activation $A(t)$ effectively
equals 1. At this point, $1 - A(t)$ equals 0 and the input no longer has
any effect. Thus, the $1 - A(t)$ multiplier causes activation to saturate
at 1. Adding a multiplier of this type (i.e., 1 minus activation) is a
standard technique we use for every excitatory term.

The next step is to account for the inhibitory input from region
B. Because this input decreases activation in region A, it carries a
negative sign on the right-hand side.

$$\frac{dA(t)}{dt} = \alpha_A I(t)[1 - A(t)] - \beta_A B(t) \qquad (2.4)$$

As before, the constant β_A measures the strength of a synapse, this
time between regions B and A. The problem with this method of
modeling inhibition is that sustained activation in region B could
drive the activation in region A to negative values. To correct this
problem, we again add a multiplier:

$$\frac{dA(t)}{dt} = \alpha_A I(t)[1 - A(t)] - \beta_A B(t) A(t) \qquad (2.5)$$

Now as the inhibitory input $B(t)$ drives the activation $A(t)$ lower and
lower, the multiplier $A(t)$ continually decreases, thereby reducing the
inhibitory effects. When $A(t)$ is effectively zero, the multiplier is
also zero, and continued inhibition has no further effect. Thus, the
multiplier $A(t)$ induces a floor at $A(t) = 0$. Adding a multiplier of
this type (i.e., equal to the total activation) is a standard technique
we use with all inhibitory inputs.

We have now accounted for all inputs to region A. Even so, note
that if all inputs to region A are turned off, the change in activation
(i.e., the derivative) is zero, meaning that the activation will neither
increase nor decrease until an input reappears. Of course, in real
neurons, activation would decay under these conditions back to a
baseline firing level. If the baseline firing level is zero, then a simple
way to model this decay is by adding one more term.

$$\frac{dA(t)}{dt} = \alpha_A I(t)[1 - A(t)] - \beta_A B(t) A(t) - \gamma_A A(t) \qquad (2.6)$$

The constant γ_A measures the speed of decay. If the spontaneous
firing rate is high, we can define a parameter A_{base} as the baseline

activation level and replace the last term with

$$-\gamma_A[A(t) - A_{base}]. \tag{2.7}$$

Virtually all equations in our models follow this same pattern. The left-hand side is the derivative of the activation. The right side includes a term for each input plus a decay term. Excitatory inputs are preceded by a plus and followed by the multiplier "1 - Activation," whereas inhibitory inputs are preceded by a minus and followed by the multiplier "Activation." This method produces differential equations that are nonlinear and whose solutions are bounded between 0 and 1 (or baseline and 1).

Following this method, it is straightforward to write an equation that describes the activation in region B with excitatory input from region A and baseline at 0:

$$\frac{dB(t)}{dt} = \alpha_B A(t)[1 - B(t)] - \beta_B B(t). \tag{2.8}$$

The simple network shown in Figure 2.1 is therefore modeled by a set of two nonlinear differential equations. Of course, real applications will typically involve more than two brain regions and, therefore, more than two differential equations. Because of their nonlinear and interconnected nature, numerical methods are required to solve these equations in most applications. Either standard algorithms could be programmed in one's language of choice (e.g., Press, Flannery, Teukolsky & Vettering, 1988) or a high-level language (e.g., MATLAB) with preprogrammed differential equation solvers could be used. For example, Figure 2.1 shows the solutions of Equations 2.6 and 2.8 produced by a standard MATLAB differential equation solver.

Each equation that results from following this algorithm has a free parameter for each term on its right-hand side. In most cases, these parameters each have a well-defined biological interpretation— either as a measure of the strength of a synapse between two brain regions or as a rate at which activation decays in the absence of input. Because of their biological foundation, a natural approach is to estimate these parameters from neuroscience data (e.g., single-cell recordings), but from a statistical perspective they can be estimated during any model-fitting exercise. The synaptic strength parameters also provide a natural vehicle for modeling learning, because it is widely assumed that many forms of learning are mediated by changes in synaptic strengths (e.g., Grimwood, Martin & Morris, 2001; Martin & Morris, 2002).

2.3   PROBLEM 3: FITTING SINGLE-CELL RECORD-ING DATA

The model derived in the last section predicts neural activations in specific brain regions. The data that are perhaps closest to these predicted values are single-unit recordings. For this reason, single-cell recording data provide an excellent opportunity to assess the validity of the network proposed in the solution of problem 1 and estimate the numerical constants of the equations that instantiate the model (e.g., the synaptic strengths). For example, in many of our applications, we use single-cell recording data to fix all numerical constants in the differential equations that describe our model. Then in other applications (e.g.,to neuroimaging or behavioral data), we leave all these constants fixed at these same values. Thus, the only free parameters in these later applications are in the unique interfaces we use to convert the neural activations predicted by the model to these new dependent measures (e.g., the fMRI BOLD signal, or percent correct in a behavioral study).

When fitting the models to single-cell recording data, however, one must be careful not to over-fit the models. This is because there is no reason to expect that any specific spike train appearing in a published article represents a gold standard. Almost invariably, moving the electrode a tiny amount uncovers a neuron with a different firing profile, sometimes profoundly different. For this reason, we rarely try to minimize a quantitative fit measure when fitting our models to single-cell recording data. Instead, our goal is typically only to roughly adjust the numerical constants so that the model captures the major qualitative properties of the data.

Although the differential equations describing the model are closely related to single-cell recording data, they are not identical. This is because, as we saw in the preceding section, the solutions of Eqs. 2.6 and 2.8 are continuous functions (i.e., see Figure 2.1), whereas single-cell recordings produce spike trains. Thus, we need an interface (or model) that converts continuous changes in activation into spike trains. This section describes three different methods, of increasing complexity, for solving this problem.

2.3.1 Poisson Process Approach

In many experiments that we may wish to model, the sensory conditions do not change quickly. For example, in delayed response tasks, a stimulus is shown for a second or two and then a prolonged delay period occurs during which no stimuli are presented. Figure 2.1 shows that when a stimulus of constant intensity is presented, activation in units that receive sensory input that is driven by this presentation quickly ramps up to a steady-state value, where it remains until the stimulus is withdrawn. At this point, activation decays to a new steady-state value. For many behaviors of interest, performance is mostly mediated by these steady-state values. The Poisson process approach to generating spikes is to solve for these steady states and then use these values to generate interarrival times by sampling from a Poisson process.

The first step is to solve for the steady states, which are just the equilibrium-level solutions of the differential equations that describe the model. For example, consider a simple cell that has a baseline activation level of A_{base} and receives a single input $I(t)$. Following the methods described in the preceding section produces the differential equation

$$\frac{dA(t)}{dt} = \alpha I(t) - \beta[A(t) - A_{base}].\qquad(2.9)$$

By definition, equilibrium or steady-state behavior occurs when the activation is no longer changing—that is, when $A(t)$ equals a constant value (call this A) and the derivative is zero. So to find the equilibrium level solution of this equation, we simply set the derivative to zero and solve for the unknown constant value A. In other words, we must solve the following equation for A:

$$0 = \alpha I(t) - \beta(A - A_{base}).\qquad(2.10)$$

Of course, this equation has a solution only if $I(t)$ is constant. There are two obvious possibilities—one in which the input has a constant nonzero value $I(t) = I$ and one in which no input is presented $[I(t) = 0]$. In the former case, the solution is

$$A = \frac{\alpha}{\beta}I + A_{base}, \qquad (2.11)$$

whereas in the latter case, the solution is $A = A_{base}$. When the activation equals these values under the respective input conditions, it will no longer increase or decrease until the input changes. Note that although this is among the simplest possible models (i.e., one cell receiving input), it still makes some rather nonobvious predictions—namely, that the steady-state firing rate of the cell depends not only on the intensity of the input and the strength of the synapse with the input unit, but also on the baseline firing level and the cell's own decay rate (i.e., β).

The equilibrium-level solutions describe the steady-state activation levels in the cell. One could expect that the firing rate of the cell should be closely related to these levels. The Poisson process approach assumes that spike trains that are representative of this model can be generated from Poisson processes in which the Poisson rate is proportional to the steady-state activation level. A Poisson process is a stochastic process in which the times between successive events are independent samples from identical exponential distributions (e.g., Cox & Miller, 1965).

Figure 2.2 illustrates how a Poisson process can be used to generate spike trains for the model described in this section. To begin, samples X_i are drawn from a uniform $(0, 1)$ distribution. These are then converted to samples T_i from an exponential distribution with rate λ, where λ is proportional to the steady-state activation level via the transformation (e.g., Ashby, 1992)

$$T_i = -\lambda^{-1}\log_e(1 - X_i). \qquad (2.12)$$

A series of spikes is then generated with the T_i defining the interspike intervals.

The Poisson process approach has the advantage of simplicity because it replaces differential equations with linear equations. However, it has the major disadvantage of ignoring the temporal dynamics that are a fundamental property of the differential equation models.

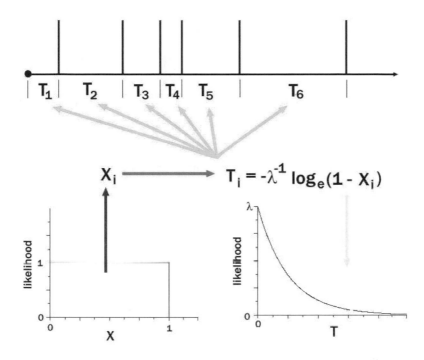

Fig. 2.2: Schematic illustrating a method for simulating a Poisson process.

In many cases, these dynamics are critical for understanding the behavior that the network is mediating. In such cases, the Poisson process approach is unacceptable. Instead, some dynamic approach for generating spikes is needed. A number of such approaches is possible.

2.3.2   Integrate-and-Fire Approach

The field of computational neuroscience has developed standard dynamic methods for generating spikes from continuous-activation models of single cells. The most common approach is to incorporate a so-called *integrate-and-fire model* (e.g., Koch, 1999). The idea is to integrate the activation and continually compare this integral to a

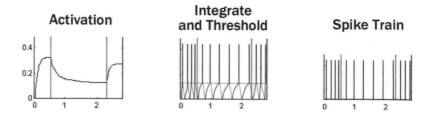

Fig. 2.3: Schematic illustrating the integrate-and-fire method for producing spike trains.

threshold. When the threshold is exceeded, a spike is generated and the integral is reset to zero and the process repeats. This process is illustrated in Figure 2.3. White noise is typically added during the integration process. Thus, this model adds two free parameters to the model of the single cell—a threshold for generating spikes and the variance of the noise process.

The integrate-and-fire model, without the thresholding process, is described by the equation

$$\frac{dA_{out}(t)}{dt} = \alpha A_{in}(t) + \varepsilon(t), \qquad (2.13)$$

where $\varepsilon(t)$ is a white noise process and $A_{in}(t)$ is the neural activation predicted by the single-cell model (i.e., the solution of the differential equation derived in the solution of problem 2). This is the equation of a nonstationary Wiener process. The nonstationary component is provided by the term $\alpha A_{in}(t)$.

The integrate-and-fire model is an incomplete model of neural activity because it assumes that the input is perfectly integrated. In real cells, input activation gradually leaks out through the cell's porous membrane. A popular generalization of the integrate-and-fire model, which corrects this shortcoming, is the leaky integrate-and-fire model (e.g., Koch, 1999). In this model, the process for generating spikes is the same, except the integrate-and-fire equation is replaced with

$$\frac{dA_{out}(t)}{dt} = \alpha A_{in}(t) + \varepsilon(t) - \beta A_{out}(t). \qquad (2.14)$$

The last term makes the model leaky because if the input stops, output activation gradually decays (or leaks) to zero.

The leaky integrate-and-fire model is closely related to the classic Ornstein-Uhlenbeck stochastic process (Cox & Miller, 1965). In fact, if $A_{in}(t) = 0$, they are equivalent. So the integrate-and-fire model could be seen as adding a Wiener process to the intracellular activation, whereas the leaky integrate-and-fire model adds an Ornstein-Uhlenbeck process.

If the methods described in the solution of problem 2 are followed when constructing the differential equation models of each neural unit, then there is no need to incorporate the decay term from the leaky integrate-and-fire model. This is because an identical decay term is already built into each equation. Thus, the models derived previously are inherently leaky. As a result, the simpler integrate-and-fire model can be used to generate spikes.

2.3.3 Dynamic Integrate-and-Fire Approach

The integrate-and-fire models work well in many applications, but they suffer from one flaw that becomes fatal in any application where the timing of spikes is critical. For example, consider the model shown in Figure 2.4. Note that there are two separate projections from region A to region C—a direct pathway and an indirect pathway through region B. In real cells, of course, the indirect path might take longer to traverse than the direct path, but the differential equations that would be used to model this network predict that activation rises immediately everywhere in all pathways at the same time. Therefore, the integrate-and-fire models also predict that the indirect path will generate spikes in region C at (almost) the same time as the direct path. Thus, any behavior that depends on a temporal difference between these two paths is described inadequately by the integrate-and-fire models.

To correct this problem, we have developed a dynamic version of the integrate-and-fire model. The method is illustrated for the network shown in Figure 2.1, except now we assume all projections are excitatory. This revised network is shown in Figure 2.5. Consider an experiment in which the input is set to some constant value for a short duration and then turned off. The first step is to set the output

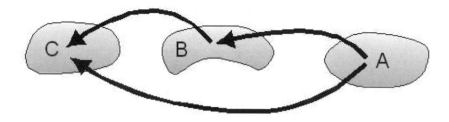

Fig. 2.4: A neural network with three regions that has two separate pathways from region A to region C.

activations from regions A and B to zero. Thus, initially, region A receives a nonzero input only from the input region. Next, activation in region A is integrated until a threshold is reached, exactly as in the standard integrate-and-fire model. When the threshold is exceeded, a square wave input is sent from region A to region B. Region B now has a nonzero input, so the activation in B is integrated until a threshold is reached, at which point a square wave input is sent from region B back to region A. This algorithm more closely mimics the natural spike generation process. To make it even more natural, delays can be incorporated to model the time it takes a spike to propagate down the cell's axon. For example, after activation in region A reaches threshold, a square wave of activation could be delivered to region B after a delay of length Δ_A, rather than immediately, and a similar delay of length Δ_B could be associated with region B. The delays Δ_I (I = A or B) would increase with the length of the axons of the cells in region I and decrease with the amount of myelinization. A simple way to add noise to this model is to make Δ_A and Δ_B random variables. A particularly attractive choice would be to determine Δ_A and Δ_B by drawing samples from an exponential distribution.

Figure 2.5 also shows an example of this spike-generation method with Δ_A and Δ_B set to zero. Note the spike-like nature of the activation produced in region B. Region B produces more spikes than region A because it is further removed from the artificial square-wave input that we assumed for the input region. Also note that, despite

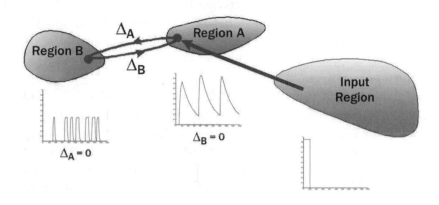

Fig. 2.5: A simple neural network and the activations it produces in the dynamic integrate-and-fire approach.

assuming that $\Delta_A = \Delta_B = 0$, the method produces temporal delays before the first spike appears that increase with the number of synapses from the initial input. For example, note that the input activation rises to a constant value at time zero and then there is a short delay before activation rises above zero in region A, and a longer delay before the same thing occurs in region B. More realistic spike trains can be produced by recording the times when the threshold is exceeded in each cell and then simply plotting a spike at each of these times.

2.4 PROBLEM 4: FITTING NEUROIMAGING DATA

Within the field of cognitive neuroscience, an extremely important challenge for future computational models is to provide quantitative fits to neuroimaging data. In humans, the most common indirect measures of neural activation are made using fMRI (e.g., Bandettini et al., 1992; Kwong et al., 1992; Ogawa et al., 1992). We say *indirect* because fMRI measures the so-called BOLD signal, rather than neural activation (Ogawa, Lee, Kay & Tank, 1990a; Ogawa, Lee, Nayak & Glynn, 1990b). Although it is commonly assumed that the BOLD signal increases with neural activation, it is known that the BOLD response is much more sluggish than the neural activation that is presumed to drive it. As a result, for example, the peak of the BOLD signal lags considerably behind the peak neural activation (i.e., by about 6 s).

In the computational models described here, the solutions of the differential equations yield continuous neural activations. Logothetis and colleagues have argued that the BOLD signals most likely are driven by the local field potentials, rather than by the spiking output of individual cells (Logothetis, 2003; Logothetis, Pauls, Augath, Trinath & Oeltermann, 2001). Local field potentials integrate the field potentials produced by small populations of cells over a submillimeter range, and they vary continuously over time. Thus, they are most closely related to the direct solutions of the differential equations that define our models (rather than, say, to the spike trains derived in the preceding section).

2.4.1   Linear Models of the BOLD Response

Because the fMRI BOLD signal is related to oxygen levels in the blood, a model of the transformation from neural activation to the fMRI BOLD signal is necessary to fit fMRI data. Several such models have been proposed. Almost all current applications assume that this transformation can be modeled as a time-invariant linear system. Although it is becoming increasingly clear that the transformation is, in fact, nonlinear (e.g., Boynton, Engel, Glover & Heeger, 1996; Buxton & Frank, 1998; Vazquez & Noll, 1998), it also appears that, under the appropriate conditions, these departures from linearity are not severe. For example, the approximation to linearity is apparently improved if the intertrial interval exceeds one second and if brief, tachistoscopic exposure durations are avoided (Vazquez & Noll, 1998). These two conditions are typically met in fMRI studies of high-level cognition.

The behavior of any linear system is completely characterized by its so-called *impulse response function*. For example, given this function, predicted BOLD signals could be computed for a given brain region by numerically convolving the neural activation that a computational model predicts in that region with the impulse response function (e.g., Chen, 1970). In the fMRI literature, the impulse response function that characterizes the transformation from neural activation to BOLD signal is known as the *hemodynamic response function* (hrf). Many models of the hrf have been proposed (Boynton, Engel, Glover & Heeger, 1996; Clark, Maisog & Haxby, 1998; Cohen, 1997; Dale & Buckner, 1997; Friston, Holmes & Ashburner, 1999; Friston, Josephs, Ress & Turner, 1998; Zarahn, Aquirre & D'Esposito, 1997).

One particularly attractive choice is to model the hrf at time t, $h(t)$, as a weighted linear combination of basis functions (Friston, Josephs, Ress & Turner, 1998):

$$h(t) = \alpha_1 b_1(t) + \alpha_2 b_2(t) + \alpha_3 b_3(t), \qquad (2.15)$$

where $b_i(t)$ is the ith basis function and α_i is its weight. Friston et al. (1998) suggested gamma probability density functions for the basis functions with means and variances equal to 4, 8, and 16, respectively. Thus,

$$b_1(t) = \frac{1}{3!} t^3 e^{-t}, \qquad (2.16)$$

$$b_2(t) = \frac{1}{7!} t^7 e^{-t}, \qquad (2.17)$$

and

$$b_3(t) = \frac{1}{15!} t^{15} e^{-t}. \qquad (2.18)$$

These three functions were selected to model peaks during the early, intermediate, and late components of the anticipated BOLD signal. The weighting parameters α_1, α_2, and α_3 might vary across participants and/or brain regions.

Once an hrf is selected, the predicted BOLD signal in a specified region of interest is computed by convolving the predicted neural activation in that region, $A(t)$ (obtained from solving the differential equation describing activation in that region) with the hrf:

$$\text{BOLD}(t) = \int_0^t h(\tau) A(t - \tau) d\tau. \qquad (2.19)$$

In our applications of Equation 2.19, we have first fixed the values of all unknown constants in the differential equations by fitting the model to single-cell recording data (using the methods of the previous section). Thus, in our applications, the only free parameters in Equation 2.19 are in the description of the hrf (e.g., the α_i in Equation 2.15). These parameters can be estimated using standard optimization algorithms, but the use of the basis function hrf model of Equation 2.15 greatly simplifies this process. For example, note that substituting Equation 2.15 into Equation 2.19 produces

$$
\begin{aligned}
\text{BOLD}(t) \;=\; & \alpha_1 \int_0^t b_1(\tau)A(t-\tau)dt \;+\; \\
& \alpha_2 \int_0^t b_2(\tau)A(t-\tau)dt \;+\; \\
& \alpha_3 \int_0^t b_3(\tau)A(t-\tau)dt. \qquad (2.20)
\end{aligned}
$$

If the parameters of the differential equations are fixed using other data (e.g., single-cell recording data), then each of these integrals involves no free parameters. As a result, if we define

$$
x_i(t) = \int_0^t b_i(\tau)A(t-\tau)d\tau, \qquad (2.21)
$$

then

$$
\text{BOLD}(t) = \alpha_1 x_1(t) + \alpha_2 x_2(t) + \alpha_3 x_3(t). \qquad (2.22)
$$

Thus, the three convolutions specified by Equation 2.21 can be computed numerically, which determines the three vectors $x_i(t)$. The parameters α_i can now be determined using standard linear regression techniques.

Despite the absence of computational models that make specific predictions about neural activation, there has nevertheless been a pressing need to test specific a priori predictions about the BOLD signal. In the absence of a detailed model, the only predictions that can typically be made are that a brain region involved in mediating some cognitive task should be active throughout the duration of that task. This idea can be modeled with a simple neural activation function that equals a constant value during the critical experimental period that defines the task (typically the time between stimulus

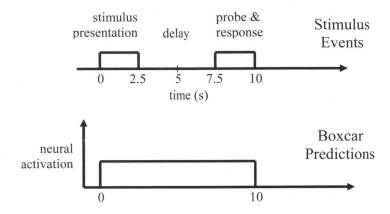

Fig. 2.6: The boxcar model. Panel (a) shows the timing of stimulus events in a hypothetical experiment. Panel (b) shows the neural activation predicted by the boxcar model for any brain region that mediates performance in this experiment.

presentation and response) and zero otherwise (e.g., Friston et al., 1995). More formally, this function $R(t) = 1/T$ for $0 < t \leq T$, and $R(t) = 0$ otherwise, where T is the assumed duration of neural activation. Because of its shape, $R(t)$ is called the *boxcar function*. An example is shown in Figure 2.6. To generate predictions from the boxcar model, one simply convolves the boxcar function with an hrf (i.e., equivalent to substituting $R(t)$ for $A(t)$ in Equation 2.19). An obvious and important first test of any computational model derived using the methods described in this chapter is to compare its ability to account for fMRI data with the traditional boxcar model.

As an example of this process, we briefly describe an application by Ashby, Ell, Valentin, and Casale (2003, 2005). Using the procedures described in this chapter, Ashby et al. (2005) derived a neurobiologically plausible model of working memory called FROST (FROntal Striatal Thalamic loops). The parameters in the differential equations that described the model were estimated by roughly fitting FROST to published single-cell recording data (Constantinidis & Steinmetz, 1996; Fuster, 1973; Fuster & Alexander, 1973; Hikosaka, Sakamoto & Sadanari, 1989; Mushiake & Strick, 1995). Using these fixed parameter values, FROST was then fit to fMRI data from a spatial delayed response task reported by Ell and colleagues (2003). During the stimulus presentation phase of this study, a target stimulus (i.e., a dot) was presented in a certain spatial location for 2.5 s (i.e., the repetition time, or TR, of the scanner). The target dot then disappeared for a delay period of either 2.5 or 5 s. During the response phase, a probe dot appeared in either the same or a different spatial location. The subject's task was to indicate with a button press whether the location of the probe dot was identical or different from the location of the target dot.

Ell and colleagues (2003) reported a sustained BOLD response during the delay period of this task in several areas predicted by FROST—namely, the posterior parietal cortex (Broadman Area 7), dorsolateral prefrontal cortex (Broadman Areas 9 and 46), the head of the caudate nucleus, the internal segment of the globus pallidus, and the medial dorsal nucleus of the thalamus. Figure 2.7 shows the observed BOLD signal in the five brain regions identified by FROST, along with the predicted BOLD signals generated by convolving the neural activations predicted by FROST with an hrf (the three-parameter delayed gamma function proposed by Boynton et al., 1996). As can be seen, FROST captures the major qualitative properties of the observed data.

As a further test, Ashby and colleagues (2003) compared the fMRI predictions of FROST with those of the traditional boxcar model (shown in Figure 2.6). First, of course, unlike a model like FROST, the boxcar model makes no predictions about which brain regions should be active during the delay period, nor does it make any predictions about single-cell recording data. Thus, models like FROST have a number of important advantages over the boxcar model even before simple goodness-of-fit is considered. In fact, the only asset of the boxcar model is its assumed ability to account quantitatively for BOLD signals in brain regions that have been somehow identified using other means. Even so, this is a significant accomplishment, and it is important to ask whether models developed using the methods described in this chapter can match this ability of the boxcar model.

To answer this question, Ashby and colleagues (2003) compared the ability of FROST and the boxcar model to account for the observed BOLD signals reported in Ell et al. (2003) in the brain regions

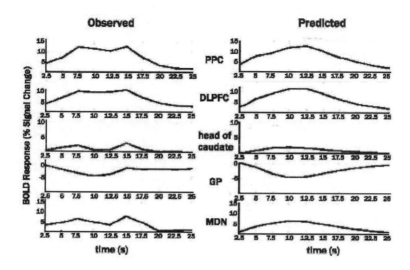

Fig. 2.7: fMRI BOLD signals in regions identified by the FROST model, and BOLD responses predicted by FROST for those regions.

identified by FROST as being important in maintaining the working memory representation of the target location. The only free parameters were from the hrf (because the boxcar function has no free parameters, and the parameters of FROST were fixed from the fits to single-cell recordings), and both models used the same hrf.

For both models, the parameters of the hrf were estimated using a least squares criterion. The best-fitting version of the boxcar model accounted for 61% of the variance in the observed BOLD signals, whereas the best-fitting version of FROST accounted for 93% of the variance. Thus, for these data at least, FROST not only made accurate a priori predictions about which brain regions should show significant delay-related activation, but it also gave a better quantitative account of the BOLD signals in these regions than the widely used boxcar model.

2.4.2   Nonlinear Models of the BOLD Response

According to the linear systems approach described by Equation 2.19, the response to a pair of stimuli presented simultaneously should equal the sum of the responses to each stimulus presented in isolation. This is the well-known superposition property that characterizes all linear systems. As mentioned earlier, superposition is approximately satisfied if the intertrial interval exceeds one second and if brief stimulus exposure durations are avoided (Vazquez & Noll, 1998). However, if stimulus events quickly follow one another, or if brief stimulus exposure durations are used, then it is well documented that the BOLD signal exhibits significant nonlinearities (Hinrichs et al., 2000; Huettel & McCarthy, 2000; Ogawa et al., 2000; Pfeuffer et al., 2003).

One reason these nonlinearities apparently occur is that, although blood flow increases with neural activity, the BOLD signal has a nonlinear dependence on flow (e.g., Mechelli et al., 2001; Miller et al., 2001). For example, the BOLD signal might saturate at high levels of blood flow, in the sense that further increases in flow cause negligible increases in the concentration of deoxyhemoglobin. In this way, a moderately strong stimulus could evoke a near-maximal fMRI response, leaving little room for further increases in response (even to a stronger stimulus).

There have been a number of attempts to model nonlinearities in the BOLD response. One of the earliest and best-known nonlinear models is the balloon model of Buxton et al. (1998), which is based on the biomechanical properties of the brain's vasculature. The BOLD signal depends on blood flow, blood volume, and blood oxygenation, and the balloon model incorporates the conflicting effects of dynamic changes in both blood oxygenation and blood volume, and it assumes that the volume flow out of the system depends on a balloon-like pressure of the vasculature. For example, when the blood flow is high, the walls of the blood vessels are under greater tension; as a result they push the blood out with greater force, which reduces the rate at which oxygen is extracted from the hemoglobin. The balloon model directly models this inherent nonlinearity. However, the balloon model makes the simplifying assumption that there is no capillary contribution to the BOLD signal—an assumption challenged by more recent models (e.g., Zheng et al., 2002).

One practical drawback to the balloon model is its complexity. Implementing the model requires a major computational effort. Fortunately, computationally simpler alternatives exist. One especially attractive choice is to construct a Volterra series to model the nonlinearities in the BOLD signal. An important theorem in nonlinear systems theory states that the output of almost any time-invariant nonlinear system can be expressed as a Volterra series of its input (e.g., Schetzen, 1980). In the present case, this means that the BOLD response can be defined by the following function (i.e., the Volterra series) of the neural activation $A(t)$:

$$\text{BOLD}(t) = \sum_{i=1}^{\infty} H_i[A(t)], \qquad (2.23)$$

where

$$H_i[A(t)] = \int_{-\infty}^{\infty} \cdots \int_{-\infty}^{\infty} h_i(\tau_1, \cdots, \tau_i) A(t - \tau_1) \cdots A(t - \tau_i) d\tau_1 \cdots d\tau_i.$$

$$(2.24)$$

The function $h_i(\tau_1, \cdots, \tau_i)$ is called the ith Volterra kernel.

Note that

$$H_1[A(t)] = \int_{-\infty}^{\infty} h_1(\tau_1) A(t - \tau_1) d\tau_1, \qquad (2.25)$$

which is the familiar convolution integral (i.e., see Equation 2.19), so $h_1(\tau)$ is just the hrf. In other words, $H_1[A(t)]$ models the linear response and the higher order kernels model the nonlinearities in the response. So the standard linear approach is to assume that $\text{BOLD}(t) = H_1[A(t)]$. Friston and colleagues (1998) argued that the nonlinearities modeled by the balloon model could be approximated by

$$\text{BOLD}(t) = H_1[A(t)] + H_2[A(t)]. \qquad (2.26)$$

Thus, we need only supplement the usual linear approach by adding a second-order correction for nonlinearity.

Now

$$H_2[A(t)] = \int_{-\infty}^{\infty} \int_{-\infty}^{\infty} h_2(\tau_1, \tau_2) A(t - \tau_1) A(t - \tau_2) d\tau_1 d\tau_2, \qquad (2.27)$$

so to follow this approach we must specify the second-order Volterra kernel $h_2(\tau_1, \tau_2)$. Friston et al. (1998) suggested

$$h_2(\tau_1, \tau_2) = \sum_{i=1}^{3} \sum_{j=1}^{3} \beta_{ij} b_i(\tau_1) b_j(\tau_2), \qquad (2.28)$$

where the $b_i(\tau)$ are the gamma basis functions of Eqs. 2.16, 2.17, and 2.18, and the β_{ij} are free parameters. The computational advantage of using basis functions to model the hrf extends to the second-order Volterra kernel because substituting Equation 2.28 into 2.27 yields

$$H_2[A(t)] = \sum_{i=1}^{3} \sum_{j=1}^{3} \beta_{ij} \int_{-\infty}^{\infty} \int_{-\infty}^{\infty} b_i(\tau_1) b_j(\tau_2) A(t-\tau_1) A(t-\tau_2) d\tau_1 d\tau_2.$$

(2.29)

If the parameters of the core neural network are estimated using other data, then none of these (nine) double integrals involves any free parameters. Thus, as in the linear case, they can be computed numerically before the parameter estimation process begins. As before, parameter estimation can now be accomplished using standard regression techniques.

Figure 2.8 shows the predicted BOLD response from this model to a simple neural activation (also shown). To generate this prediction, all nonlinear coefficients were set to zero, except β_{11}, which was set to 4. Also shown is the linear model (i.e., Equation 2.20) that provides the best fit to the nonlinear BOLD response. Although the linear model shows systematic deviations from the nonlinear model, the fit is reasonably good and would probably be satisfactory for most cognitive experiments. With more complex neural activations, the difference between the linear and nonlinear predictions would increase. For example, as mentioned earlier, when stimulus events closely follow one another, the nonlinearities in the BOLD response become especially pronounced.

2.5   PROBLEM 5: FITTING BEHAVIORAL DATA

The models derived in this chapter predict how neural activations change in specific brain regions under different experimental conditions. Of course, neural activations are not behaviors, so to fit the models to behavioral data, some assumptions must be added that describe how neural activation is related to behavior. In most cases, this process involves at least two steps. The first is to identify which brain regions in the hypothesized network control the behavioral response. This problem is similar to problem 1 in the sense that neither has an algorithmic solution. Instead, a solution depends on one's

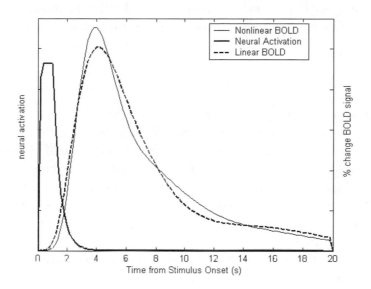

Fig. 2.8: Hypothetical neural activation from a simple experiment and the BOLD response predicted by the nonlinear model described in Equations 2.25, 2.26, and 2.29. Also shown is the best fitting BOLD response from the linear hrf model.

knowledge of the relevant neuroscience literatures. For example, the FROST model of working memory (Ashby et al., 2005) includes differential equations that describe neural activation in parietal cortex, prefrontal cortex, thalamus, caudate nucleus, and globus pallidus. Yet it makes sense, for a variety of reasons that are beyond the scope of this chapter, to assume that the integrity of a working memory depends primarily on neural activation within prefrontal cortex.

Once the critical neural structure is identified, the second step is to decide how activation in this region controls behavior. There are many possibilities, but we have had success with two especially simple assumptions. The first assumes that the behavioral response is correct if the activation on a critical unit exceeds a threshold. This is an obvious model for any kind of task that requires a YES/NO or GO/NO GO response. For tasks in which subjects must select among several alternatives, a natural assumption is that different neural units within the critical region control different responses, and the unit with the greatest activation determines the behavioral response.

2.5.1   Threshold Model

As mentioned before, in tasks requiring a YES/NO or GO/NO GO response, it is natural to assume that a YES or GO response occurs if activation on some critical neural unit exceeds a threshold. Of course, all real data have inherent variability. If accuracy is the dependent variable of interest, then experimental conditions are arranged so that subjects do not always emit the same response to the same stimulus; if the focus is on response time (RT), then the data exhibit trial-by-trial variability no matter what the experimental conditions. The models highlighted in this chapter can only account for such variability if we somehow add noise to the network.

There are many ways to add noise to the models proposed here. Unfortunately, there is a tradeoff among these methods between intuitive plausibility and mathematical tractability. The most intuitively appealing method is to add noise to the input, and perhaps also within each unit, and let it propagate through the network. This makes the differential equations stochastic. Although there is a well-developed mathematical theory of stochastic differential equations (e.g., Øksendal, 2000), the computational problems associated with finding numerical solutions are extreme—mostly because of the discontinuous nature of standard (white) noise processes.

A second choice that is less intuitively appealing, but more mathematically tractable, is to allow the network to be deterministic and then add a stochastic noise process to the output of the critical neural unit that determines the response. For example, suppose we assume that the subject responds YES if the activation $A(t)$ (obtained by solving the differential equation describing the critical unit) exceeds a threshold τ sometime before a response deadline occurs. If a noise process $\varepsilon(t)$ is added to $A(t)$, then the decision rule becomes

$$\text{Respond YES if } A(t) + \varepsilon(t) > \tau. \tag{2.30}$$

A variety of different models can be used for the noise process $\varepsilon(t)$, including white noise, a Wiener process, or an Ornstein-Uhlenbeck process (e.g., Cox & Miller, 1965). In any case, however, the resulting stochastic process $A(t) + \varepsilon(t)$ is nonstationary (i.e., nonergodic or inhomogeneous) because $A(t)$ changes with time, which changes the statistical properties of the process. As a result, analytic predictions of either accuracy or RT will be difficult to derive. Even so, some excellent numerical methods for deriving predictions have been developed (e.g, Diederich & Busemeyer, 2003; Smith, 2000), so this method of adding noise is a viable option.

A third method for adding noise, which is the most psychologically implausible of the three, but which leads to simple analytic predictions, is to assume that on each trial a single sample from a noise distribution is added to the output activation of the critical unit. Thus, the decision rule in Equation 2.30 becomes

$$\text{Respond YES if } A(t) + \varepsilon > \tau, \qquad (2.31)$$

where ε is a sample from some noise distribution. A common approach would be to assume that ε is normally distributed with mean 0 and variance σ_ε^2. In this case, analytic predictions about accuracy and RT can be derived in a straightforward manner.

To begin, note that the noise ε has no effect on the shape of the activation function $A(t)$. This is because ε has a single value on each trial, so the effect of adding noise is to displace the activation function $A(t)$ up or down on each trial by a random amount. For this reason, the maximum value of $A(t) + \varepsilon$ occurs at the same time point on every trial (i.e., assuming the same stimulus conditions). Call this time t_R. Thus, if $A(t) + \varepsilon$ ever exceeds the threshold τ, it must exceed the threshold at time t_R. Thus,

$$
\begin{aligned}
P(\text{YES}) &= P[A(t) + \varepsilon > \tau], \text{for some time } t \\
&= P[A(t_R) + \varepsilon > \tau] \\
&= P[\varepsilon > \tau - A(t_R)] \\
&= P\left[Z > \frac{\tau - A(t_R)}{\sigma_\varepsilon}\right] \\
&= 1 - P\left[Z \leq \frac{\tau - A(t_R)}{\sigma_\varepsilon}\right], \qquad (2.32)
\end{aligned}
$$

where Z has a standard z-distribution. Thus, this probability can be computed from z-tables. If all parameters needed to compute $A(t_R)$

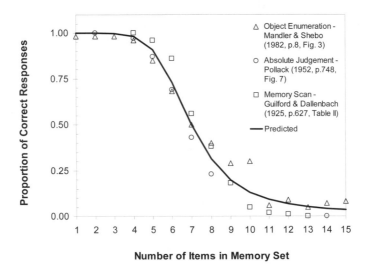

Fig. 2.9: Some classic working memory span data and fits by the FROST model using the threshold model as an interface.

were estimated from previous fits to neuroscience data, the only free parameters here are τ and σ_ε^2.

We (Ashby et al., 2005) previously used this threshold model to fit the FROST model of working memory to the most classic of all working memory span data—namely, the data that formed the basis of Miller's famous magical number 7 ± 2. Figure 2.9 (adapted from Batchelder, 2000) summarizes data from three very different working memory experiments—classic memory span (Guilford & Dallenbach, 1925), span of apprehension or object enumeration (Mandler & Shebo, 1982), and absolute identification of pure tones (Pollack, 1952). Figure 2.9 shows the proportion of correct responses as a function of set size for all three experiments. The magical number seven results if the criterion for working memory capacity is defined as the number of items for which accuracy is 50%.

Without going into details of the application, we (Ashby et al., 2005) assumed that each to-be-remembered item would be encoded by activity in its own prefrontal cortical unit, and that the subject would correctly retrieve this item if the activation in its associated unit exceeds a threshold τ at the time of retrieval. The free parameters in this decision model are τ and the noise variance σ_ε^2. Fits of this model to the classic data shown in Figure 2.9 are indicated by the solid curve.[1] As can be seen, FROST provides an excellent account of these behavioral data, accounting for 99.7% of the variance in the mean memory span data.

The threshold model can also be used to make RT predictions, although in the case of RT, the stochastic noise model described by Equation 2.30 is usually a better alternative. In some simple cases, however, the static noise model may suffice. The derivation here closely follows that presented by Ashby (1982). We assume that a YES response occurs as soon as the threshold τ is first exceeded. Thus, the cumulative RT distribution function on YES trials is given by

$$P(RT \leq t|\text{YES}) = \frac{P[A(t) + \varepsilon > \tau, A(t_R) + \varepsilon > \tau]}{P[A(t_R) + \varepsilon > \tau]}$$

$$= \frac{P[A(t) + \varepsilon > \tau]}{P[A(t_R) + \varepsilon > \tau]}. \tag{2.33}$$

Now the denominator of Equation 2.33 is given in Equation 2.32, whereas the numerator is equal to

$$P[A(t) + \varepsilon > \tau] = 1 - P\left[Z \leq \frac{\tau - A(t)}{\sigma_\varepsilon}\right]. \tag{2.34}$$

Equations 2.32 to 2.34 specify the RT distribution in any experimental condition in which activation functions can be predicted.

2.5.2   Max Activation Model

The threshold model makes sense only if there are two response alternatives. In experiments with more than two alternatives, a plausible assumption is that different units control different responses, and that

---

[1] A third parameter was estimated in these fits. This extra parameter measured the strength of lateral inhibition between prefrontal cortical units. This parameter could not be estimated from single-cell recording data because the available single-cell data were all derived from tasks in which there was only one item in the memory set.

the behavioral response is determined by the unit with the greatest activation. As with the threshold model, a variety of different noise models could be used. However, the computational problems with the more psychologically plausible models are even more severe in the max activation model because of the greater number of response alternatives. Even so, under appropriate distributional assumptions, the single-noise-sample-per-trial model remains tractable.

Suppose there are n alternative responses. Let $A_i(t)$ denote the output activation of the unit that controls response i, let ε_i denote the value of the noise added to $A_i(t)$, and let t_R denote the response time. Then the max rule is to

$$\text{Respond } i \text{ if } A_i(t_R) + \varepsilon_i = \max_{k=1}^{n}[A_k(t_R) + \varepsilon_k], \qquad (2.35)$$

Computing the probability that response i is emitted is, in general, a difficult problem. However, the solution is well known in the special case in which the ε_k are all independent and identically distributed with double exponential distributions (Yellott, 1977). In this case, the probability reduces to the familiar Luce-Shepard choice rule (Luce, 1963; Shepard, 1957):

$$P(i) = \frac{A_i(t_R)}{\sum\limits_k A_k(t_R)}. \qquad (2.36)$$

A slight generalization of this model, which adds one free parameter, is to assume that the probability of response i is given by

$$P(i) = \frac{A_i^{\gamma}(t_R)}{\sum\limits_k A_k^{\gamma}(t_R)}. \qquad (2.37)$$

The exponent γ, which was introduced to the model by Ashby and Maddox (1993), is inversely related to response variability. For example, as γ approaches infinity, the model predicts that the subject will respond i on all trials for which the activation is greatest on unit i. In contrast, when $\gamma = 0$, the model responds at chance performance no matter what the neural activations. For this reason, γ is inversely related to the amount of internal noise, σ_{ε}^2 (i.e., see Ashby & Maddox, 1993).

We (Ashby et al., 2003) have also used the max activation rule to fit the FROST model to some human behavioral data from a task designed to be as similar as possible to the delayed response tasks used in many single-cell recording studies and in the Ell et al. (2003) neuroimaging study. The major constraint was to increase difficulty enough so that errors were common. On each trial, a target dot and 0, 1, or 2 distractor dots of different colors were briefly displayed at random locations. After a delay of 0, 2, 4, or 6 seconds, the target dot and 49 distractor dots of the same color as the target were displayed. The subject's task was to point to the location of the target dot. Experiment 1 varied the number of initial distractors (i.e., from 0 to 2), whereas Experiment 2 was identical to the one-distractor condition of Experiment 1, except the target had the same color on 75% of the trials.

The proportions of correct responses at each delay are plotted in Figure 2.10 for both experiments. Also shown are the fits of FROST using the max activation model (i.e., Equation 2.37). The critical variable in FROST is the amount of activation in the PFC working memory unit associated with the spatial location of the target dot. The model predicts a correct response so long as this activation is substantially larger than the activations produced by the 49 distractor dots. The data from Experiments 1 and 2 were fit simultaneously (the data had 20 degrees of freedom). As in our other applications, the numerical constants in the basic FROST circuit were determined by first fitting the model to single-cell recording data. As a result, FROST had only four free parameters in this application.[2] As can be seen, FROST provides an excellent account of these behavioral data, accounting for more than 97% of the variance in these 20 data points. This is especially impressive given that only four free parameters were estimated to fit these 20 data points.

---

[2] The four parameters were as follows: (a) the response variability parameter γ from Equation 2.37, (b) the summed magnitude of PFC activations induced by all 49 distractor dots, (c) the strength of PFC lateral inhibition, and (d) a parameter that modulated the strength of lateral inhibition in Experiment 2 depending on the target selection probability (i.e., so that the inhibition of more probable targets on less probable targets was greater than the opposite inhibition).

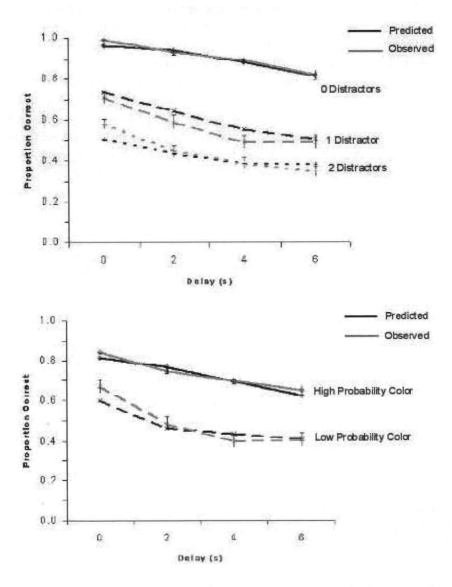

Fig. 2.10: (a) Experiment 1 and (b) Experiment 2. Human delayed response data and fits by the FROST model using the max activation model as an interface.

2.6   CONCLUSIONS

The cognitive neuroscience revolution has carried with it a dramatic increase in the variety of data sources that are now routinely considered. Whereas the older purely cognitive theories generally were concerned only with behavioral measures of response accuracy and response time, today's theories might also be challenged with neuropsychological patient data, functional neuroimaging data, EEGs and ERPs, animal lesion results, and single-cell recording data. Such incredible diversity requires a new approach to model building. The methods described in this chapter were developed as a first attempt to meet this challenge.

This chapter focuses on fitting three different types of data: single-cell recordings, fMRI, and behavioral data. However, the same models could also be used to fit other kinds of data. One important application is to model neuropsychological patient data. For example, lesions can be modeled by setting the output of the lesioned brain region to zero or, perhaps more realistically, by reducing the gain on this output.

If the goal is to model a qualitatively different type of data than was discussed in this chapter, then a new interface is needed that carries the neural activations predicted by the core neural network to this new dependent variable. For example, an obvious extension of the methods presented here would be to ERPs. In traditional ERP analyses, the goal is to solve the so-called *inverse problem*—that is, to determine which brain regions produced the pattern of electrical charges observed on the scalp. In our case, however, the brain regions and their activations would be known (i.e., specified by the model), so our problem would be to solve the less difficult forward problem – to determine the pattern of electrical charges on the scalp that would follow from a given set of neural activations. The forward problem poses a significant challenge, and a complete discussion is beyond the scope of this chapter. Even so, significant progress has been made toward its solution (e.g., Ferguson & Stroink, 1997), so it seems reasonable to expect that an acceptable interface could be developed that would allow the network models described here to be fit to ERP data.

Another advantage of the models proposed here is that, because they are closely related to the underlying neuroscience, they are easy to augment with other neuroscience models. For example, we recently proposed a model of how dopamine modulates glutamate activity in frontal cortex (Ashby & Casale, 2003). This model makes much more detailed neuroscience assumptions than the models described in this chapter (e.g., about how dopamine has different modulatory effects on NMDA versus AMPA receptor activations). Models produced using our standard approach could be generalized by incorporating more detailed neuroscience models of this type into the differential equations that describe activation in frontal areas. The resulting augmented model could then be used to predict how changes in cortical dopamine affect the behavior of interest.

In summary, the methods described here represent a new approach to the computational modeling of cognitive processes. Our goal in developing these methods was to bridge the gaps among neuroanatomy, behavioral neuroscience, brain imaging, and cognition. Although it is far too early to decide how successful we have been, it is true that the application of these methods has forced us to consider carefully and attempt to integrate a far more extensive and diverse set of results than in our previous modeling efforts, which used more traditional, purely cognitive methods. In this sense, at least, the approach described here has already been successful.

ACKNOWLEDGMENTS

Preparation of this chapter was supported in part by Public Health Service Grant MH3760. We thank Michael Casale, Shawn Ell, and Elliott Waldron for their invaluable participation in the development of the methods described in this chapter.

References

Amini, B., Clark, J. W. & Canavier, C. C. (1999). Calcium dynamics underlying pacemaker-like and burst firing oscillations in midbrain dopaminergic neurons: A computational study. *Journal of Neurophysiology, 82*, 2249–2261.

Ashby, F. G. (1982). Deriving exact predictions from the cascade model. *Psychological Review, 89*, 599–607.

Ashby, F. G. (1992). *Multidimensional models of perception and cognition*, chapter Multivariate probability distributions, (pp. 1–34). Hillsdale, NJ: Lawrence Erlbaum Associates, Inc.

Ashby, F. G. & Casale, M. B. (2003). A model of dopamine modulated cortical activation. *Neural Networks, 16*, 973–984.

Ashby, F. G. & Ell, S. W. (2002). *Steven's handbook of experimental psychology: Methodology in experimental psychology* (3rd Ed.), Volume 4, chapter Single versus multiple systems of learning and memory, (pp. 655–692). New York: Wiley.

Ashby, F. G., Ell, S. W., Valentin, V. V. & Casale, M. B. (2003). A neurocomputational model of working memory and executive attention. Unpublished manuscript.

Ashby, F. G., Ell, S. W., Valentin, V. V. & Casale, M. B. (2005). FROST: A distributed neurocomputational model of working memory. *Journal of Cognitive Neuroscience, 17*, 1728–1743.

Ashby, F. G. & Maddox, W. T. (1993). Relations between prototype, exemplar, and decision bound models of categorization. *Journal of Mathematical Psychology, 37*, 372–400.

Bandettini, P. A., Wong, E. C., Hinks, R. S., Tikofsky, R. S. & Hyde, J. S. (1992). Time course EPI of human brain function during task activation. *Magnetic Resonance Medicine, 25*, 390–397.

Batchelder, B. L. (2000). The magical number 4 = 7: Span theory on capacity limitations. *Behavioral and Brain Sciences, 24*, 116–117.

Boynton, G. M., Engel, S. A., Glover, G. H. & Heeger, D. J. (1996). Linear systems analysis of functional magnetic resonance imaging in human v1. *Journal of Neuroscience, 16*, 4207–4221.

Brunel, N. & Wang, X.-J. (2001). Effects of neuromodulation in a cortical network model of object working memory dominated by recurrent inhibition. *Journal of Computational Neuroscience, 11(1)*, 63–85.

Buxton, R. B. & Frank, L. R. (1998). A model for coupling between cerebral blood flow and oxygen metabolism during neural stimulation. *Journal of Cerebral Blood Flow and Metabolism, 17*, 64–72.

Buxton, R. B., Wong, E. C. & Frank, L. R. (1998). Dynamics of blood flow and oxygenation changes during brain activation: the balloon model. *Magnetic Resonance in Medicine, 39*, 855–864.

Canavier, C. C. & Wilson, C. J. (1999). Sodium dynamics underlying burst firing and putative mechanisms for the regulation of the firing pattern in midbrain dopamine neurons: A computational approach. *Journal of Computational Neuroscience, 6*, 49–69.

Chen, C. (1970). *Introduction to linear systems theory*. New York: Holt, Rinehart and Winston.

Clark, V. P., Maisog, J. M. & Haxby, J. V. (1998). FMRI studies of face memory using random stimulus sequences. *Journal of Neurophysiology, 79*, 3257–3265.

Cohen, M. S. (1997). Parametric analysis of fMRI data using linear systems methods. *Neuroimage, 6*, 93–103.

Constantinidis, C. & Steinmetz, M. (1996). Neuronal activity in posterior parietal area 7a during the delay periods of a spatial memory task. *Journal of Neurophysiology, 76*, 1352–1354.

Cox, D. R. & Miller, H. D. (1965). *The theory of stochastic processes*. London: Methuen.

Dale, A. M. & Buckner, R. L. (1997). Selective averaging of rapidly presented individual trials using fMRI. *Human Brain Mapping, 5*, 329–340.

Diederich, A. & Busemeyer, J. R. (2003). Simple matrix methods for analyzing diffusion models of choice probability, choice response time, and simple response time. *Journal of Mathematical Psychology, 47*, 304–322.

Durstewitz, D., Kelc, M. & Gunturkun, O. (1999). A neurocomputational theory of the dopaminergic modulation of working memory functions. *Journal of Neuroscience, 19*, 2807–2822.

Durstewitz, D., Seamans, J. K. & Sejnowski, T. J. (2000). Dopamine-mediated stabilization of delay-period activity in a network model of prefrontal cortex. *Journal of Neurophysiology*, *83*, 1733–1750.

Ell, S. W., Ashby, F. G. & Miller, M. B. (2003). An analysis of delay-related activity in spatial working memory using event-related fMRI. Unpublished manuscript.

Ferguson, A. S. & Stroink, G. (1997). Factors affecting the accuracy of the boundary element method in the forward problem, I: Calculating surface potentials. *IEEE Transactions on Biomedical Engineering*, *44*, 1139–1155.

Friston, K. J., Holmes, A. P. & Ashburner, J. (1999). Statistical parametric mapping (SPM). http://www.fil.ion.ucl.ac.uk/spm/.

Friston, K. J., Holmes, A. P., Worsley, K., Poline, J., Frith, C. & Frackowiak, R. (1995). Statistical parametric maps in functional imaging: a general linear approach. *Human Brain Mapping*, *2*, 189–210.

Friston, K. J., Josephs, O., Ress, G. & Turner, R. (1998). Nonlinear event-related responses in fMRI. *Magnetic Resonance in Medicine*, *39*, 41–52.

Fuster, J. M. (1973). Unit activity in prefrontal cortex during delayed-response performance: Neuronal correlates of transient memory. *Journal of Neurophysiology*, *36*, 61–78.

Fuster, J. M. & Alexander, G. E. (1973). Firing changes in cells of the nucleus medialis dorsalis associated with delayed response behavior. *Brain Research*, *61*, 79–91.

Grimwood, P. D., Martin, S. J. & Morris, R. G. M. (2001). *Synapses*, chapter Synaptic plasticity and memory, (pp. 519–570). Baltimore, MD: Johns Hopkins.

Guilford, J. P. & Dallenbach, K. M. (1925). The determination of memory span by the method of constant stimuli. *American Journal of Psychology*, *36*, 621–628.

Hikosaka, O., Sakamoto, M. & Sadanari, U. (1989). Functional properties of monkey caudate neurons III. activities related to expectation of target and reward. *Journal of Neurophysiology*, *61*, 814–831.

Hinrichs, H., Scholz, M., Tempelmann, C., Woldorff, M., Dale, A. M. & Heinze, H. J. (2000). Deconvolution of event-related fMRI responses in fast-rate experimental designs: Tracking amplitude variations. *Journal of Cognitive Neuroscience*, *12(6)*, 76–89.

Huettel, S. A. & McCarthy, G. (2000). Evidence for a refractory period in the hemodynamic response to visual stimuli as measured by MRI. *Neuroimage*, *11*, 547–553.

Koch, C. (1999). *Biophysics of computation*. New York: Oxford.

Kwong, K. K., Belliveau, J. W., Chesler, D. A., Goldberg, I. E., Weiskoff, R. M., Poncelet, B. P., Kennedy, D. N., Hoppel, B. E., Cohen, M. S., Turner, R., Cheng, H. M., Brady, T. J. & Rosen, B. R. (1992). Dynamic magnetic resonance imaging of human brain activity during primary sensory stimulation. *Proceedings of the National Academy of Sciences*, *89*, 5675–5679.

Logothetis, N. K. (2003). The underpinnings of the BOLD functional magnetic resonance imaging signal. *The Journal of Neuroscience*, *23*, 3963–3971.

Logothetis, N. K., Pauls, J., Augath, M., Trinath, T. & Oeltermann, A. (2001). Neurophysiological investigation of the basis of the fMRI signal. *Nature*, *412*, 150–157.

Luce, R. D. (1963). *Handbook of mathematical psychology*, Volume 1, chapter Detection and recognition, (pp. 103–190). New York: Wiley.

Mandler, G. & Shebo, B. J. (1982). Subitizing: An analysis of its component processes. *Journal of Experimental Psychology: General*, *111*, 1–22.

Martin, S. J. & Morris, R. G. (2002). New life in an old idea: The synaptic plasticity and memory hypothesis revisited. *Hippocampus*, *12*, 609–636.

Mechelli, A., Price, C. J. & Friston, K. J. (2001). Nonlinear coupling between evoked rCBF and BOLD signals: A simulation study of hemodynamic responses. *Neuroimage*, *14*, 862–872.

Miller, K. L., Luh, W. M., Liu, T. T., Martinez, A., Obata, T., Wong, E. C., Frank, L. R. & Buxton, R. B. (2001). Nonlinear temporal dynamics of the cerebral blood flow response. *Human Brain Mapping*, *13*, 1–12.

Mushiake, H. & Strick, P. (1995). Pallidal neuron activity during sequential arm movements. *Journal of Neurophysiology*, *74*, 2754–2758.

Ogawa, S., Lee, T. M., Kay, A. R. & Tank, D. W. (1990a). Brain magnetic resonance imaging with contrast dependent on blood oxygenation. *Proceedings of the National Academy of Sciences*, *87*, 9868–9872.

Ogawa, S., Lee, T. M., Nayak, A. S. & Glynn, P. (1990b). Oxygenation-sensitive contrast in magnetic resonance imaging of rodent brain at high magnetic fields. *Magnetic Resonance in Medicine*, *16*, 9–18.

Ogawa, S., Lee, T. M., Stepnoski, R., Chen, W., Zhu, X. H. & Ugurbil, K. (2000). An approach to probe some neural systems interaction by functional MRI at neural time scale down to milliseconds. *Proceeding of the National Academy of Sciences USA*, *97*, 1102611031.

Ogawa, S., Tank, D. W., Menon, R., Ellermann, J. M., Kim, S.-G., Merkle, H. & Ugurbil, K. (1992). Intrinsic signal changes accompanying sensory stimulation: functional brain mapping with magnetic resonance imaging. *Proceedings of the National Academy of Sciences*, *89*, 5951–5955.

Øksendal, B. (2000). *Stochastic differential equations* (Fifth Ed.). Berlin: Springer.

Pfeuffer, J., McCullough, J. C., Van de Moortele, P.-F., Ugurbil, K. & Hu, X. (2003). Spatial dependence of the nonlinear BOLD response at short stimulus duration. *Neuroimage*, *18*, 990–1000.

Pollack, I. (1952). The information of elementary auditory displays. *Journal of the Acoustical Society of America*, *24*, 745–749.

Press, W. H., Flannery, B. P., Teukolsky, S. A. & Vettering, W. T. (1988). *Numerical recipes in C.* New York: Cambridge.

Rumelhart, D. E. & McClelland, J. L. E. (1986). *Parallel distributed processing. Volume 1: Foundations.* Cambridge, MA: MIT Press.

Schetzen, M. (1980). *The Volterra and Wiener theories of nonlinear systems.* New York: Wiley.

Shepard, R. N. (1957). Stimulus and response generalization: A stochastic model relating generalization to distance in psychological space. *Psychometrika*, *22*, 325–345.

Smith, P. L. (2000). Stochastic dynamic models of response time and accuracy: A foundational primer. *Journal of Mathematical Psychology*, *44*, 408–463.

Vazquez, A. & Noll, D. (1998). Non-linear aspects of the blood oxygenation response in functional MRI. *Neuroimage*, *8*, 108–118.

Yellott, J. I. J. (1977). The relationship between Luce's choice axiom, Thurstone's theory of comparative judgment, and the double exponential distribution. *Journal of Mathematical Psychology*, *15*, 109–144.

Zarahn, E., Aquirre, G. & D'Esposito, M. (1997). A trial-based experimental design for fMRI. *Neuroimage*, *6*, 122–138.

Zheng, Y., Martindale, J., Johnston, D., Jones, M., Berwick, J. & Mayhew, J. (2002). A model of the hemodynamic response and oxygen delivery to brain. *Neuroimage*, *16*, 617–637.

3

Modeling the Role of Acetylcholine and Hippocampal Theta Rhythm in Memory-Guided Behavior

Michael E. Hasselmo, Jill McGaughy, and Christiane Linster
Boston University

Computational modeling provides an effective means of linking data across different levels of experimental techniques. Currently, extensive physiological and molecular data concerns cellular mechanisms of cholinergic modulation within cortical structures. However, these data have not been extensively linked to the behavioral evidence for a role of acetylcholine in memory function or attentional mechanisms. This chapter describes a computational modeling framework that simultaneously addresses detailed experimental data at both cellular and behavioral levels, providing a means to bridge the gap between experimental data at a cellular level and the behavior of complete organisms (Hasselmo, 1995, 1999). This chapter also provides a description of how the different physiological effects of acetylcholine could interact to alter specific functional properties of the cortex. As a central theme, the chapter focuses on how acetylcholine enhances the response to afferent sensory input while decreasing the internal processing based on previously formed cortical representations. These same circuit-level effects can be categorized with different colloquial terms at a behavioral level, sometimes being interpreted as an enhancement of attention, sometimes as an enhancement of memory encoding. The same regulatory influences on circuit-level dynamics could underlie all these behavioral effects. This chapter first describes the basic change in circuit dynamics and then reviews specific physiological effects of acetylcholine in the context of this framework. Finally, we discuss how the loss of cholinergic modulation shifts network dynamics toward those appropriate for the consolidation of previously encoded information.

3.1   ACETYLCHOLINE ENHANCES INPUT RELATIVE TO FEEDBACK

This chapter focuses on a single general framework for interpreting the effects of acetylcholine within cortical structures. As summarized in Figure 3.1, acetylcholine appears to enhance the strength of input relative to feedback in the cortex. The physiological effects of acetylcholine serve to enhance the influence of feed-forward afferent input to the cortex while decreasing background activity due to spontaneous spiking and the spread of activity via excitatory feedback connections within cortical circuits. By enhancing the response to sensory input, high levels of acetylcholine make cortical circuits more responsive to specific features of sensory stimuli, enhancing attention to the environment. Similarly, high levels of acetylcholine enhance the encoding of memory for specific stimuli by making cortical circuits respond to the specific features of sensory stimuli, allowing more effective and accurate encoding of sensory events.

This basic theoretical framework is applied in discussing a number of effects of acetylcholine within cortical structures. The change in dynamics results from three primary sets of effects on a physiological level: (a) modulation of intrinsic properties of pyramidal cells, (b) selective modulation of excitatory synaptic transmission, and (c) modulation of inhibitory neuron depolarization and synaptic transmission. The physiological effects of acetylcholine are described within this functional framework in the following sections.

3.2   ACETYLCHOLINE ENHANCES SPIKING RESPONSE TO AFFERENT INPUT

The physiological effects of acetylcholine on cortical pyramidal cells act to enhance the spiking response to excitatory afferent input, consistent with the enhanced response to input summarized in Figure 3.1. Early studies using single-unit recordings from the neocortex showed that application of cholinergic agonists to the cortex would cause a strong increase in neurons' firing rate (Krnjevic & Phillis, 1963). This

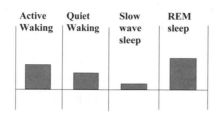

Fig. 3.1: General theory of acetylcholine effects in cortical circuits. This circuit diagram summarizes the predominant effect of acetylcholine within cortical circuits, an increase in the influence of afferent input relative to internal processing. This is due to three sets of effects. (a) Intrinsic properties. Acetylcholine causes depolarization of pyramidal cells, and reduction in spike-frequency accommodation, allowing pyramidal cells to respond more robustly to external afferent input. (b) Modulation of inhibition. Acetylcholine depolarizes inhibitory interneurons, decreasing background spiking activity, while suppressing inhibitory synaptic transmission, allowing a stronger response to afferent input due to reduced inhibitory feedback. (c) Modulation of excitatory synaptic transmission. When acetylcholine is present, activation of nicotinic receptors enhances thalamic afferent input, whereas muscarinic suppression reduces excitatory recurrent processing in cortex.

increase in firing rate was demonstrated to result from a slow depolarization of cortical pyramidal cells due to blockade of a potassium current, causing the membrane potential to move away from the reversal potential of potassium (Krnjevic, Pumain & Renaud, 1971; Benardo & Prince, 1982; Cole & Nicoll, 1984; Barkai & Hasselmo, 1994). This slow depolarization of membrane potential enhances the spiking response to excitatory synaptic input (see Figure 3.2).

Another physiological effect that enhances the spiking response to afferent input is the suppression of spike frequency accommodation, also shown in Figure 3.2. Pyramidal cells normally respond to a sustained current injection with a high initial firing rate that gradually slows down. This results from activation of a voltage-sensitive potassium current (the M current) and also from voltage-dependent calcium influx causing activation of calcium-sensitive potassium currents (the AHP current Constanti & Galvan, 1983; Constanti & Sim, 1987; Madison & Nicoll, 1984; Madison, Lancaster & Nicoll, 1987; Schwindt, Spain, Foehring, Stafstrom, Chubb & Crill, 1988). Activation of muscarinic receptors decreases activation of both of these potassium currents, allowing neurons to fire in a more sustained manner in response to input. This reduction in spike frequency accommodation appears in neocortical structures (McCormick & Prince, 1986) as well as the piriform cortex (Tseng & Haberly, 1989; Barkai & Hasselmo, 1994) and hippocampal region CA1 (Madison & Nicoll, 1984). This effect allows neurons to continue to generate spiking responses to sustained afferent input, which could be very important for maintaining responsiveness to sensory input in attentional tasks. In particular, behavioral accuracy in continuous performance tasks requires neurons to remain responsive to subtle sensory input over extended periods of time. Suppression of spike frequency accommodation could prevent spontaneous background activity from reducing the sensitivity of cortical pyramidal cells to afferent input. Similarly, more sustained spiking activity would be important for maintaining responses necessary for encoding new memories.

3.3   ACETYLCHOLINE SELECTIVELY SUPPRESSES EXCITATORY FEEDBACK BUT DOES NOT SUPPRESS AFFERENT INPUT

Along with the enhancement of response to afferent input caused by depolarization of neurons, acetylcholine appears to reduce the internal processing of information by cortical structures, due to suppression of excitatory synaptic transmission at excitatory feedback connections within cortical circuits. This suppression of excitatory glutamatergic transmission initially appears paradoxical when contrasted with the depolarization of excitatory pyramidal cells. In the framework of computational modeling, these competing effects of acetylcholine make sense when it is emphasized that the cholinergic suppression of excitatory transmission is selective for the excitatory feedback connections. As described later, acetylcholine allows afferent input to maintain a strong influence on cortical circuits.

The selective cholinergic suppression of excitatory feedback, but

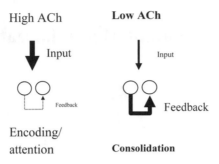

Fig. 3.2: Intrinsic effects which enhance spiking response to afferent input. (a) Acetylcholine causes direct depolarization of pyramidal cell membrane potential (Krnjevic et al., 1971; Krnjevic, 1984; Cole and Nicoll, 1984; Barkai and Hasselmo, 1994), making cells more likely to generate spikes. (b) In addition, acetylcholine allows cells to generate spikes more persistently, due to cholinergic reduction in spike frequency accommodation (Madison and Nicoll, 1984; Tseng and Haberly, 1989; Barkai and Hasselmo, 1994).

not afferent input to the cortex, has been demonstrated in a number of different regions using a number of different techniques. This differential cholinergic modulation was first demonstrated in slice preparations of the piriform cortex (Hasselmo & Bower, 1992). Earlier studies demonstrated cholinergic suppression of excitatory synaptic transmission in tangential slices of the piriform cortex (Williams & Constanti, 1988), but those slices did not allow comparison of different synapses in different layers. As shown in Figure 3.3, the use of coronal slices allowed direct comparison of the cholinergic effects on excitatory afferent input synapses from the olfactory bulb in Layer Ia of piriform cortex versus excitatory feedback connections in Layer Ib (Hasselmo & Bower, 1992). As summarized in Figure 3.3, acetylcholine and muscarine caused selective suppression of excitatory feedback potentials in Layer Ib while having a much weaker effect on afferent input in Layer Ia (Hasselmo & Bower, 1992). This effect has been confirmed in anesthetized preparations in vivo, in which direct stimulation of the cholinergic innervation of piriform cortex suppresses feedback from posterior piriform cortex to anterior pir-

Membrane potential depolarization

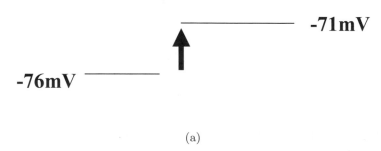

(a)

Reduced spike frequency accomodation

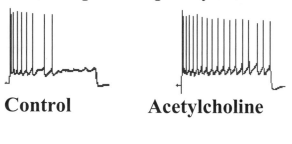

(b)

Fig. 3.3: (a) Membrane potential depolarization (b) Reduced spike frequency accommodation

iform cortex, but does not influence the afferent input to piriform cortex from the lateral olfactory tract (Linster, Wyble & Hasselmo, 1999; Linster & Hasselmo, 2001).

Subsequently, a similar selectivity of cholinergic suppression has been demonstrated in the neocortex. In particular, in slice preparations of somatosensory cortex, cholinergic modulation causes suppression of excitatory transmission at feedback connections from higher order somatosensory cortex, while having less effect on synaptic potentials elicited in layer IV by stimulation of subcortical white matter (Hasselmo & Cekic, 1996). The differential regulation of different pathways was demonstrated further in thalamocortical slice preparations (Gil, Connors & Amitai, 1997), where activation of nicotinic receptors enhanced thalamic input to the neocortex, whereas that of muscarinic receptors suppressed both intracortical and thalamocortical synaptic transmission. Similarly, in the primary auditory cortex, acetylcholine suppressed intracortical synaptic potentials (Hsieh, Cruikshank & Metherate, 2000) while having no effect on or enhancing thalamocortical connections (Metherate & Ashe, 1993; Hsieh, Cruikshank & Metherate, 2000). Cholinergic modulation has also been demonstrated to suppress intracortical synaptic transmission in primary visual cortex (Brocher, Artola & Singer, 1992) and frontal cortex (Vidal & Changeux, 1993). In studies of visual cortex using optical imaging, cholinergic modulation appeared to regulate the intracortical spread of activity while having a much weaker effect on thalamic input (Kimura, Fukuda & Tsumoto, 1999; Kimura, 2000). The nicotinic enhancement of thalamic input to the neocortex has also been demonstrated for the medial dorsal thalamic input to prefrontal cortex (Vidal & Changeux, 1993; Gioanni et al., 1999). Thus, the differential suppression of intracortical feedback connections with sparing of afferent input connections that was demonstrated in piriform cortex appears to generalize to most neocortical regions, supporting the functional framework illustrated in Figure 3.1.

The selective suppression of excitatory synaptic transmission at feedback but not feedforward synapses has also been demonstrated at connections within the hippocampal formation, as described in a recent review (Hasselmo, 1999). The suppression of excitatory synaptic transmission by acetylcholine was described in a number of early studies in slice preparations of the hippocampal formation. Muscarinic suppression of excitatory transmission was reported at connections including the medial entorhinal input to the middle molecular layer of the dentate gyrus (Yamamoto & Kawai, 1967; Kahle & Cotman, 1989) as well as the Schaffer collaterals projecting from hippocampal region CA3 to region CA1 (Hounsgaard, 1978; Valentino & Dingledine, 1981). Similar suppression of Schaffer collateral synaptic potentials was obtained in anesthetized animals with microintophoretic application of acetylcholine (Rovira, Cherubini & Ben-Ari, 1982), stimulation of the medial septum (Rovira, Ben-Ari, Cherubini, Krnjevic & Ropert, 1983), and sensory stimulation that activates hippocampal theta rhythm (Herreras, Solis, Munoz, Martin del Rio & Lerma, 1988a; Herreras, Solis, Herranz, Martin del Rio & Lerma, 1988b). Cholinergic modulation has also been demonstrated to suppress excitatory synaptic transmission in the amygdala (Yajeya et al., 2000).

The differential modulation of excitatory synaptic transmission has been explicitly demonstrated in slice preparations of the hippocampal formation. Within the dentate gyrus, the synaptic inputs to the outer molecular layer from lateral entorhinal cortex show little decrease in the presence of cholinergic agonists (Yamamoto & Kawai, 1967; Kahle & Cotman, 1989). Within hippocampal region CA1, there is strong suppression of excitatory transmission in the stratum radiatum, where Schaffer collateral inputs terminate (Hounsgaard, 1978; Valentino & Dingledine, 1981; Hasselmo & Schnell, 1994), but there is a much weaker suppression of synaptic potentials in the stratum lacunosum-moleculare, where input from entorhinal cortex layer III terminates (Hasselmo & Schnell, 1994). In hippocampal region CA3, excitatory recurrent connections in stratum radiatum are strongly suppressed (Hasselmo, Schnell & Barkai, 1995; Vogt & Regehr, 2001), whereas the effect at synapses from dentate gyrus terminating in stratum lucidum appears much weaker (Hasselmo, Schnell & Barkai, 1995). There was some evidence for suppression of the mossy fiber input from dentate gyrus, but this appeared to be due to secondary cholinergic activation of inhibitory interneurons, because there was no cholinergic suppression of mossy fiber input in the presence of GABAB receptor blockers (Vogt & Regehr, 2001).

The selectivity of the cholinergic suppression of synaptic transmission is summarized in Figure 3.3. This general suppression of excitatory feedback would act to reduce feedback within the hippocampus and from hippocampus to other cortical areas during high acetylcholine levels. But none of these articles shows total suppression—the influence of hippocampus is reduced but not removed, and there is still sufficient feedback to allow retrieval of relevant stored information.

These specific data are consistent with recordings showing changes in feedback transmission in awake, behaving animals. Recordings from the entorhinal cortex suggest that during active waking the influence of hippocampus on entorhinal cortex is weak, as determined by the low rates of spiking activity in deep layers of entorhinal cortex, which receive output from the hippocampus, in contrast to the higher rates of activity in the superficial layers of entorhinal cortex, which send input to the hippocampus (Chrobak & Buzsaki, 1994). In contrast to this weak hippocampal feedback during active waking, the spiking activity in deep entorhinal layers is much higher during quiet waking and slow wave sleep (Chrobak & Buzsaki, 1994). In addition, stimulation of entorhinal input pathways causes very small amplitude-evoked potentials in the entorhinal cortex during active waking, whereas the same stimulation amplitude will evoke much larger evoked potentials in the entorhinal cortex during slow-wave sleep (Winson & Abzug, 1978; Buzsaki, 1986). A weaker cholinergic influence on perforant path input to the dentate gyrus is supported by the fact that EPSPs evoked in the dentate gyrus by angular bundle stimulation are larger during the high acetylcholine levels of active waking than during the lower acetylcholine levels of slow-wave sleep (Winson & Abzug, 1978). In anesthetized animals, sensory stimulation activating theta rhythm appears to increase the sensory response within the dentate gyrus (Herreras, Solis, Herranz, Martin del Rio & Lerma, 1988b), although this may be due to a cholinergic increase in post-synaptic excitability because stimulation of the medial septum causes increases in population spike activity in the dentate gyrus, but does not have a systematic effect on EPSPs (Mizumori, McNaughton & Barnes, 1989).

3.4   CHOLINERGIC MODULATION OF INHIBITORY INTERNEURONS SUPPRESSES BACKGROUND ACTIVITY WHILE ENHANCING RESPONSE TO INPUT

Acetylcholine also regulates the functional properties of cortical circuits through modulation of inhibitory interneurons. As summarized in Figure 3.4, experimental data in the hippocampus demonstrates that acetylcholine simultaneously depolarizes inhibitory interneurons while suppressing the evoked release of GABA at inhibitory synaptic terminals (Pitler & Alger, 1992; Behrends & ten Bruggencate, 1993). In whole-cell clamp recordings, the cholinergic agonist carbachol suppresses spontaneous GABAA inhibitory synaptic potentials, suggesting a direct suppression of the release of synaptic vesicles containing GABA (Pitler & Alger, 1992). However, carbachol also increases the number of miniature synaptic potentials presumed to result from the spontaneous spiking of inhibitory interneurons (Pitler & Alger, 1992). This coincides with other evidence showing that application of acetylcholine causes direct increases in spiking activity of inhibitory interneurons (McCormick & Prince, 1986). This evidence includes recordings from inhibitory interneurons in cortical structures that demonstrate direct depolarization of inhibitory interneurons by activation of cholinergic receptors in the hippocampus (Chapman & Lacaille, 1999; Frazier, Rollins, Breese, Leonard, Freedman & Dunwiddie, 1998; McQuiston & Madison, 1999a, 1999b). The activation of muscarinic receptors causes depolarization in many individual interneurons (McQuiston & Madison, 1999b). Similarly, activation of nicotinic receptors depolarizes interneurons with different receptor properties in different neurons (McQuiston & Madison, 1999a). The direct depolarization of interneurons is consistent with the fact that nicotinic receptor activation causes an increase in GABA currents in hippocampal pyramidal cells and interneurons (Alkondon & Albuquerque, 2001).

Thus, acetylcholine appears to increase spiking activity in inhibitory interneurons, while decreasing synaptic transmission from these neurons. These effects appear somewhat paradoxical; but as demonstrated in Figure 3.4, computational modeling provides a framework for understanding such a combination. The influence of these two effects was analyzed in a circuit model evaluating the steady-state response to different levels of afferent input A. The cholinergic depolarization of interneurons has the effect of reducing the background firing rate of pyramidal cells during weak afferent input. In contrast, the cholinergic suppression of GABAergic transmission has the effect of enhancing the steady-state response to strong afferent input. Thus, these cholinergic effects reduce background activity, but heighten the response to supra-threshold stimuli. Overall, these modulation effects on inhibition could enhance the sensitivity of cortical circuits to specific sensory input, important for performance in attention tasks as well as encoding tasks. The reduction in background firing could enhance the detection of subtle sensory input (assuming

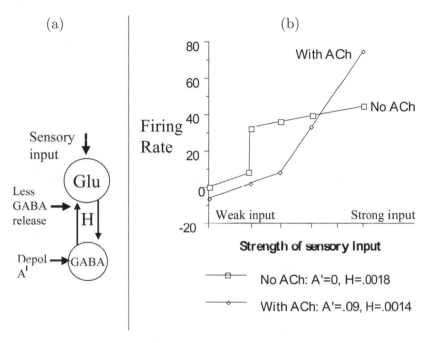

Fig. 3.4: Schematic diagram of cholinergic modulation of inhibition. (a) Basic circuit diagram depicting feedback inhibition. A population of excitatory neurons (labeled by Glu) receives depolarizing afferent input A. These neurons send excitatory output to inhibitory interneurons (labeled GABA). Modulatory effects of acetylcholine include direct suppression of inhibitory synaptic transmission (H) and direct depolarization of inhibitory interneuron membrane potential (represented by depolarizing input A). (b) Analysis of this circuit demonstrates that these effects of acetylcholine decrease background activity while enhancing the response to strong afferent input. The equilibrium (steady state) of the network is plotted for different levels of afferent input A. When acetylcholine is not present (A=0, H=0.0018), the network responds to weak afferent input and only shows slight increases as afferent input increases. When acetylcholine is present, causing depolarization of interneurons (A=0.09) and suppression of inhibitory transmission (H=0.0014), the network shows little response to weak afferent input, but an enhanced response to strong afferent input (Patil & Hasselmo, 1999).

that the input strongly activates a subset of cells). In addition, this reduction in background firing activity would prevent activation of the calcium-dependent potassium currents underlying spike frequency accommodation. Thus, depolarization of interneurons could enhance the ability of cortical circuits to maintain responses to sensory input over extended periods, whereas the suppression of inhibitory transmission would reduce inhibition when a signal activates the cortex.

Evidence for selective cholinergic regulation of cortical circuitry has also been demonstrated in rat visual neocortex circuits. In particular, nicotinic depolarization of low-threshold spiking interneurons could inhibit activity in upper layers (and dendritic inputs to Layer V pyramidal cells), whereas muscarinic hyperpolarization of fast spiking interneurons could release inhibition at the soma of layer V pyramidal cells and increase spiking activity (Xiang, Huguenard & Prince, 1998, 2002). Acetylcholine also causes suppression of inhibitory synaptic potentials in visual cortex while depolarizing pyramidal cells (Murakoshi, 1995). These combined effects could play a similar role in reducing background activity while enhancing responses to suprathreshold stimulation. These studies emphasize the potential importance of selective modulation of different network properties.

3.5　EVIDENCE FOR DIFFUSE MODULATORY STATE CHANGES CAUSED BY ACETYLCHOLINE

The computational models described here assume that acetylcholine causes diffuse modulatory state changes within cortical structures. The following sections address evidence for this modulatory influence, including anatomical studies of cholinergic fibers indicating diffuse modulatory influences on cortical function and microdialysis studies showing dramatic changes in acetylcholine level in cortex during different stages of waking and sleep. This evidence for a diffuse effect is consistent with data showing a relatively slow time course of changes in physiological effects of acetylcholine.

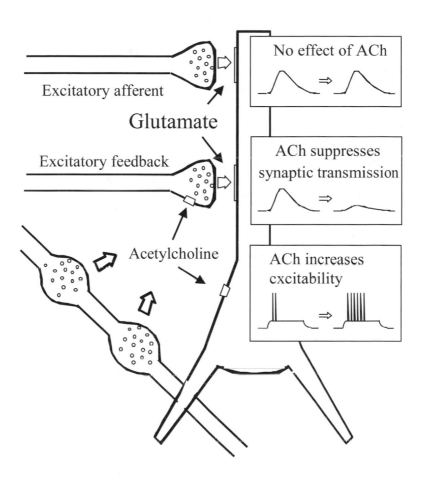

Fig. 3.5: Acetylcholine selectively suppresses excitatory synaptic transmission at feedback synapses, but not afferent input and feedforward
connections. This diagram shows synaptic transmission in the piriform
cortex at afferent fiber synapses on distal dendrites (top) and excitatory feedback synapses on proximal dendrites (middle). Activation of
cholinergic receptors selectively suppresses glutamatergic transmission
(Hasselmo and Bower, 1992; Linster, Wyble, and Hasselmo, 1999) at
excitatory feedback synapses (middle), but not excitatory afferent fibers
(top). Acetylcholine simultaneously enhances the spiking response of
neurons to current injection (shown) or synaptic input (Patil and Hasselmo, 1999; Linster et al., 1999).

3.5.1   Anatomical Support for Volume Transmission

In the computational modeling work presented here and previously
(Hasselmo, Anderson & Bower, 1992; Hasselmo & Schnell, 1994; Patil
& Hasselmo, 1999; Linster & Hasselmo, 2001), we model acetylcholine
effects as being diffuse and relatively homogeneous within cortical
circuits. That is, we assume that volume transmission provides a
general activation of cholinergic receptors at a number of receptor
sites, rather than focused effects localized at individual synaptic contacts (Descarries, Gisiger & Steriade, 1997). Anatomical evidence
supports this concept of volume transmission for acetylcholine. In
particular, the axonal varicosities on cholinergic fibers predominantly
are not accompanied by specific post-synaptic densities (Umbriaco,
Watkins, Descarries, Cozzari & Hartman, 1994; Umbriaco, Garcia,
Beaulieu & Descarries, 1995), suggesting that the release sites of
acetylcholine are not associated with specific clusters of cholinergic
receptors. For example, in the hippocampus, only 7% of the axonal varicosities on cholinergic fibers are associated with junctional
specialization, whereas all GABAergic varicosities showed synaptic
specializations (Umbriaco, Garcia, Beaulieu & Descarries, 1995). In
the parietal cortex, less than 15% of cholinergic varicosities were associated with post-synaptic junctions (Umbriaco, Watkins, Descarries, Cozzari & Hartman, 1994). These data support the concept of
volume transmission for acetylcholine within the hippocampus and
neocortex. The number of cholinergic neurons within the basal forebrain is on the order of 105 in the rat (Mesulam, Mufson, Wainer
& Levey, 1983a; Mesulam, Mufson, Levey & Wainer, 1983b). It is
unlikely that the small number of cholinergic neurons could be involved in encoding the information of individual memories. Instead,
this small number of neurons could work in a more cohesive manner
to set different functional properties during longer functional stages
of waking and sleep.

3.5.2   Microdialysis Studies of Acetylcholine

Consistent with this framework, microdialysis studies demonstrate
striking changes in the levels of acetylcholine within the cortex during different behaviors (Giovannini et al., 2001) and during different stages of waking and sleep (Jasper & Tessier, 1971; Kametani

& Kawamura, 1990; Marrosu et al., 1995). In particular, acetylcholine levels are higher during active waking in freely moving rats (Kametani & Kawamura, 1990) and cats (Marrosu et al., 1995) as summarized in Figure 3.1. In experiments on rats, active waking is defined as periods of time during which the rat is actively exploring the environment, scurrying along the walls or across the floor, sniffing novel objects, and rearing up extensively. In EEG recordings from hippocampus and entorhinal cortex, this period is characterized by large amplitude oscillations in the theta frequency range (Bland & Colom, 1993; Buzsaki, 1989; Chrobak & Buzsaki, 1994), whereas the neocortex displays high-frequency, low-amplitude activity with local synchronization (Steriade, Amzica & Contreras, 1996) and some periods of theta in certain regions (Maloney, Cape, Gotman & Jones, 1997). The increase in acetylcholine during waking is particularly strong when a rat is initially exposed to a novel environment, apparently in association with both the increase in fear elicited by such an environment, as well as the increase in attention to stimuli within the environment (Giovannini et al., 2001). Cortical acetylcholine levels rise dramatically during performance of tasks requiring sustained attention for detection of a stimulus (Arnold, Burk, Hodgson, Sarter & Bruno, 2002; Himmelheber, Sarter & Bruno, 2000).

In contrast, acetylcholine levels decrease during periods of "quiet waking," during which animals are immobile or performing consummatory behaviors such as eating or grooming (Marrosu et al., 1995). Recordings of the EEG in this phase of behavior show irregular EEG activity with periodic appearance of brief, large-amplitude events termed *sharp waves* (Buzsaki, 1986; Chrobak & Buzsaki, 1994). Acetylcholine levels decrease even more dramatically during slow-wave sleep, to levels less than one third of those observed during active waking (Jasper & Tessier, 1971; Kametani & Kawamura, 1990; Marrosu et al., 1995). Slow-wave sleep is defined by the characteristic EEG phenomena occurring during this phase of sleep, particularly the large-amplitude, low-frequency oscillations found in neocortical structures and commonly termed slow waves (Steriade, 1994, 2001). Thus, there are striking changes in acetylcholine levels within cortical circuits that are correlated with striking changes in behavior and electroencephalographic dynamics within these structures. Computational modeling can help to elucidate how the changes in acetylcholine concentration could contribute to the change in EEG dynamics and functional properties of cortical circuits during these different periods.

3.5.3 Slow Time Course of Modulatory Changes Caused by Acetylcholine

The large-scale regulation of functional state via volume transmission is also supported by the relatively long time course of cholinergic modulatory effects. Experimental data demonstrate that activation of muscarinic cholinergic receptors causes physiological changes that take several seconds to reach their maximum and persist for a minimum of 10-20 seconds, both for measurements of membrane potential depolarization (Cole & Nicoll, 1984; Krnjevic, Pumain & Renaud, 1971) and for cholinergic modulation of excitatory synaptic transmission (Hasselmo & Fehlau, 2001). This slow time course means that even weak, temporally variable diffusion of acetylcholine within the extracellular space will build up over many seconds to cause strong and tonic changes in functional state within broad cortical regions. Thus, these considerations support the modeling of acetylcholine as a diffuse and relatively homogeneous regulation of circuit properties.

3.6 FUNCTIONAL DATA

The theoretical framework presented in Figure 3.1 raises this question: What is the functional purpose of the alteration in circuit dynamics induced by cholinergic modulation? Why would it be necessary to selectively enhance the afferent input relative to feedback excitation? This section reviews behavioral evidence demonstrating the potential role of this change in circuit dynamics, showing how acetylcholine effects may enhance attention to external stimuli and may enhance encoding of new input. This raises another question: If this enhancement of attention and encoding is important, then why should circuit dynamics not remain in this state at all times? The existence of a selective modulator for changing these dynamics suggests that the absence of these dynamics are important for some function. The last section here will review how the low acetylcholine state may be important for a separate function. In this state, excitatory feedback is strong, whereas afferent input is relatively weak. Additional physiological and behavioral data suggest that low levels of acetylcholine may set appropriate dynamics for the consolidation of previously encoded information.

3.6.1   Acetylcholine and the Enhancement of Encoding

As noted earlier, the enhanced response to afferent input with the reduction of feedback can play a role in enhancing performance in attention tasks. But this same change in dynamics could also be important for the encoding of new information in memory. Traditionally, researchers have attempted to distinguish and differentiate the role of acetylcholine in attention from the role in encoding. However, in this section, we review how these may not be separable functions. The same enhancement of afferent input relative to feedback excitation may be interpreted as enhancing attention when it occurs in neocortical structures, whereas this same effect in medial temporal structures such as the hippocampus could serve to enhance the encoding of new memories.

Numerous human memory studies demonstrate that the blockade of muscarinic acetylcholine receptors by systemic administration of the drug scopolamine interferes with the encoding of new verbal information while having little effect on retrieval of previously stored information (Beatty, Butters & Janowsky, 1986; Crow & Grove-White, 1973; Drachman & Leavitt, 1974; Ghonheim & Mewaldt, 1975; Hasselmo, 1995; Hasselmo & Wyble, 1997; Peterson, 1977; Sherman, Atri, Hasselmo, Stern & Howard, 2003). Scopolamine appears to primarily affect episodic memory, while sparing semantic and procedural memory (Broks, Preston, Traub, Poppleton, Ward & Stahl, 1988; Caine, Weingartner, Ludlow, Cudahy & Wehry, 1981) and short-term memory phenomena such as the recency component of a serial position curve (Crow & Grove-White, 1973) and digit span (Beatty, Butters & Janowsky, 1986; Drachman & Leavitt, 1974).

A selective impairment of encoding has also been demonstrated in experiments testing memory function in animals. In particular, one series of experiments used a task with an encoding phase during which a monkey viewed a series of visual objects, followed by a later recognition phase during which they were tested for their recognition of these items (Aigner & Mishkin, 1986; Aigner, Walker & Mishkin, 1991). In these experiments, systemic injections of scopolamine impaired the encoding of new objects while having little effect when administered during the recognition phase for objects encoded without scoplamine. These encoding effects appeared to be focused in the parahippocampal regions, because encoding of stimuli in this task was impaired by local infusions of scopolamine into the perirhinal (and entorhinal) regions, but not by infusions into the dentate gyrus or inferotemporal cortex (Tang, Mishkin & Aigner, 1997). Microdialysis showed a 41% increase in acetylcholine levels in perirhinal cortex during performance of this visual recognition task (Tang & Aigner, 1996).

In rats, effects of muscarinic receptor blockade by scopolamine have been observed in tasks where the rat must encode episodic memories—events occurring at a specific place and time. For example, injections of scopolamine impaired the encoding of platform location in a task in which the platform was moved on a day-by-day basis (Buresova, Bolhuis & Bures, 1986; Whishaw, 1985). In the eight-arm radial maze task, the encoding of previously visited arms appeared to be impaired in a similar manner by systemic scopolamine injections, as well as by lesions of the fornix, which destroys the cholinergic innervation of the hippocampus (Cassel & Kelche, 1989). The effects of scopolamine were stronger when a delay was interposed between response and test (Bolhuis, Strijkstra & Kramers, 1988). Scopolamine had an effect when it was present during encoding—for example, the first four arm visits before a delay, but did not affect retrieval when injected during the delay (Buresova, Bolhuis & Bures, 1986).

Scopolamine has also been shown to impair learning in various conditioning tasks. In eye-blink conditioning tasks, the rate of learning was significantly slowed by electrolytic lesions of the medial septum (Berry & Thompson, 1979) as well as by ibotenic acid lesions of the medial septum (Allen, Padilla & Gluck, 2002). Systemic scopolamine also slowed the learning of classical conditioning in eye-blink conditioning tasks in rabbits (Salvatierra & Berry, 1989; Solomon, Solomon, Schaaf & Perry, 1983b) and in humans (Solomon et al., 1983a). These effects have been modeled in a hippocampal simulation (Myers, Ermita, Hasselmo & Gluck, 1998). The slowing of eye-blink conditioning showed a direct correlation with reductions in hippocampal theta rhythm (Berry & Thompson, 1979; Salvatierra & Berry, 1989). The hippocampal theta rhythm appearing during alert immobility in these types of experiments was sensitive to cholinergic blockade (Kramis, Vanderwolf & Bland, 1975). A similar correlation with theta rhythm has been shown in experiments where presentation of the stimulus during periods of theta rhythm enhances the rate of learning (Berry & Seager, 2001; Seager, Johnson, Chabot, Asaka & Berry, 2002). Scopolamine also impairs appetitive jaw movement conditioning (Seager, Asaka & Berry, 1999), and scopolamine has also been shown to impair encoding of fear conditioning (Anagnostaras, Maren & Fanselow, 1995; Anagnostaras, Maren, Sage, Goodrich & Fanselow, 1999; Young, Bohenek & Fanselow, 1995) even when injected directly into the hippocampus (Gale, Anagnostaras & Fanselow, 2001), but appears to enhance consolidation of fear conditioning when injected after training (Young, Bohenek & Fanselow, 1995). This enhancement of consolidation by cholinergic blockade supports the hypothesis presented later that low levels of acetylcholine are important for consolidation.

Acetylcholine also appears important for encoding of sensory representations in neocortical structures such as the auditory cortex. Experimental recordings from individual neurons in auditory cortex showed a tuning curve focused on specific frequencies. These tuning curves were altered by conditioning and could also be altered by auditory stimulation combined with microiontophoretic application of acetylcholine (Metherate, Ashe & Weinberger, 1990; Metherate & Weinberger, 1990). Cholinergic modulation has also been shown to cause long-term alterations in responses to somatosensory stimulation (Dykes, 1997; Tremblay, Warren & Dykes, 1990).

3.6.2 Cholinergic Suppression of Feedback may Prevent Interference

The cholinergic suppression of excitatory transmission might appear somewhat paradoxical when considering encoding. Why would a substance that is important for learning cause suppression of excitatory transmission? As noted above, it is important to emphasize the selectivity of this suppression for intrinsic but not afferent fibers. The importance of this selective suppression of transmission has been analyzed in computational models of associative memory function (Hasselmo, Anderson & Bower, 1992; Hasselmo & Bower, 1993; DeRosa & Hasselmo, 2000; Linster & Hasselmo, 2001). These models demonstrate that cholinergic suppression of transmission prevents retrieval of previously encoded associations from interfering with the encoding of new associations. For example, if an association A-B has been encoded, then subsequent presentation of an association A-C could cause retrieval of the A-B association. This would cause the new association A-C to suffer from interference from the A-B association and cause associations between C and B. Recent experiments have tested behavioral predictions of these computational models (DeRosa & Hasselmo, 2000; DeRosa, Hasselmo & Baxter, 2001). In one experiment, rats were initially trained to respond to odor A when presented with the odor pair A-B. Then in a separate phase of the experiment, the rat had to learn to respond to odor C when presented with odor pair A-C and, during the same period, had to learn to respond to odor D when presented with odor pair D-E. In a counterbalanced design, rats received injections of scopolamine, methylscopolamine, or saline after learning of A-B and before learning of A-C and D-E. Injections of scopolamine during encoding caused a greater impairment in the learning of overlapping odor pairs (A-C) than non-overlapping odor pairs (D-E). Thus, scopolamine appears to enhance proactive interference, consistent with its blockade of the cholinergic suppression of excitatory synaptic transmission at intrinsic synapses in the piriform cortex. Saporin lesions of the horizontal limb of the diagonal band, resulting in cholinergic denervation of piriform cortex, heightened the sensitivity to scopolamine in this paradigm (DeRosa, Hasselmo & Baxter, 2001). This model is further supported by experimental data showing that electrical stimulation of the olfactory cortex can modulate the activity of neurons in the HDB, thus providing a pathway for regulation of cholinergic activity (Linster & Hasselmo, 2000). Cholinergic blockade also increases the generalization between similar odorants seen in odor-guided digging tasks (Linster, Garcia, Hasselmo & Baxter, 2001). Similar effects have been obtained in an experiment performed on human subjects, in which scopolamine caused greater impairments in the encoding of overlapping versus non-overlapping word pairs (Atri, Sherman, Norman, Kirchhoff, Nicolas, Greicius, Cramer, Breiter, Hasselmo & Stern, 2003; Kirchhoff, Hasselmo, Norman, Nicolas, Greicius, Breiter & Stern, 2000). These data suggest that interference effects may underlie the impairments caused by lesions of the medial septum, including impairments of reversal learning (M'Harzi, Palacios, Monmaur, Willig, Houcine & Delacour, 1987), and delayed alternation (Numan, Feloney, Pham & Tieber, 1995). Interference effects could also contribute to the impairment of eight-arm radial maze performance caused by scopolamine (Bolhuis, Strijkstra & Kramers, 1988; Buresova, Bolhuis & Bures, 1986).

3.6.3 Acetylcholine Enhances Long-term Potentiation

Activation of acetylcholine receptors also enhances synaptic modification in long-term potentiation experiments. This enhancement would naturally be important for the encoding of new information. Physiological experiments in brain slice preparations have demonstrated enhancement of LTP by cholinergic agonists at a number of different synaptic pathways, including the perforant path input to the dentate gyrus (Burgard & Sarvey, 1990), the Schaffer collateral input to region CA1 (Blitzer, Gil & Landau, 1990; Huerta & Lisman, 1993), excitatory synaptic connections in primary visual cortex (Brocher, Artola & Singer, 1992), and association fiber connections in the piriform cortex (Hasselmo & Barkai, 1995; Patil, Linster, Lubenov & Hasselmo, 1998). In slice studies of region CA1, it has been shown that LTP is most strongly enhanced by stimulation in phase with spontaneous oscillatory activity (Huerta & Lisman, 1993). Drugs that block these neuromodulatory effects on LTP appear to impair memory function: muscarinic receptor antagonists such as scopolamine block the cholinergic enhancement of LTP (Burgard & Sarvey, 1990; Huerta & Lisman, 1993; Patil, Linster, Lubenov & Hasselmo, 1998), and these antagonists also impair encoding as described earlier. These results demonstrate that modulators could contribute to encoding of new information through enhancement of long-term potentiation.

3.6.4 Acetylcholine Enhances Sustained Spiking Activity

Acetylcholine also appears to influence the firing activity of cortical circuits by enhancing intrinsic mechanisms for sustained spiking activity in individual neurons. Data from slice preparations of entorhinal cortex demonstrate this cellular mechanism for sustained spiking activity. In physiological recordings from non-stellate cells in slice preparations (Klink & Alonso, 1997a, 1997b), application of the cholinergic agonist carbachol causes long-term depolarizations, which have been termed *plateau potentials*. If the cells generate an action potential during cholinergic modulation, either due to cholinergic depolarization or current injection, these neurons show sustained spiking activity. This sustained spiking activity appears to result from activation of a non-specific cation current (termed I_{NCM}) which is sensitive to muscarinic receptor activation as well as the intracellular concentration of calcium (Shalinsky, Magistretti, Ma & Alonso, 2002). This intrinsic capacity for self-sustained spiking activity of individual neurons could underlie the sustained spiking activity observed during performance of delayed non-match and delayed match to sample tasks in the entorhinal cortex of rats (Young, Otto, Fox & Eichenbaum, 1997) and monkeys (Suzuki, Miller & Desimone, 1997). Simulations demonstrate how these phenomena could directly arise from I_{NCM} in individual entorhinal neurons (Fransen, Alonso & Hasselmo, 2002). These phenomena include stimulus selective spiking activity during the delay period, as well as enhancement of spiking response to stimuli that match the previously presented sample stimulus. In addition, incorporation of these effects in a network of excitatory and inhibitory neurons can create other phenomena such as match suppression and non-match enhancement and suppression (Suzuki, Miller & Desimone, 1997). Recent data demonstrate that cholinergic modulation of neurons in entorhinal cortex layer V causes activation of a current capable of maintaining graded levels of spiking activity, potentially relevant to the maintenance of analog representations of external stimuli (Egorov, Hamam, Fransen, Hasselmo & Alonso, 2002).

If cholinergic activation of I_{NCM} is important to provide intrinsic mechanisms for self-sustained spiking activity, then blockade of this cholinergic activation should prevent sustained spiking activity during the delay period and match enhancement. This effect of muscarinic antagonists could underlie the behavioral impairments in delayed matching tasks seen with systemic injections of muscarinic antagonists (Bartus & Johnson, 1976; Penetar & McDonough, 1983).

In addition to this role in short-term memory function, sustained activity in entorhinal cortex could also be very important for effective encoding of long-term representations through synaptic modification in the hippocampal formation. Thus, the blockade of sustained spiking activity in entorhinal cortex could contribute to the encoding impairment caused by injections of scopolamine (Aigner & Mishkin, 1986; Aigner, Walker & Mishkin, 1991; Anagnostaras, Maren & Fanselow, 1995; Anagnostaras, Maren, Sage, Goodrich & Fanselow, 1999; Buresova, Bolhuis & Bures, 1986; Tang, Mishkin & Aigner, 1997).

3.6.5   Acetylcholine and the Enhancement of Attention

Behavioral data support the functional framework presented here for the role of acetylcholine within cortical structures. In particular, the enhancement of afferent input relative to internal processing could enhance performance in attention tasks. The performance in attention tasks often depends on the sensitivity to specific weak stimuli over an extended period of time. Performance in these tasks is enhanced if the neuronal response to the stimulus is strong (allowing rapid and accurate behavioral responses), whereas the background noise in neural systems should be relatively weak (thereby preventing generation of incorrect responses at inappropriate times in the task).

The cholinergic influence on circuit dynamics illustrated in Figure 3.1 has the net effect of enhancing the response to external sensory stimuli relative to background noise. This was demonstrated in a spiking network simulation of piriform cortex (Linster & Hasselmo, 2001). This model implements selective suppression of excitatory feedback synaptic transmission, as well as modulation that reduces feedback inhibition (analogous to the suppression of GABAergic transmission shown experimentally). These effects serve to enhance the response of the network to the pattern of input while reducing the amount of background spiking activity (Linster & Hasselmo, 2001). These effects are analogous to what has been reported in single-unit recordings from neurons in the primary visual cortex, which shows that local application of acetylcholine enhances the response of neurons to visual input (Sato, Hata, Masui & Tsumoto,

1987) and enhances the direction selectivity of individual neurons (Murphy & Sillito, 1991). Thus, the change in network dynamics enhances response to sensory stimulation relative to background noise.

These changes in dynamics could underlie the role of acetylcholine in attention. A wide range of studies have shown impairments of attention associated with infusions of muscarinic antagonists such as scopolamine in humans (Wesnes & Warburton, 1984). In addition, many studies in rats have shown impairments of attention processes associated with lesions of the cholinergic basal forebrain (Bucci, Holland & Gallagher, 1998; Chiba, Bucci, Holland & Gallagher, 1995; McGaughy, Kaiser & Sarter, 1996; McGaughy & Sarter, 1998; McGaughy, Decker & Sarter, 1999; Turchi & Sarter, 1997). Intrabasalis infusions of the immunotoxin severely impaired sustained attention (McGaughy, Kaiser & Sarter, 1996). Multiple cortical infusions of the toxin (McGaughy & Sarter, 1998) or smaller doses of the toxin into the nucleus basalis of Meynert (McGaughy, Decker & Sarter, 1999) produced qualitatively similar although less severe impairment in sustained attention. In all studies, the degree of attentional impairment was correlated with the extent of cortical deafferentation (McGaughy, Decker & Sarter, 1999; McGaughy, Kaiser & Sarter, 1996; McGaughy & Sarter, 1998).

The framework illustrated in Figures 3.1, 3.2 and 3.3 can be used to account for the importance of cholinergic modulation in sustained attention performance as described below (Arnold, Burk, Hodgson, Sarter & Bruno, 2002; McGaughy & Sarter, 1995). Effective performance in that task requires discrimination of neural activity induced by a brief light stimulus, in contrast with the activity associated with the absence of a stimulus. Cholinergic modulation of cellular and synaptic properties could contribute to this task in two ways. First, the depolarization of interneurons and the suppression of excitatory feedback transmission could reduce spontaneous background activity as well as any response to distractor stimuli, such as a flashing house light (McGaughy & Sarter, 1995), thereby reducing false alarms. Second, the depolarization of pyramidal cells and the suppression of GABAergic transmission could enhance the magnitude of response to sensory stimuli, which will increase the propensity of the target light stimulus for pushing network activity over threshold, resulting in correct detection of the target light stimulus (increasing hits relative to misses). Excessive cholinergic modulation could cause too much depolarization of pyramidal cells and too strong a response to afferent input, resulting in the generation of false alarms.

In summary, converging neuroscientific data continue to provide support for the hypothesis that corticopetal cholinergic afferents originating in the nucleus basalis of Meynert are critical to attentional processing.

3.6.6   Low Levels of Acetylcholine Set Appropriate Dynamics for Consolidation

If acetylcholine plays such an important role in attention and encoding, then why is it not present at high concentrations at all times? Or why could the modulatory effects of acetylcholine not be maintained as the baseline parameters for cortical circuits? The ability of acetylcholine to selectively regulate these parameters suggests that the low acetylcholine state has functional importance. In this section, we review the hypothesis that low levels of acetylcholine are important for the consolidation of previously encoded information (for more detailed review, see Hasselmo, 1999). This consolidation would take place during quiet waking and slow wave sleep, when levels of acetylcholine are low and cortical network dynamics include EEG phenomena such as slow waves (Steriade, 1994, 2001) and quiet waking (Buzsaki, 1989).

The hypothesis that consolidation occurs during slow-wave sleep and quiet waking has been discussed for many years (Buzsaki, 1989; Wilson & McNaughton, 1994). This hypothesis proposes that initial encoding of memories occurs within the hippocampal formation during active waking. Subsequently, during quiet waking or slow wave sleep, in the absence of specific sensory input, random activity in the hippocampus causes reactivation of memory representations. Some research has focused on recordings of hippocampal place cells, showing that when pairs of place cells code adjacent positions during a period of active waking, these neurons show greater correlations of firing during subsequent slow-wave sleep, compared with slow-wave sleep preceding the training session (Wilson & McNaughton, 1994). Another set of experiments have focused on the predominant flow of activity during different behavioral states (as symbolized by the arrows in Figure 3.6). These experiments demonstrate that during active waking, when theta rhythm is present in the hippocampus, there is extensive neuronal activity in the layer of entorhinal cortex that provides input to the hippocampus (layer II), but not in the entorhinal layers receiving output from the hippocampus (layers V and VI Chrobak & Buzsaki, 1994). In contrast, during quiet waking and slow wave sleep, EEG phenomena termed sharp waves originate among the strong excitatory recurrent collaterals in hippocampal region CA3 and spread back through region CA1 to deep, output layers of entorhinal cortex (Chrobak & Buzsaki, 1994). This suggests that hippocampus could be inducing coactivation of neurons in neocortical regions, which could form new cross-modal associations. During this stage, slow waves are prominent in the cortical EEG arising from neocortical and thalamocortical circuits (Steriade, 2001). These slow waves include both delta waves and lower frequency oscillations, which with sleep spindles are also postulated to contribute to the consolidation of memory traces acquired during the state of wakefulness (Steriade, 2001).

The sharp waves observed in the hippocampus during quiet waking and slow-wave sleep could directly arise from the change in dynamics caused by a drop in acetylcholine levels during these behavioral states. As summarized in Figure 3.6, lower levels of acetylcholine would release glutamatergic feedback synapses from the cholinergic suppression described before (Hasselmo & Schnell, 1994; Hounsgaard, 1978; Rovira, Cherubini & Ben-Ari, 1982; Valentino & Dingledine, 1981), resulting in strong excitatory feedback. Slow-wave sleep would be characterized by a great increase in the effect of excitatory recurrent connections in region CA3 and excitatory feedback connections from CA3 to CA1 and entorhinal cortex. This drop in cholinergic modulation could thereby underlie the increase in sharp wave activity observed during slow-wave sleep (Buzsaki, 1989; Chrobak & Buzsaki, 1994). In fact, muscarinic antagonists such as atropine put the hippocampus into a sharp wave state (Buzsaki, 1986). In addition, this spread of activity should be influenced by synaptic modification during the previous waking period. Thus, the release of suppression of excitatory transmission could contribute to the greater tendency of cells to fire together during slow-wave sleep if they fired during the previous waking period (Wilson & McNaughton, 1994).

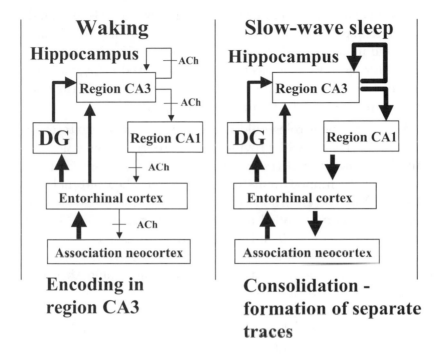

Fig. 3.6: Schematic of cholinergic modulation of hippocampal dynamics during active waking and slow wave sleep. Left: During active waking, high levels of acetylcholine set appropriate dynamics for encoding. Sensory information from neocortical structures flows through the entorhinal cortex and dentate gyrus (DG) into hippocampal region CA3, where cholinergic enhancement of synaptic modification helps in formation of an intermediate term representation binding together different elements of an episodic memory. Feedback connections to region CA1, entorhinal cortex and association cortex are strong enough to mediate immediate retrieval, but cholinergic suppression of these connections (ACh) prevents them from dominating over the feedforward connectivity. Right: During quiet waking or slow wave sleep, much lower levels of acetylcholine release the suppression of excitatory feedback. This strong excitatory feedback mediates reactivation of memories stored in region CA3 during EEG phenomena termed sharp waves. These waves of activity flow back through region CA1 to entorhinal cortex. This will enable the slow consolidation of long-term episodic memory in hippocampal region CA1, entorhinal cortex and association neocortex, and may underlie modification of semantic memory within circuits of association neocortex.

The loss of cholinergic modulation during slow-wave sleep should also enhance the spread of excitatory activity in response to stimulation. This could underlie the increase in magnitude of evoked synaptic potentials during slow-wave sleep, which is observed in region CA1 and entorhinal cortex after stimulation of the input connections to the hippocampal formation (Winson & Abzug, 1978).

What functional role could this enhancement of excitatory feedback have? This would provide the appropriate dynamics for the formation of additional traces within regions CA3 and CA1, and it could allow the hippocampus to further strengthen internal connections and train the entorhinal cortex or association neocortex on the basis of previously encoded associations (Buzsaki, 1989; Hasselmo, Wyble & Wallenstein, 1996; Hasselmo, 1999; Wilson & McNaughton, 1994). As shown in Figure 3.6, the spontaneous reactivation of neurons coding an association in the hippocampus would then be able to drive cells in entorhinal cortex and neocortex without any assistance from sensory input. The reduction of cholinergic suppression might provide the opportunity for this strong feedback influence. The physiological activity during slow wave sleep has been proposed to be appropriate for modification of synaptic components (Trepel & Racine, 1998). Behavioral data suggest that slow-wave sleep may be important for the declarative component of behavioral tasks, which correspond most closely to episodic memories. Subjects are better at retrieval of word lists if they learn the list before falling asleep and are tested on retrieval after being awakened in the middle of the night than if they learn the list after many hours sleep and are tested in the morning (Stickgold, 1998).

What is the functional purpose of suppressing feedback to entorhinal cortex during active waking? To begin with, this suppression should not be total, because recently stored memories from the hippocampus are still accessible for retrieval. But the strength of connections necessary for the strong transmission of stored memories back to region CA1 and entorhinal cortex would allow them to dominate over afferent input. This could distort the initial perception of sensory information, causing interference during learning in temporal structures—and if the retrieval activity is sufficiently dominant—causing hallucinations such as those observed under the influence of cholinergic antagonists at high doses (Perry & Perry,

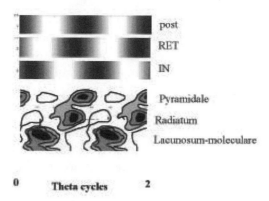

Fig. 3.7: Top: Phases for maximum function in performance measure linking theta rhythmic changes in hippocampal physiology to behavioral function. Bottom: Current source density data showing phases in region CA1 of hippocampus (Brankack et al., 1993)

1995). Thus, partial cholinergic suppression of excitatory feedback might allow cued retrieval without hallucinatory retrieval.

3.7   CHOLINERGIC INDUCTION OF THETA RHYTHM OSCILLATIONS

During active waking, acetylcholine also contributes to the induction of theta rhythm oscillations in the hippocampal formation and associated cortical structures (Bland & Colom, 1993; Buzsaki, Leung & Vanderwolf, 1983). The hippocampal theta rhythm is a 3-10 Hz oscillation that appears prominently in the electroencephalograph (EEG) recorded at the hippocampal fissure. This theta rhythm shows clear dependence on behavior, with a large increase in the amplitude of theta rhythm during locomotion and exploration (Buzsaki, Leung & Vanderwolf, 1983) and also during attention to behaviorally relevant stimuli such as predators or the tone in appetitive or eye-blink conditioning paradigm (Seager, Johnson, Chabot, Asaka & Berry, 2002). Lesions that block theta rhythm impair performance in a range of memory tasks, including spatial alternation, eight-arm radial maze, and spatial reversal.

Recent research in our laboratory has focused on the possible functional role of the theta rhythm within the hippocampus. Theta rhythm results from oscillatory changes in synaptic currents in different layers of region CA1 of the hippocampus, as shown by current source density analysis (Bragin, Jando, Nadasdy, Hetke, Wise & Buzsaki, 1995; Brankack, Stewart & Fox, 1993). This current source density analysis is summarized in Figure 3.7. In particular, at the trough the EEG recorded in the hippocampal fissure, there is a strong current sink in stratum lacunosum-moleculare, the layer that receives excitatory synaptic input from the entorhinal cortex. In contrast, during this phase, there is a strong current source in the cell body layer, stratum pyramidale, reflecting the outward currents resulting from inhibition at the cell bodies. At the opposite phase of the theta rhythm, there is a current sink in stratum radiatum, associated with strong synaptic input from region CA3.

The mechanisms of generation of hippocampal theta rhythm have been studied extensively by a number of researchers (Buzsaki, Leung & Vanderwolf, 1983; Stewart & Fox, 1990). However, few researchers have described models of the functional role of hippocampal theta rhythm. In recent work, we described a model of the functional role of hippocampal theta rhythm (Cannon, Hasselmo & Koene, 2002; Hasselmo, Bodelon & Wyble, 2002a; Hasselmo, Hay, Ilyn & Gorchetchnikov, 2002b; Hasselmo, Cannon & Koene, 2002c). This theta theory provides a functional framework in which a behavioral performance measure is maximized by the relative phases of different oscillatory dynamics within different regions of the hippocampus and associated structures. The next section describes a simple model of the proposed functional role of theta rhythm.

3.7.1 Modeling the Function of Hippocampal Theta Rhythm.

In previous work, we have described how the phase of oscillatory changes in different parameters during theta rhythm could provide maximal encoding and retrieval function (Hasselmo, Bodelon & Wyble, 2002a; Hasselmo & Eichenbaum, 2005). These descriptions focused on performing reversal of prior learning, using a phase-dependent learning rule that could transition between Hebbian long-term potentiation (strengthening) of connections on one phase and Hebbian long-term depression (weakening) on another phase. This is consistent with physiological data on changes at different phases of the theta rhythm oscillation, in which stimulation on the peak of the local theta wave causes LTP, and stimulation at the trough of the local theta wave causes LTD (Holscher, Anwyl & Rowan, 1997; Huerta & Lisman, 1995; Hyman, Wyble, Goyal, Rossi & Hasselmo, 2003). This process allows forgetting of previous memories to maximize the learning of new memories—for instance, in a spatial reversal task (Hasselmo, Bodelon & Wyble, 2002a). However, in many circumstances, it is not desirable to forget previous learning. Therefore, it is worth considering circumstances where synaptic modification stays positive and LTD does not occur. These conditions require slightly different phase relationships. In particular, they appear to require that there be some overlap in the influence of afferent input and synapses mediating associative retrieval. We reintroduce a simple model of these effects to describe how phase relationships differ with the assumption that synaptic connections are not weakened.

A simple example

To make the functional role of theta rhythm clear, we provide an extremely simple example of its possible role in reducing interference during learning of new paired associates. In a typical paired associate memory task, subjects are given a set of word pairs A-B, such as leather-holster, and are tested on retrieval (e.g. what word was associated with leather?). They are then trained repeatedly on a second set of overlapping word pairs A-C, such as leather-boot, and are tested on a second retrieval (e.g. What word was most recently associated with leather?). If we consider each word A, B and C to be represented by column vectors a_A a_B and a_C and retrieval activity by a_{out}, the performance on the second retrieval phase can be measured by:

$$M = \Sigma[a_C^T a_{post} - a_B^T a_{post}]. \tag{3.1}$$

Now consider a simple heteroassociative memory (e.g., Kohonen, 1984), that stores the word pairs and is then cued with the input a_A to generate the response a_{out}. In most models, interference during encoding is prevented by using specialized dynamics for encoding and retrieval. The simplified example presented here focuses on showing the interference effects that could occur in a neural system, and how theta rhythmicity could solve these problems. Note that in this example we always assume vectors of unit length.

Consider a network with two populations a_{post} and a_{pre} with all initial weights $W(0) = 0$. The network receives afferent input representing the two words and undergoes Hebbian synaptic modification analogous to Hebbian long-term potentiation:

$$a_{post} = a_B + W a_A \qquad a_{pre} = a_A \qquad (3.2)$$

$$\Delta W = a_{post} a_{pre} = a_B a_A^T \qquad (3.3)$$

Note that when a second overlapping paired associate is stored in the network, synaptic modification includes interference from retrieval of the first paired associate:

$$a_{post} = a_C + W a_A = a_C + a_B a_A^T a_A = a_C + a_B \qquad (3.4)$$

$$\Delta W = (a_C + a_B) a_A^T, W = (a_C + a_B) a_A^T + a_B a_A^T \qquad (3.5)$$

Subsequently, retrieval cued by input of word A will not effectively differentiate the recent word, resulting in poor performance shown by the performance measure.

$$a_{post} = W a_A = a_C + a_B + a_B \qquad (3.6)$$

$$M = \Sigma[a_C^T a_{post} - a_B^T a_{post}] = -1 \qquad (3.7)$$

Oscillatory dynamics

This simple example can be used to illustrate the potential functional role of theta rhythm in providing appropriate dynamics for encoding and retrieval within neural circuitry of the hippocampal formation. The interference from previous retrieval during encoding can be prevented by assuming oscillatory functions for each component of this model. Previous work used oscillatory modulation of synaptic transmission at input synapses (IN) representing phasic sinks in stratum lacunosum-moleculare and synapses representing retrieval (RET) in stratum radiatum of region CA1.

$$\theta_{\mathrm{IN}}(t) = x/2 * \sin(t + \phi_{\mathrm{IN}}) + (1 - x/2) \qquad (3.8)$$

$$\theta_{\mathrm{RET}}(t) = x/2 * \sin(t + \phi_{\mathrm{RET}}) + (1 - x/2) \qquad (3.9)$$

In previous work, the oscillatory modulation of long-term potentiation was modeled with a traditional sine wave going positive to negative.

$$\theta_{\mathrm{LTP}}(t) = \sin(t + \phi_{\mathrm{LTP}}) \qquad (3.10)$$

In the description here, we instead consider a situation where there is no decay of synaptic weight, so that long-term potentiation is also constrained to remain positive at all times. Thus, we use the form:

$$\theta_{\mathrm{LTP}}(t) = x/2 * \sin(t + \phi_{\mathrm{LTP}}) + (1 - x/2) \qquad (3.11)$$

Learning of the first pattern takes the form:

$$a_{\mathrm{post}} = \theta_{\mathrm{IN}} a_B + \theta_{\mathrm{RET}} W a_A \qquad a_{\mathrm{pre}} = a_A \qquad (3.12)$$

$$\Delta W = \int_0^{2\pi} \theta_{\mathrm{LTP}}(\theta_{\mathrm{IN}} a_B + \theta_{\mathrm{RET}} W a_A) a_A^T \qquad (3.13)$$

We assume first pattern learning reaches a maximum strength of $W(0) = k$. Then learning of the second pattern takes the form:

$$a_{\mathrm{post}} = \theta_{\mathrm{IN}} a_C + \theta_{\mathrm{RET}} k a_B a_A^T a_A \qquad (3.14)$$

$$\Delta W = \int_0^{2\pi} \theta_{\mathrm{LTP}}(\theta_{\mathrm{IN}} a_C + \theta_{\mathrm{RET}} k a_B) a_A^T \qquad (3.15)$$

The use of LTP constrained to all positive values is motivated by context-dependent retrieval in paired associate tasks. In an actual paired associate task, subjects would be able to retrieve both B and C in a context-dependent manner, suggesting that B is not forgotten. In this case, correct retrieval of C or B depends on an association of the experimental context with the specific paired associate. Here we represent context-dependent cue activity as oscillatory input biased toward one response $\theta_{\mathrm{IN}} a_C$. The retrieval activity of the network is also regulated by oscillations in the activation of the post-synaptic population θ_{DEP} as follows:

$$a_{\mathrm{post}} = \int_0^{2\pi} \theta_{\mathrm{DEP}}[\theta_{\mathrm{IN}} a_C + \theta_{\mathrm{RET}} W a_A] \qquad (3.16)$$

If we use the new assumption that synaptic modification remains positive at all times, the integral solution to Equation 3.1 takes the form:

$$M \;\; = \;\; (1/4)\pi\{[\cos(\phi_{\text{somaCA1}} - \phi_{\text{ECIII}}) + 2] +$$
$$(1/4)\pi[\cos(\phi_{\text{somaCA1}} - \phi_{\text{CA3}}) + 2]$$
$$[\cos(\phi_{\text{LTP}} - \phi_{\text{EC}}) - \cos(\phi_{\text{LTP}} - \phi_{\text{CA3}})]\} \qquad (3.17)$$

Computing this performance measure with a reference point of $\phi_{LTP} = 0$ degrees gives a notion of how performance varies based on the relative values of LTP and EC. Finding the maximum of the performance measure at a resolution of 1 degree, demonstrates that the best function is found with $\phi_{EC} = 28$ degrees, $\phi_{CA3} = 152$ degrees, and with $\phi_{somaCA1} = 107$ degrees. Thus, the analysis of this system of equations suggests that the best function is obtained when the peak of LTP induction follows the peak of entorhinal input by 28 degrees (with the additive form of the phase parameter ϕ_{EC} used in the equations, a positive value means the phase $\phi_{EC} = 28$ degrees comes earlier than the LTP oscillation with $\phi_{LTP} = 0$). This computation is consistent with the offsets of phase observed in current source density data (Brankack et al., 1993), as shown in Figure 3.7, and with the offsets in phase of induction of long-term potentiation (Judge & Hasselmo, 2004).

This form of the equation reaches a maximum when postsynaptic depolarization is in phase with the retrieval spread RET. The phase relationships of post-RET are plotted in the top of Figure 3.1, which demonstrates their general consistency with the timing of synaptic currents recorded electrophysiologically in the hippocampus (see Figure 3.7). If we assume that the oscillatory modulation of LTP induction must stay positive (no LTD), then the phase relationships for maximum function are shifted slightly relative to each other, similar to the data at the bottom of Figure 3.1. Note that the modulation of postsynaptic depolarization is constrained to stay positive, although spiking activity in the dendrites during encoding might cause an explicit suppression of repeated patterns during retrieval due to a refractory period after dendritic spiking (Golding, Staff & Spruston, 2002).

The cues for retrieval are presumed to be held in working memory and delivered from neocortical areas such as prefrontal cortex. The same steps described earlier can be used to demonstrate that this would require rhythmic activity in prefrontal cortex, which is in phase with the hippocampal retrieval activity. Specifically, phasic activity in prefrontal cortex working memory would appear in equations as θ_{PFC} with the same maximal phase as demonstrated before for θ_{DEP}.

$$a_{\text{post}} = \int_0^{2\pi} [\theta_{\text{IN}}\theta_{\text{PFC}}a_A + \theta_{\text{RET}}W\theta_{\text{PFC}}a_A] \qquad (3.18)$$

Ongoing experiments in our laboratory have shown that at least in some periods prefrontal and hippocampal theta rhythm are synchronized (Hyman, Wyble, Goyal, Rossi & Hasselmo, 2003).

Theta rhythm interactions can also facilitate the context-dependent selective retrieval of sequences of activity, with an increase in entorhinal activity spread correlated with a decrease in region CA3 activity spread. This mechanism would involve forward associations between elements of a sequence being encoded in ECIII and temporal context being encoded in the interactions of entorhinal cortex layer II with dentate gyrus and region CA3. This can be expressed as

$$a_{\text{cal}}(t)_s = \eta^{(s-o)/t}b_s * \mu^t\mu^{(c-s)}b_s = b_{o+t}, \qquad (3.19)$$

where the retrieval activity a_{cal} contains sequential items b_s in a sequence. The activity for each item results from input from ECIII reflecting forward spread from a cue item b_o to each item s with strength of spread η increasing within each theta cycle $\eta^{(s-o)/t}$. In addition, the activity depends on input from CA3 reflecting temporal context scaled by μ to the distance of the item s from current context c. The strength of temporal context decreases according to μ^t. Note that $0 < \mu < \eta < 1$. If thresholds are set properly, this system selectively retrieves items s, which followed the cue o with an index increasing sequentially with time (index: $o + t$).

Electrophysiological Data

The use of oscillatory variables to regulate dynamics is directly motivated by experimental evidence from electrophysiological recordings within the hippocampal formation of awake behaving rats. In fact, the oscillatory variables described earlier appear to resemble evidence from current source density showing phasic changes in magnitude

of synaptic input in different layers of the hippocampal region CA1
(Brankack, Stewart & Fox, 1993). In particular, the phase of input
IN could correspond to the excitatory afferent input from entorhinal
cortex causing current sinks in stratum lacunosum moleculare of region CA1, the phase of retrieval RET could correspond to afferent
input from region CA3 causing current sinks in stratum radiatum of
region CA1 (Brankack, Stewart & Fox, 1993), and the phase of post-
synaptic depolarization DEP could correspond to the phase of rhythmic somatic depolarization (Fox, 1989; Kamondi, Acsady, Wang &
Buzsaki, 1998) appearing when inhibition is weak within stratum
pyramidale of region CA1. The phase relationships for maximum
performance are summarized in Figure 3.1, and the bottom of the
figure shows how these phase relationships match the current source
density data showing the relative timing of current sinks determined
by current source density analysis in region CA1 of the hippocampal
formation.

These phase relationships are behaviorally relevant, because lesions of region CA1 of the hippocampus have been shown to selectively impair performance in paired associate memory tasks in humans (Rempel-Clower, Zola, Squire & Amaral, 1996). In rats, lesions
of the fornix that remove much of the amplitude of theta rhythm impair the ability to learn reversal tasks, in which a previously rewarded
behavior must be replaced with an opposite behavior. For example,
rats with fornix lesions have difficult learning to make a right turn
response after initially learning a left turn response (Markowska,
Olton, Murray & Gaffan, 1989; M'Harzi, Palacios, Monmaur, Willig,
Houcine & Delacour, 1987).

3.7.2   Context-Dependent Retrieval for Memory-Guided Behavior

Lesions of the hippocampus cause impairments in memory-guided
tasks, including delayed spatial alternation, delayed match to position, and the eight-arm radial maze (Markowska, Olton, Murray &
Gaffan, 1989; Eichenbaum & Cohen, 2001; Ennaceur, Neave & Aggleton, 1996). Many models have addressed hippocampal memory
function, but few have explicitly modeled the actions of a virtual rat
in these types of tasks. Ongoing research in our laboratory uses the

MATLAB program and the CATACOMB simulation package (Cannon, Hasselmo & Koene, 2002) to analyze cortical mechanisms involved in memory-guided behavior in these tasks.

A number of models have addressed memory-guided behavior, but do not simultaneously address neurophysiological phenomena such as theta rhythm (Redish & Touretzky, 1998; Sharp, Blair & Brown, 1996). The modeling work described earlier has been extended in recent modeling work to provide an explicit description of the use of context-dependent retrieval for memory-guided behavior. In particular, previous models from this lab used an interaction of a reverse spread of activity from the goal and forward retrieval activity to select next desired destination in the form of region CA1 activity (Hasselmo, Cannon & Koene, 2002c; Hasselmo, Hay, Ilyn & Gorchetchnikov, 2002b). However, general goal-directed behavior is spared by hippocampal lesions and appears to involve prefrontal cortical circuits. Therefore, we now use a model of prefrontal cortical circuitry to address the interaction of goal and current state, to obtain selection of the next action. This network implementation of goal-directed function has features resembling aspects of temporal difference learning and action selection in reinforcement learning (Sutton & Barto, 1998). The hippocampal simulation interacts with this representation of prefrontal cortex.

In addition, the new simulations address context-dependent retrieval of full sequences of activity, which is necessary for memory-guided behavior in spatial alternation. This requires both encoding of the sequential associations between elements of an episode, as well as encoding of temporal context analogous to that described by Howard and colleagues (Howard & Kahana, 2002; Howard, Fotedar, Datey & Hasselmo, 2005). Activity necessary for both aspects can be provided by sustained activity in entorhinal cortex due to cholinergic activation of intrinsic regenerating cation currents (Fransen, Alonso & Hasselmo, 2002). As described previously (Hasselmo, Cannon & Koene, 2002c; Jensen & Lisman, 1996), these currents allow slow behavioral transitions to cause sequential spiking, which falls within the window of spike-timing-dependent synaptic plasticity (Bi & Poo, 1998; Levy & Steward, 1983). Gradual decay of these representations also allows formation of associations between a gradually changing temporal context (Howard & Kahana, 2002) and individual behav-

ioral events. This representation of temporal context has been used
to model verbal memory function (Howard & Kahana, 2002) and
can be used to model the moderate location specificity of neurons in
entorhinal cortex (Howard, Fotedar, Datey & Hasselmo, 2005).

Previous simulations of the hippocampus have demonstrated forward retrieval of individual sequences (Jensen & Lisman, 1996; Levy,
1996; Lisman, 1999). The simulation presented here addresses the
additional problem of selective episodic retrieval without interference
from other episodes. In the new simulations, sequential retrieval of
all possible previous episodes occurs due to associations within the
circuit. Selection of a single current episode without interference from
other episodes involves the convergence of sequential retrieval with
temporal context in region CA1 of the simulation. This utilizes dynamical interactions during theta rhythm that match features of the
physiological data on theta rhythm obtained with current source density analysis (Brankack, Stewart & Fox, 1993). The sequential read
out of previous episodes resembles theta phase precession (Skaggs,
McNaughton, Wilson & Barnes, 1996), but has the additional feature
of context-dependent retrieval, which matches evidence for place cell
responses specific to prior or future responses in spatial alternation
(Wood, Dudchenko, Robitsek & Eichenbaum, 2000).

3.7.3 Prefrontal Mechanisms of Goal-Directed Selection of Next Action

In the new model, the goal-directed selection of next movement is
mediated by a simulation of prefrontal cortex. Performance of most
behavioral tasks requires learning of rules associated with these tasks.
Thus, effective simulation of hippocampal-dependent behavior requires a sophisticated model of rule learning in prefrontal cortex as
well. Recent simulations have extended a similar framework to modeling of neocortical function. In these simulations, goal-dependent
feedback spreads through local circuits representing the sequential
states of the external environment as well as proprioceptive feedback
of motor actions that induce transitions between different sequential states. When this backward flow of activity reaches the current
state, the convergence of the forward flow from current state input
and the backward forward flow from the goal representation acti-

vates the appropriate motor output. This provides an explicit neural implementation of the action-selection process based on action-value representations in reinforcement learning (Sutton & Barto, 1998). The function of this circuit continues to require separate phases of encoding sensory input from a phase for goal-dependent feedback activity. In particular, this simulation has been used to model generation of task-dependent behavior in the standard spatial alternation task.

3.8 CONCLUDING REMARKS

Acetylcholine has a number of different physiological effects on cortical circuits that often appear inconsistent. Computational modeling provides a unifying theoretical framework for understanding these different physiological effects, as summarized in this chapter. Modeling demonstrates that the combined physiological effects of acetylcholine serve to enhance the influence of afferent input on neuronal spiking activity, while reducing the influence of internal and feedback processing. Computational models demonstrate how these network properties can be interpreted functionally as both enhancing attention to sensory stimuli and enhancing the encoding of new memories. Acetylcholine also plays a strong role in the induction of theta rhythm oscillations in the hippocampus. Computational modeling indicates how a rapid shift in dynamics between strong input and strong recurrent excitation could mediate transitions between encoding and retrieval during each cycle of the hippocampal theta rhythm. Thus, the oscillatory dynamics induced by cholinergic modulation could underlie rapid changes in functional dynamics within cortical structures.

ACKNOWLEDGMENTS

Supported by NIH Grants MH60013, MH61492 and DA 16454 (as part of the NIH/NSF Collaborative Research in Computational Neuroscience Program) and NSF Science of Learning Center SBE 0354378.

References

Aigner, T. G. & Mishkin, M. (1986). The effects of physostigmine and scopolamine on recognition memory in monkeys. *Behavioral Neuroscience, 45*, 81–87.

Aigner, T. G., Walker, D. L. & Mishkin, M. (1991). Comparison of the effects of scopolamine administered before and after acquisition in a test of visual recognition memory in monkeys. *Behavioral and Neural Biology, 55*, 61–67.

Alkondon, M. & Albuquerque, E. X. (2001). Nicotinic acetylcholine receptor alpha7 and alpha4beta2 subtypes differentially control GABAergic input to CA1 neurons in rat hippocampus. *Journal of Neurophysiology, 86*, 3043–3055.

Allen, M. T., Padilla, Y. & Gluck, M. A. (2002). Ibotenic acid lesions of the medial septum retard delay eyeblink conditioning in rabbits (Oryctolagus cuniculus). *Behavioral Neuroscience, 116*, 733–738.

Anagnostaras, S. G., Maren, S. & Fanselow, M. S. (1995). Scopolamine selectively disrupts the acquisition of contextual fear conditioning in rats. *Neurobiology of Learning and Memory, 64*, 191–194.

Anagnostaras, S. G., Maren, S., Sage, J. R., Goodrich, S. & Fanselow, M. S. (1999). Scopolamine and pavlovian fear conditioning in rats: Dose-effect analysis. *Neuropsychopharmacology, 21*, 731–744.

Arnold, H. M., Burk, J. A., Hodgson, E. M., Sarter, M. & Bruno, J. P. (2002). Differential cortical acetylcholine release in rats performing a sustained attention task versus behaviorl control tasks that do not explicitly tax attention. *Neuroscience, 114*, 451–460.

Atri, A., Sherman, S. J., Norman, K. A., Kirchhoff, B. A., Nicolas, M. M., Greicius, M. D., Cramer, S., Breiter, H. C., Hasselmo, M. E. & Stern, C. E. (2003). Blockade of central cholinergic receptors impairs new learning and increases proactive interference in a word paired-associate memory task. *Behavioral Neuroscience, 118(1)*, 223–236.

Barkai, E. & Hasselmo, M. E. (1994). Modulation of the input/output function of rat piriform cortex pyramidal cells. *Journal of Neurophysiology, 72*, 644–658.

Bartus, R. T. & Johnson, H. R. (1976). Short term memory in the rhesus monkey: Disruption from the anticholinergic scopolamine. *Pharmacology Biochemistry and Behavior, 5*, 39–40.

Beatty, W. W., Butters, N. & Janowsky, D. S. (1986). Patterns of memory failure after scopolamine treatment: Implications for cholinergic hypotheses of dementia. *Behavioral and Neural Biology, 45*, 196–211.

Behrends, J. C. & ten Bruggencate, G. (1993). Cholinergic modulation of synaptic inhibition in the guinea pig hippocampus in vitro: Excitation of GABAergic interneurons and inhibition of GABA release. *Journal of Neurophysiology, 69*, 626–629.

Benardo, L. S. & Prince, D. A. (1982). Ionic mechanisms of cholinergic excitation in mammalian hippocampal pyramidal cells. *Brain Research, 249*, 333–344.

Berry, S. D. & Seager, M. A. (2001). Hippocampal theta oscillations and classical conditioning. *Neurobiology of Learning and Memory, 76*, 298–313.

Berry, S. D. & Thompson, R. F. (1979). Medial septal lesions retard classical conditioning of the nicitating membrane response in rabbits. *Science, 205*, 209–211.

Bi, G. Q. & Poo, M. M. (1998). Synaptic modifications in cultured hippocampal neurons: Dependence on spike timing, synaptic strength, and postsynaptic cell type. *Journal of Neuroscience, 18(24)*, 10464–10472.

Bland, B. H. & Colom, L. V. (1993). Extrinsic and intrinsic properties underlying oscillation and synchrony in limbic cortex. *Progress in Neurobiology, 41*, 157–208.

Blitzer, R. D., Gil, O. & Landau, E. M. (1990). Cholinergic stimulation enhances long-term potentiation in the CA1 region of rat hippocampus. *Neuroscience Letters, 119*, 207–210.

Bolhuis, J. J., Strijkstra, A. M. & Kramers, R. J. (1988). Effects of scopolamine on performance of rats in a delayed-response radial maze task. *Physiology and Behavior, 43*, 403–409.

Bragin, A., Jando, G., Nadasdy, Z., Hetke, J., Wise, K. & Buzsaki, G. (1995). Gamma (40-100 Hz) oscillation in the hippocampus of the behaving rat. *Journal of Neuroscience, 15*, 47–60.

Brankack, J., Stewart, M. & Fox, S. E. (1993). Current source density analysis of the hippocampal theta rhythm: Associated sustained potentials and candidate synaptic generators. *Brain Research, 625(2)*, 310–327.

Brocher, S., Artola, A. & Singer, W. (1992). Agonists of cholinergic and noradrenergic receptors facilitate synergistically the induction of long-term potentiation in slices of rat visual cortex. *Brain Research, 573*, 27–36.

Broks, P., Preston, G. C., Traub, M., Poppleton, P., Ward, C. & Stahl, S. M. (1988). Modelling dementia: Effects of scopolamine on memory and attention. *Neuropsychologia, 26*, 685–700.

Bucci, D. J., Holland, P. C. & Gallagher, M. (1998). Removal of cholinergic input to rat posterior parietal cortex disrupts incremental processing of conditioned stimuli. *Journal of Neuroscience, 18*, 8038–8046.

Buresova, O., Bolhuis, J. J. & Bures, J. (1986). Differential effects of cholinergic blockade on performance of rats in the water tank navigation task and in a radial water maze. *Behavioral Neuroscience, 100*, 476–482.

Burgard, E. C. & Sarvey, J. M. (1990). Muscarinic receptor activation facilitates the induction of long-term potentiation (LTP) in the rat dentate gyrus. *Neuroscience Letters, 116*, 34–39.

Buzsaki, G. (1986). Hippocampal sharp waves: Their origin and significance. *Brain Research, 398*, 242–252.

Buzsaki, G. (1989). Two-stage model of memory trace formation: A role for "noisy" brain states. *Neuroscience, 31*, 551–570.

Buzsaki, G., Leung, L. W. & Vanderwolf, C. H. (1983). Cellular bases of hippocampal EEG in the behaving rat. *Brain Research*, *287(2)*, 139–171.

Caine, E. D., Weingartner, H., Ludlow, C. L., Cudahy, E. A. & Wehry, S. (1981). Qualitative analysis of scopolamine-induced amnesia. *Psychopharmology*, *74*, 74–80.

Cannon, R. C., Hasselmo, M. E. & Koene, R. A. (2002). From biophysics to behavior: Catacomb2 and the design of biologically plausible models for spatial navigation. *Neuroinformatics*, *1(1)*, 3–42.

Cassel, J. C. & Kelche, C. (1989). Scopolamine treatment and fimbria-fornix lesions: Mimetic effects on radial maze performance. *Physiology and Behavior*, *46*, 347–353.

Chapman, C. A. & Lacaille, J. C. (1999). Intrinsic theta-frequency membrane potential oscillations in hippocampal CA1 interneurons of stratum lacunosum-moleculare. *Journal of Neurophysiology*, *81*, 1296 1307.

Chiba, A. A., Bucci, D. J., Holland, P. C. & Gallagher, M. (1995). Basal forebrain cholinergic lesions disrupt increments but not decrements in conditioned stimulus processing. *Journal of Neuroscience*, *(15)*, 7315–7322.

Chrobak, J. J. & Buzsaki, G. (1994). Selective activation of deep layer (V-VI) retrohippocampal cortical neurons during hippocampal sharp waves in the behaving rat. *Journal of Neuroscience*, *14*, 6160–6170.

Cole, A. E. & Nicoll, R. A. (1984). Characterization of a slow cholinergic postsynaptic potential recorded in vitro from rat hippocampal pyramidal cells. *Journal of Physiology - London*, *352*, 173–188.

Constanti, A. & Galvan, M. (1983). M-current in voltage clamped olfactory cortex neurones. *Neuroscience Letters*, *39*, 65–70.

Constanti, A. & Sim, J. A. (1987). Calcium-dependent potassium conductance in guinea-pig olfactory cortex neurons in vitro. *Journal of Physiology - London*, *387*, 173–194.

Crow, T. J. & Grove-White, I. G. (1973). An analysis of the learning deficit following hyoscine administration to man. *British Journal of Pharmacology, 49*, 322–327.

DeRosa, E. & Hasselmo, M. E. (2000). Muscarinic cholinergic neuromodulation reduces proactive interference between stored odor memories during associative learning in rats. *Behavioral Neuroscience, 114*, 32–41.

DeRosa, E., Hasselmo, M. E. & Baxter, M. G. (2001). Contribution of the cholinergic basal forebrain to proactive interference from stored odor memories during associative learning in rats. *Behavioral Neuroscience, 115*, 314–327.

Descarries, L., Gisiger, V. & Steriade, M. (1997). Diffuse transmission by acetylcholine in the CNS. *Progress in Neurobiology, 53*, 603–625.

Drachman, D. A. & Leavitt, J. (1974). Human memory and the cholinergic system. *Archives of Neuroloy, 30*, 113–121.

Dykes, R. W. (1997). Mechanisms controlling neuronal plasticity in somatosensory cortex. *Canadian Journal of Physiology and Pharmacology, 75*, 535–545.

Egorov, A. V., Hamam, B. N., Fransen, E., Hasselmo, M. E. & Alonso, A. A. (2002). Graded persistent activity in entorhinal cortex neurons. *Nature, 420*, 173–178.

Eichenbaum, H. & Cohen, N. J. (2001). *From Conditioning to Conscious Recollection: Memory Systems of the Brain.* Oxford: Oxford University Press.

Ennaceur, A., Neave, N. & Aggleton, J. P. (1996). Neurotoxic lesions of the perirhinal cortex do not mimic the behavioural effects of fornix transection in the rat. *Behaviour Brain Research, 80*, 9–25.

Fox, S. E. (1989). Membrane potential and impedence changes in hippocampal pyramidal cells during theta rhythm. *Experimental Brain Research, 77*, 283–294.

Fransen, E., Alonso, A. A. & Hasselmo, M. E. (2002). Simulations of the role of the muscarinic-activated calcium-sensitive non-specific cation current I(NCM) in entorhinal neuronal activity during delayed matching tasks. *Journal of Neuroscience*, *22*, 1081–1097.

Frazier, C. J., Rollins, Y. D., Breese, C. R., Leonard, S., Freedman, R. & Dunwiddie, T. V. (1998). Acetylcholine activates an alpha-bungarotoxin-sensitive nicotinic current in rat hippocampal interneurons, but not pyramidal cells. *Journal of Neuroscience*, *18*, 1187–95.

Gale, G. D., Anagnostaras, S. G. & Fanselow, M. S. (2001). Cholinergic modulation of pavlovian fear conditioning: Effects of intrahippocampal scopolamine infusion. *Hippocampus*, *11*, 371–376.

Ghonheim, M. M. & Mewaldt, S. P. (1975). Effects of diazepan and scopolamine on storage, retrieval, and organisational processes in memory. *Psychopharmacology*, *44*, 257–262.

Gil, Z., Connors, B. W. & Amitai, Y. (1997). Differential regulation of neocortical synapses by neuromodulators and activity. *Neuron*, *19*, 679–686.

Gioanni, Y., Rougeot, C., Clarke, P. B., Lepouse, C., Thierry, A. M. & Vidal, C. (1999). Nicotinic receptors in the rat prefrontal cortex: Increase in glutamate release and facilitation of mediodorsal thalamo-cortical transmission. *European Journal of Neuroscience*, *11*, 18–30.

Giovannini, M. G., Rakovska, A., Benton, R. S., Pazzagli, M., Bianchi, L. & Pepeu, G. (2001). Effects of novelty and habituation on acetylcholine, GABA, and glutamate release from the frontal cortex and hippocampus of freely moving rats. *Neuroscience*, *106*, 43–53.

Golding, N. L., Staff, N. P. & Spruston, N. (2002). Dendritic spikes as a mechanism for cooperative long-term potentiation. *Nature*, *418(6895)*, 326–331.

Hasselmo, M. E. (1995). Neuromodulation and cortical function: Modeling the physiological basis of behavior. *Behaviour Brain Research*, *67*, 1–27.

Hasselmo, M. E. (1999). Neuromodulation: Acetylcholine and memory consolidation. *Trends in Cognitive Sciences, 3*, 351–359.

Hasselmo, M. E., Anderson, B. P. & Bower, J. M. (1992). Cholinergic modulation of cortical associative memory function. *Journal of Neurophysiology, 67*, 1230–1246.

Hasselmo, M. E. & Barkai, E. (1995). Cholinergic modulation of activity-dependent synaptic plasticity in rat piriform cortex. *Journal of Neuroscience, 15*, 6592–6604.

Hasselmo, M. E., Bodelon, C. & Wyble, B. P. (2002a). A proposed function for hippocampal theta rhythm: Separate phases of encoding and retrieval enhance reversal of prior learning. *Neural Computation, 14(4)*, 793–817.

Hasselmo, M. E. & Bower, J. M. (1992). Cholinergic suppression specific to intrinsic not afferent fiber synapses in rat piriform (olfactory) cortex. *Journal of Neurophysiology, 67*, 1222–1229.

Hasselmo, M. E. & Bower, J. M. (1993). Acetylcholine and memory. *Trends in Neuroscience, 16*, 218–222.

Hasselmo, M. E., Cannon, R. C. & Koene, R. A. (2002c). *The parahippocampal region: Organisation and role in cognitive functions*, chapter A simulation of parahippocampal and hippocampal structures guiding spatial navigation of a virtual rat in a virtual environment: A functional framework for theta theory, (pp. 139–161). Oxford: Oxford University Press.

Hasselmo, M. E. & Cekic, M. (1996). Suppression of synaptic transmission may allow combination of associative feedback and self-organizing feedforward connections in the neocortex. *Behaviour Brain Research, 79*, 153–161.

Hasselmo, M. E. & Eichenbaum, H. (2005). Hippocampal mechanisms for the context-dependent retrieval of episodes. *Neural Networks*. In press.

Hasselmo, M. E. & Fehlau, B. P. (2001). Differences in time course of cholinergic and GABAergic modulation of excitatory synaptic potentials in rat hippocampal slice preparations. *Journal of Neurophysiology, 86*, 1792–1802.

Hasselmo, M. E., Hay, J., Ilyn, M. & Gorchetchnikov, A. (2002b). Neuromodulation, theta rhythm and rat spatial navigation. *Neural Networks, 15*, 689–707.

Hasselmo, M. E. & Schnell, E. (1994). Laminar selectivity of the cholinergic suppression of synaptic transmission in rat hippocampal region CA1: Computational modeling and brain slice physiology. *Journal of Neuroscience, 14*, 3898–3914.

Hasselmo, M. E., Schnell, E. & Barkai, E. (1995). Dynamics of learning and recall at excitatory recurrent synapses and cholinergic modulation in hippocampal region CA3. *Journal of Neuroscience, 15*, 5249–5262.

Hasselmo, M. E. & Wyble, B. P. (1997). Free recall and recognition in a network model of the hippocampus: Simulating effects of scopolamine on human memory function. *Behaviour Brain Research, 89*, 1–34.

Hasselmo, M. E., Wyble, B. P. & Wallenstein, G. V. (1996). Encoding and retrieval of episodic memories: Role of cholinergic and GABAergic modulation in the hippocampus. *Hippocampus, 6*, 693–708.

Herreras, O., Solis, J. M., Herranz, A. S., Martin del Rio, R. & Lerma, J. (1988b). Sensory modulation of hippocampal transmission. II. Evidence for a cholinergic locus of inhibition in the Schaffer-CA1 synapse. *Brain Research, 461*, 303–313.

Herreras, O., Solis, J. M., Munoz, M. D., Martin del Rio, R. & Lerma, J. (1988a). Sensory modulation of hippocampal transmission. I. Opposite effects on CA1 and dentate gyrus synapsis. *Brain Research, 461*, 290–302.

Himmelheber, A., Sarter, M. & Bruno, J. (2000). Increases in cortical acetylcholine release during sustained attention performance in rats. *Cognitive Brain Research, 9*, 313–325.

Holscher, C., Anwyl, R. & Rowan, M. J. (1997). Stimulation on the positive phase of hippocampal theta rhythm induces long-term potentiation that can be depotentiated by stimulation on the negative phase in area CA1 in vivo. *Journal of Neuroscience, 17(16)*, 6470–6477.

Hounsgaard, J. (1978). Presynaptic inhibitory action of acetylcholine in area ca1 of the hippocampus. *Experimental Neurology, 62*, 787–797.

Howard, M. W., Fotedar, M. S., Datey, A. V. & Hasselmo, M. E. (2005). The temporal context model in spatial navigation and relational learning: Toward a common explanation of medial temporal lobe function across domains. *Psychological Review, 112(1)*, 75–116.

Howard, M. W. & Kahana, M. J. (2002). A distributed representation of temporal context. *Journal of Mathematical Psychology, 46(3)*, 269–299.

Hsieh, C. Y., Cruikshank, S. J. & Metherate, R. (2000). Differential modulation of auditory thalamocortical and intracortical synaptic transmission by cholinergic agonist. *Brain Research, 880*, 51–64.

Huerta, P. T. & Lisman, J. E. (1993). Heightened synaptic plasticity of hippocampal CA1 neurons during a cholinergically induced rhythmic state. *Nature, 364*, 723–725.

Huerta, P. T. & Lisman, J. E. (1995). Bidirectional synaptic plasticity induced by a single burst during cholinergic theta oscillation in CA1 in vitro. *Neuron, 15(5)*, 1053–1063.

Hyman, J. M., Wyble, B. P., Goyal, V., Rossi, C. A. & Hasselmo, M. E. (2003). Stimulation in hippocampal region CA1 in behaving rats yields LTP when delivered to the peak of theta and LTD when delivered to the trough. *Journal of Neuroscience, 23(37)*, 11725–11731.

Jasper, H. H. & Tessier, J. (1971). Acetylcholine liberation from cerebral cortex during paradoxical (REM) sleep. *Science, 172*, 601–602.

Jensen, O. & Lisman (1996). Novel lists of 7 +/- 2 known items can be reliably stored in an oscillatory short-term memory network: Interaction with long-term memory. *Learning Memory, 3(2-3)*, 257–263.

Judge, S. J. & Hasselmo, M. E. (2004). Theta rhythmic stimulation of stratum lacunosum-moleculare in rat hippocampus contributes to associative LTP at a phase offset in stratum radiatum. *Journal of Neurophsyiology, 92(3)*, 1615–1624.

Kahle, J. S. & Cotman, C. W. (1989). Carbachol depresses the synaptic responses in the medial but not the lateral perforant path. *Brain Research, 482*, 159–163.

Kametani, H. & Kawamura, H. (1990). Alterations in acetylcholine release in the rat hippocampus during sleep-wakefulness detected by intracerebral dialysis. *Life Sciences, 47*, 421–426.

Kamondi, A., Acsady, L., Wang, X. J. & Buzsaki, G. (1998). Theta oscillations in somata and dendrites of hippocampal pyramidal cells in vivo: Activity-dependent phase-precession of action potentials. *Hippocampus, 8(3)*, 244–261.

Kimura, F. (2000). Cholinergic modulation of cortical function: A hypothetical role in shifting the dynamics in cortical network. *Neuroscience Research, 38(1)*, 19–26.

Kimura, F., Fukuda, M. & Tsumoto, T. (1999). Acetylcholine suppresses the spread of excitation in the visual cortex revealed by optical recording: Possible differential effect depending on the source of input. *European Journal of Neuroscience, 11(10)*, 3597–3609.

Kirchhoff, B. A., Hasselmo, M. E., Norman, K. A., Nicolas, M. M., Greicius, M. D., Breiter, H. C. & Stern, C. E. (2000). Effect of cholinergic blockade on paired associate learning in humans. *Soc. Neuroscience. Abstr, 26*, 263.18.

Klink, R. & Alonso, A. (1997a). Muscarinic modulation of the oscillatory and repetitive firing properties of entorhinal cortex layer II neurons. *Journal of Neurophysiology, 77*, 1813–1828.

Klink, R. & Alonso, A. (1997b). Ionic mechanisms of muscarinic depolarization in entorhinal cortex layer II neurons. *Journal of Neurophysiology, 77*, 1829–1843.

Kohonen, T. (1984). *Self-organization and Associative Memory.* New York: Springer-Verlag.

Kramis, R., Vanderwolf, C. H. & Bland, B. H. (1975). Two types of hippocampal rhythmical slow activity in both the rabbit and the rat: Relations to behavior and effects of atropine, diethyl ether, urethane, and pentobarbital. *Experimental Neurology, 49(1)*, 58–85.

Krnjevic, K. & Phillis, J. W. (1963). Acetylcholine-sensitive cells in the cerebral cortex. *Journal of Physiology - London, 166*, 296–327.

Krnjevic, K., Pumain, R. & Renaud, L. (1971). The mechanism of excitation by acetylcholine in the cerebral cortex. *Journal of Physiology - London, 215*, 247–268.

Levy, W. B. (1996). A sequence predicting CA3 is a flexible associator that learns and uses context to solve hippocampal-like tasks. *Hippocampus, 6*, 579–590.

Levy, W. B. & Steward, O. (1983). Temporal contiguity requirements for long-term associative potentiation depression in the hippocampus. *Neuroscience, 8(4)*, 791–797.

Linster, C., Garcia, P. A., Hasselmo, M. E. & Baxter, M. G. (2001). Selective loss of cholinergic neurons projecting to the olfactory system increases perceptual generalization between similar, but not dissimilar, odorants. *Behavioral Neuroscience, 115*, 826–833.

Linster, C. & Hasselmo, M. E. (2000). Neural activity in the horizontal limb of the diagonal band of broca can be modulated by electrical stimulation of the olfactory bulb and cortex in rats. *Neuroscience Letters, 282*, 157–160.

Linster, C. & Hasselmo, M. E. (2001). Neuromodulation and the functional dynamics of piriform cortex. *Chemical Senses, 26*, 585–594.

Linster, C., Wyble, B. P. & Hasselmo, M. E. (1999). Electrical stimulation of the horizontal limb of the diagonal band of broca modulates population EPSP's in piriform cortex. *Journal of Neurophsyiology*, *81*, 2737–2742.

Lisman, J. E. (1999). Relating hippocampal circuitry to function: Recall of memory sequences by reciprocal dentate-CA3 interactions. *Neuron*, *22*, 233–242.

Madison, D. V., Lancaster, B. & Nicoll, R. A. (1987). Voltage clamp analysis of cholinergic action in the hippocampus. *Journal of Neuroscience*, *7*, 733–741.

Madison, D. V. & Nicoll, R. A. (1984). Control of the repetitive discharge of rat ca1 pyramidal neurones in vitro. *Journal of Physiology - London*, *354*, 319–331.

Maloney, K. J., Cape, E. G., Gotman, J. & Jones, B. E. (1997). High frequency gamma electroencephalogram activity in association with sleep-wake states and spontaneous behaviors in the rat. *Neuroscience*, *76*, 541–555.

Markowska, A. L., Olton, D. S., Murray, E. A. & Gaffan, D. (1989). A comparative analysis of the role of fornix and cingulate cortex in memory: Rats. *Experimental Brain Research*, *74(1)*, 187–201.

Marrosu, F., Portas, C., Mascia, M. S., Casu, M. A., Fa, M., Giagheddu, M., Imperato, A. & Gessa, G. L. (1995). Microdialysis measurement of cortical and hippocampal acetylcholine release during sleep-wake cycle in freely moving cats. *Brain Research*, *671*, 329–332.

McCormick, D. A. & Prince, D. A. (1986). Mechanisms of action of acetylcholine in the guinea-pig cerebral cortex in vitro. *Journal of Physiology - London*, *375*, 169–194.

McGaughy, J., Kaiser, T. & Sarter, M. (1996). Behavioral vigilance following infusions of 192 IgG-saporin into the basal forebrain: Selectivity of the behavioral impairment and relation to cortical AChE-positive fiber density. *Behavioral Neuroscience*, *110*, 247–265.

McGaughy, J. & Sarter, M. (1995). Behavioral vigilance in rats: Task validation and effects of age, amphetamine and benzodiazepine receptor ligands. *Psychopharmacology, 117,* 340–357.

McGaughy, J. & Sarter, M. (1998). Sustained attention performance in rats with intracortical infusions of 192 IgG-saporin-induced cortical cholinergic deafferentation: Effects of physostigmine and FG 7142. *Behavioral Neuroscience, 110,* 247–265.

McGaughy, M., Decker, M. W. & Sarter, M. (1999). Enhancement of sustained attention performance by the nicotinic receptor agonist ABT-418 in intact but not basal forebrain-lesioned rats. *Psychopharmacology, 144,* 175–182.

McQuiston, A. R. & Madison, D. V. (1999a). Nicotinic receptor activation excites distinct subtypes of interneurons in the rat hippocampus. *Journal of Neuroscience, 19,* 2887–2896.

McQuiston, A. R. & Madison, D. V. (1999b). Muscarinic receptor activity has multiple effects on the resting membrane potentials of CA1 hippocampal interneurons. *Journal of Neuroscience, 19,* 5693–5702.

Mesulam, M. M., Mufson, E. J., Levey, A. I. & Wainer, B. H. (1983b). Cholinergic innervation of cortex by the basal forebrain: Cytochemistry and cortical connections of the septal area, diagonal band nuclei, nucleus basalis (substantia innominata and hypothalamus) in the rhesus monkey. *Journal of Comparative Neurology, 214,* 170–197.

Mesulam, M. M., Mufson, E. J., Wainer, B. H. & Levey, A. I. (1983a). Central cholinergic pathways in the rat: An overview based on an alternative nomenclature (Ch1-Ch6). *Neuroscience, 10,* 1185–1201.

Metherate, R. & Ashe, J. H. (1993). Nucleus basalis stimulation facilitates thalamocortical synaptic transmission in the rat auditory cortex. *Synapse, 14(2),* 132–143.

Metherate, R., Ashe, J. H. & Weinberger, N. M. (1990). Acetylcholine modifies neuronal acoustic rate level functions in guinea pig auditory cortex by an action at muscarinic receptors. *Synapse, 6*, 364–368.

Metherate, R. & Weinberger, N. M. (1990). Cholinergic modulation of responses to single tones produces tone-specific receptive-field alterations in cat auditory-cortex. *Synapse, 6*, 133–145.

M'Harzi, M., Palacios, A., Monmaur, P., Willig, F., Houcine, O. & Delacour, J. (1987). Effects of selective lesions of fimbria-fornix on learning set in the rat. *Physiology and Behavior, 40*, 181–188.

Mizumori, S. J., McNaughton, B. L. & Barnes, C. A. (1989). A comparison of supramammillary and medial septal influences on hippocampal field potentials and single-unit activity. *Journal of Neurophsyiology, 61(1)*, 15–31.

Murakoshi, T. (1995). Cholinergic modulation of synaptic transmission in the rat visual cortex in vitro. *Vision Research, 35(1)*, 25–35.

Murphy, P. C. & Sillito, A. M. (1991). Cholinergic enhancement of direction selectivity in the visual cortex of the cat. *Neuroscience, 40(1)*, 13–20.

Myers, C. E., Ermita, B. R., Hasselmo, M. & Gluck, M. A. (1998). Further implications of a computational model of septohippocampal cholinergic modulation in eyeblink conditioning. *Psychobiology, 26*, 1–20.

Numan, R., Feloney, M. P., Pham, K. H. & Tieber, L. M. (1995). Effects of medial septal lesions on an operant go/no-go delayed response alternation task in rats. *Physiology and Behavior, 58*, 1263–1271.

Patil, M. M. & Hasselmo, M. E. (1999). Modulation of inhibitory synaptic potentials in the piriform cortex. *Journal of Neurophysiology, 81*, 2103–2118.

Patil, M. M., Linster, C., Lubenov, E. & Hasselmo, M. E. (1998). Cholinergic agonist carbachol enables associative long-term potentiation in piriform cortex slices. *Journal of Neurophysiology, 80*, 2467–2474.

Penetar, D. M. & McDonough, J. H. (1983). Effects of cholinergic drugs on delayed match to sample performance of rhesus monkeys. *Pharmacology Biochemistry and Behavior*, *19*, 963–967.

Perry, E. K. & Perry, R. H. (1995). Acetylcholine and hallucinations: Disease-related compared to drug-induced alterations in human consciousness. *Brain and Cognition*, *28*, 240–258.

Peterson, R. C. (1977). Scopolamine-induced learning failures in man. *Psychopharmacologia*, *52*, 283–289.

Pitler, T. A. & Alger, B. E. (1992). Cholinergic excitation of GABAergic interneurons in the rat hippocampal slice. *Journal of Physiology - London*, *450*, 127–142.

Redish, A. D. & Touretzky, D. S. (1998). The role of the hippocampus in solving the Morris water maze. *Neural Computation*, *10*, 73–111.

Rempel-Clower, N. L., Zola, S. M., Squire, L. R. & Amaral, D. G. (1996). Three cases of enduring memory impairment after bilateral damage limited to the hippocampal formation. *Journal of Neuroscience*, *16(16)*, 5233–5255.

Rovira, C., Ben-Ari, Y., Cherubini, E., Krnjevic, K. & Ropert, N. (1983). Pharmacology of the dendritic action of acetylcholine and further observations on the somatic disinhibition in the rat hippocampus in situ. *Neuroscience*, *8*, 97–106.

Rovira, C., Cherubini, E. & Ben-Ari, Y. (1982). Opposite actions of muscarinic and nicotinic agents on hippocampal dendritic negative fields recorded in rats. *Neuropharmacology*, *21(9)*, 933–936.

Salvatierra, A. T. & Berry, S. D. (1989). Scopolamine disruption of septo-hippocampal activity and classical conditioning. *Behavioral Neuroscience*, *103(4)*, 715–721.

Sato, H., Hata, Y., Masui, H. & Tsumoto, T. (1987). A functional role of cholinergic innervation to neurons in the cat visual cortex. *Journal of Neurophysiology*, *58*, 765–80.

Schwindt, P. C., Spain, W. J., Foehring, R. C., Stafstrom, C. E., Chubb, M. C. & Crill, W. E. (1988). Slow conductances in neurons from cat sensorimotor cortex and their role in slow excitability changes. *Journal of Neurophysiology*, *59*, 450–467.

Seager, M. A., Asaka, Y. & Berry, S. D. (1999). Scopolamine disruption of behavioral and hippocampal responses in appetitive trace classical conditioning. *Behaviour Brain Research*, *100*, 143–151.

Seager, M. A., Johnson, L. D., Chabot, E. S., Asaka, Y. & Berry, S. D. (2002). Oscillatory brain states and learning: Impact of hippocampal theta-contingent training. *Proceedings of the National Academy of Sciences of the United States of America*, *99*, 1616–1620.

Shalinsky, M. H., Magistretti, J., Ma, L. & Alonso, A. A. (2002). Muscarinic activation of a cation current and associated current noise in entorhinal-cortex layer-II neurons. *Journal of Neurophysiology*, *88(3)*, 1197–1211.

Sharp, P. E., Blair, H. T. & Brown, M. (1996). Neural network modeling of the hippocampal formation spatial signals and their possible role in navigation: A modular approach. *Hippocampus*, *6*, 720–734.

Sherman, S. J., Atri, A., Hasselmo, M. E., Stern, C. E. & Howard, M. W. (2003). Scopolamine impairs human recognition memory: Data and modeling. *Behavioral Neuroscience*, *117(3)*, 526–539.

Skaggs, W. E., McNaughton, B. L., Wilson, M. A. & Barnes, C. A. (1996). Theta phase precession in hippocampal neuronal populations and the compression of temporal sequences. *Hippocampus*, *6*, 149–172.

Solomon, P. R., Groccia-Ellison, M. E., Flynn, D., Mirak, J., Edwards, K. R., Dunehew, A. & Stanton, M. E. (1983a). Disruption of human eyeblink conditioning after central cholinergic blockade with scopolamine. *Behavioral Neuroscience*, *107(2)*, 271–279.

Solomon, P. R., Solomon, S. D., Schaaf, E. V. & Perry, H. E. (1983b). Altered activity in the hippocampus is more detrimental to classical conditioning than removing the structure. *Science*, *220(4594)*, 329–331.

Steriade, M. (1994). Sleep oscillations and their blockage by activating systems. *Journal of Psychiatry Neuroscience*, *19*, 354–358.

Steriade, M. (2001). Impact of network activities on neuronal properties in corticothalamic systems. *Journal of Neurophysiology*, *86*, 1–39.

Steriade, M., Amzica, F. & Contreras, D. (1996). Synchronization of fast (30-40 Hz) spontaneous cortical rhythms during brain activation. *Journal of Neuroscience*, *16*, 392–417.

Stewart, M. & Fox, S. E. (1990). Do septal neurons pace the hippocampal theta rhythm? *Trends in Neuroscience*, *13(5)*, 163–168.

Stickgold, R. (1998). Sleep: Off-line memory reprocessing. *Trends in Cognitive Sciences*, *2*, 484–492.

Sutton, R. S. & Barto, A. G. (1998). *Reinforcement Learning: An Introduction*. Cambridge, MA: MIT Press.

Suzuki, W. A., Miller, E. K. & Desimone, R. (1997). Object and place memory in the macaque entorhinal cortex. *Journal of Neurophysiology*, *78*, 1062–1081.

Tang, Y. & Aigner, T. G. (1996). Release of cerebral acetylcholine increases during visually mediated behavior in monkeys. *NeuroReport*, *7*, 2231–2235.

Tang, Y., Mishkin, M. & Aigner, T. G. (1997). Effects of muscarinic blockade in perirhinal cortex during visual recognition. *Proceedings of the National Academy of Sciences of the United States of America*, *94*, 12667–12669.

Tremblay, N., Warren, R. A. & Dykes, R. W. (1990). Electrophysiological studies of acetylcholine and the role of the basal forebrain in the somatosensory cortex of the cat. II. cortical neurons excited by somatic stimuli. *Journal of Neurophysiology*, *64(4)*, 1212–1222.

Trepel, C. & Racine, R. J. (1998). Long-term potentiation in the neocortex of the adult, freely moving rat. *Cerebral Cortex*, *8*, 719–729.

Tseng, G. F. & Haberly, L. B. (1989). Deep neurons in piriform cortex. II. membrane properties that underlie unusual synaptic responses. *Journal of Neurophysiology*, *62(2)*, 386–400.

Turchi, J. & Sarter, M. (1997). Cortical acetylcholine and processing capacity: Effects of cortical cholinergic deafferentation on crossmodal divided attention in rats. *Cognitive Brain Research*, *6*, 147–158.

Umbriaco, D., Garcia, S., Beaulieu, C. & Descarries, L. (1995). Relational features of acetylcholine, noradrenaline, serotonin and GABA axon terminals in the stratum radiatum of adult rat hippocampus (CA1). *Hippocampus*, *5(6)*, 605–620.

Umbriaco, D., Watkins, K. C., Descarries, L., Cozzari, C. & Hartman, B. K. (1994). Ultrastructural and morphometric features of the acetylcholine innervation in adult rat parietal cortex: An electron microscopic study in serial sections. *Journal of Comparative Neurology*, *348*, 351–373.

Valentino, R. J. & Dingledine, R. (1981). Presynaptic inhibitory effect of acetylcholine in the hippocampus. *Journal of Neuroscience*, *1*, 784–792.

Vidal, C. & Changeux, J. P. (1993). Nicotinic and muscarinic modulations of excitatory synaptic transmission in the rat prefrontal cortex in vitro. *Neuroscience*, *56*, 23–32.

Vogt, K. E. & Regehr, W. G. (2001). Cholinergic modulation of excitatory synaptic transmission in the CA3 area of the hippocampus. *Journal of Neuroscience*, *21(1)*, 75–83.

Wesnes, K. & Warburton, D. M. (1984). Effects of scopolamine and nicotine on human rapid information processing performance. *Psychopharmacology*, *82*, 147–150.

Whishaw, I. Q. (1985). Cholinergic receptor blockade in the rat impairs locale but not taxon strategies for place navigation in a swimming pool. *Behavioral Neuroscience, 99*, 979–1005.

Williams, S. H. & Constanti, A. (1988). Quantitative effects of some muscarinic agonists on evoked surface-negative field potentials recorded from the guinea-pig olfactory cortex slice. *British Journal of Pharmacology, 93*, 846–854.

Wilson, M. A. & McNaughton, B. L. (1994). Reactivation of hippocampal ensemble memories during sleep. *Science, 265*, 676–679.

Winson, J. & Abzug, C. (1978). Dependence upon behavior of neuronal transmission from perforant pathway through entorhinal cortex. *Brain Research, 147*, 422–427.

Wood, E. R., Dudchenko, P. A., Robitsek, R. J. & Eichenbaum, H. (2000). Hippocampal neurons encode information about different types of memory episodes occurring in the same location. *Neuron, 27(3)*, 623.

Xiang, Z., Huguenard, J. R. & Prince, D. A. (1998). Cholinergic switching within neocortical inhibitory networks. *Science, 281*, 985–988.

Xiang, Z., Huguenard, J. R. & Prince, D. A. (2002). Synaptic inhibition of pyramidal cells evoked by different interneuronal subtypes in layer v of rat visual cortex. *Journal of Neurophysiology, 88*, 740–750.

Yajeya, J., De La Fuente, A., Criado, J. M., Bajo, V., Sanchez-Riolobos, A. & Heredia, M. (2000). Muscarinic agonist carbachol depresses excitatory synaptic transmission in the rat basolateral amygdala in vitro. *Synapse, 38(2)*, 151–160.

Yamamoto, C. & Kawai, N. (1967). Presynaptic action of acetylcholine in thin sections from the guinea-pig dentate gyrus in vitro. *Experimental Neurology, 19*, 176–187.

Young, B. J., Otto, T., Fox, G. D. & Eichenbaum, H. (1997). Memory representation within the parahippocampal region. *Journal of Neuroscience, 17(13)*, 5183–5195.

Young, S. L., Bohenek, D. L. & Fanselow, M. S. (1995). Scopolamine impairs acquisition and facilitates consolidation of fear conditioning: Differential effects for tone vs context conditioning. *Neurobiology of Learning and Memory, 63*, 174–180.

4

Modeling Amnesia: Connectionist and Mathematical Approaches

Jaap M. J. Murre, Martijn Meeter, and Antonio G. Chessa
University of Amsterdam

How are memories acquired and how are they lost in amnesia? Which brain areas are involved and how do they interact? In 1881, Théodule Ribot discovered that recent memories, although apparently strongly encoded and most reliably accessed, are nonetheless the first ones to be lost in many forms of amnesia, whereas remote memories are more resistant to brain damage. Over a century of research has produced a large body of data that aims to further elucidate these questions. Important contributions have come from neurology, psychiatry, neurobiology, experimental psychology, and neuropsychology and consist of studies with brain-damaged patients, experimental animals, and healthy subjects. From a modeling point of view, this data set is very heterogeneous, with a low sampling rate and a high error rate. Is it still worthwhile to attempt to model these data?

Perhaps because of this reason, the field of memory disorders has long been dominated by verbal theories. In recent years, computational models of amnesia have started to appear. In these and in computational models in general, two lines can be detected.

In a first line, the role of modeling remains limited to existence proofs, showing that certain mechanisms proposed in the literature can in fact work when implemented in a consistent manner and that they can explain many of the existing studies. This first step follows on the formulation of verbal theories that are typically vague, with many hidden assumptions and unspecified mechanisms. For a model to work, the assumptions must be made explicit and the mechanisms specified. This initial phase is typically focused on defending uncovered assumptions and proposing underlying mechanisms, and it usually involves running simulations that provide existence proofs.

They demonstrate that the model based on these assumptions and mechanisms *can* indeed work.

So, we see that since the 1950s, many theories have been published that address aspects of the formation of long-term memory and its decline with amnesia (e.g., Milner, 1957, 1989; Mishkin, 1982; Nadel & Moscovitch, 1997; Squire & Zola-Morgan, 1991; Squire, Cohen & Nadel, 1984; Teyler & DiScenna, 1986; Wickelgren, 1979, 1987). The more recent connectionist models by (Alvarez & Squire, 1994), (Mc-Clelland et al., 1995), (Murre, 1996, 1997), and (Nadel et al., 2000) have their roots in these verbal theories and, through their implementation, provide existence proofs, demonstrating that many of the earlier ideas are indeed viable.

The second line of modeling is one in which a model is applied to specific data sets by precisely fitting them. Whereas models in the first line thus only reproduce data qualitatively, models of the second kind do that in a quantitative way. The latter usually have a rigorous mathematical form, and care is taken not to make models overly flexible. Although such modeling has a long history in the memory literature (e.g., Estes, 1950), it is only recently that such models have made their appearance in research on amnesia.

In this chapter, we review two models of amnesia from these two lines of modeling. After an introduction to consolidation theory, we discuss an example of a connectionist approach to modeling amnesia that follows the first line and offers a proof of principle for consolidation theory. This model is then abstracted, generalized, and extended to a mathematical model that aims to take another step—namely, to provide quantitatively accurate descriptions of learning and forgetting both in healthy subjects and in those with memory disorders. We discuss both models in three contexts: (a) in the context of normal learning and forgetting; (b) in the context of the amnesic syndromes, and retrograde amnesia in particular; and (c) in the context of semantic dementia, a disorder of memory that has received much attention recently and that is in many ways a mirror image of the classic amnesic syndrome.

4.1   CONSOLIDATION THEORY

Most computational models of amnesia assume that the neocortex
and hippocampus play different roles in long-term memory storage.
The hippocampus and adjacent temporal lobe structures (e.g., entorhinal and perirhinal cortexes, parahippocampal gyrus, etc.) receive extensive inputs from many parts of the cerebral cortex. Figure 4.1 gives a partial view of the resulting neuroanatomical hierarchy.

A prevalent view on the formation of long-term memory may be
called Consolidation Theory. It proposes that, although initially the
retrieval of a recently experienced event is reliant on the hippocampal
system, repeated reinstatement of the hippocampal-neocortical representation gradually results in the formation of a more permanent—
hippocampus-independent—memory representation in the neocortex.
Many theorists have proposed that consolidation takes place during
sleep, and recent evidence makes the case for it quite strong (Stickgold, James & Hobson, 2000; Wilson & McNaughton, 1994). We
return to this issue later. Why the brain might employ two different
systems for the storage of memory remains an unanswered question.
Two reasons may derive from a connectivity problem in the brain
and from a generalization problem with rapid learning.

We have argued that the neocortex does not have sufficient connectivity to rapidly form the required point-to-point connections that
make up an arbitrary memory episode, at least not in the short time
that an individual experiences an event (Murre & Sturdy, 1995).
Functional point-to-point connections may instead be set up by re-
cruiting intermediate neurons (Murre & Raffone, 2006), but such a
process must be slow and cannot normally be expected to take place
in a single learning trial, because it requires repeated reinstatement
of the cortical neural ensemble that represents the episode. The hippocampus may serve as a rapid storage device that facilitates the
repeated reinstatements needed to build up long-distance cortical
connections' intermediate neurons (Meeter & Murre, in pressb).

McClelland et al. (1995) put forward an alternative hypothesis
for the different roles of hippocampus and cortex. In their view,
memory consolidation helps prevent catastrophic interference in sequential learning. Their hypothesis finds support in computer simulations in which newly acquired knowledge must be integrated into

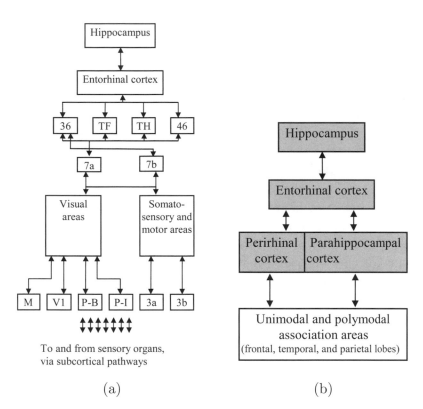

(a)   (b)

Fig. 4.1: Schematic overview of neuroanatomy. (a) Illustration of how
the hippocampus is located at the top of the neuroanatomical hierarchy
by Felleman and Van Essen (1991). Shown is a small part of a combination of the maps of the visual and somatosensory areas. (b) Similar
hierarchy according to Squire (1992; Squire and Zola-Morgan, 1991),
but simplified even further.

the existing knowledge database. They used a back-propagation network (Rumelhart, Hinton & Williams, 1986) and contrasted *focused learning*, where semantic memory can rapidly acquire new facts, with *interleaved learning*, where learning of new facts (temporarily stored in a hippocampus) is interleaved with additional learning of already learned facts. Focused learning will lead to catastrophic interference, causing overwriting of old facts by newly learned facts. McClelland et al. (1995) showed, for example, that learning about penguin might lead to the forgetting of robin and other birds. They also showed that with interleaved learning catastrophic interference is avoided, and new facts are smoothly integrated in memory.

Both hypotheses show, from both a neuroanatomical and a functional point of view, why the human brain may have evolved a learning system with different roles for the hippocampus and neocortex. Damage to different parts of this system then causes characteristic forms of amnesia. Damage to the hippocampus causes a loss of recent memories and the ability to form new memories. Damage to the neocortex causes a general loss of remote memories.

4.2   THE TRACELINK MODEL

The neocortex of the model by McClelland et el. (1995) is a three-layer back-propagation network. The hippocampus is not implemented as a neural network, but patterns are simply stored until they are selected (randomly) for interleaved learning. When we developed the TraceLink model, our aim was to also simulate the details of the consolidation process. Would such a mechanism still work if it were implemented completely in a neural network? It turns out that it does, but while working on this we encountered some surprising behaviors that influenced the final design.

The neural architecture of Figure 4.1 is simplified even further for the purposes of modeling. A schematic drawing of resulting architecture of the TraceLink model (Murre, 1994, 1996, 1997; Meeter & Murre, in pressb) is shown in Figure 4.2. Its three main components are (a) a trace system, (b) a link system, and (c) a modulatory system. The role of the trace system is analogous to that of the neocortex in the models discussed earlier, and the role of the link system is analogous to that of the medial temporal lobe or hippocampus. The

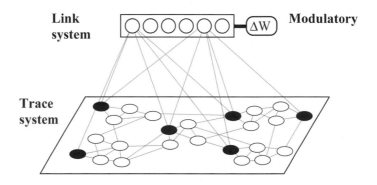

Fig. 4.2: Overview of the TraceLink model, showing the link system, the trace system, and the modulatory system (indicated by a Δ W sign, symbolizing control of learning rate on the connection weights in the system). Only a few nodes and a few connections have been drawn in order to prevent clutter.

neurons in TraceLink fire stochastically: They have a higher probability of firing (i.e., signaling a 1) when they receive a higher net input. Each node in the trace system is connected to other trace nodes and to and from a random subset of the nodes in the link system. As in the model by Alvarez and Squire (1994), the learning rate in the trace system is lower than that of the link system. The link system's function is to interconnect trace nodes without direct cortico-cortical connections. In addition, link nodes are also interconnected within the link system (i.e., there are link-link connections).

The modulatory system includes certain basal forebrain nuclei—especially the medial septum with its cholinergic inputs to the hippocampus via the fornix (see also Hasselmo, 1995, 1999) and several areas that have a more indirect, controlling function. The role of the system is to trigger increased plasticity in the link system so that it can rapidly record a new episodic representation. We did not include a detailed implementation of this system with the TraceLink model as discussed here, but instead opted to dedicate a separate model to

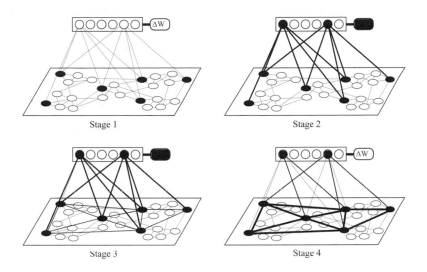

Fig. 4.3: Normal episodic learning in Murre's TraceLink model. *Stage 1*: A new memory representation activates a number of trace elements (shown as filled black circles). *Stage 2*: Several link elements are activated and the relevant trace-link connections are strengthened (shown as thicker connections). Also, the modulatory system has been activated. *Stage 3*: Weak trace-trace connections are developing. The modulatory system is weakly activated. *Stage 4*: Strong trace-trace connections have been formed. Trace-link connections have decayed and the modulatory system does not necessarily respond to the stimulus.

this system (see Meeter, Murre & Talamini, in press).

During normal acquisition, a memory representation passes through four stages (see Figure 4.3). These have no deep theoretical meaning, but are merely an expository convenience.

- *Stage 1.* External and internal information—anything that is included in the to-be-remembered episode—activates a number of nodes in the trace system (filled circles).

- *Stage 2.* Via the trace system, a set of link nodes is activated. We assume that this is a fast process, occurring in seconds to

possibly tens of minutes in case of entirely new contexts (Leutgeb, Leutgeb, Treves, Moser & Moser, in press). If the episode
is sufficiently novel or interesting, the modulatory system is
activated. This allows strengthening of connections between
activated link nodes and trace nodes through Hebbian learning
(Hebb, 1949), shown by the thickening of the connections.

- *Stage 3.* This stage represents the initial consolidation process.
  Repeated activation takes place, leading to the gradual formation of trace-to-trace connections. These are initially weak. It is
  the purpose of the TraceLink model to study how they grow in
  strength with each consolidation episode, where consolidation
  is implemented as the repeated reactivation of already learned
  representations. Consolidation is driven by randomly activating a number of nodes in the link system. These then activate
  nodes in the trace system as well. In most cases, the activations
  stabilize after a while, having retrieved one of the stored patterns (technically, the system has moved to an attractor). Consolidation occurs by further strengthening of trace-trace connections. Trace-link connections are not strengthened further
  at this time (see the models of Hasselmo, 1995, 1999; Meeter,
  Murre & Talamini, in press).

- *Stage 4.* In the final stage, multiple consolidation trials have
  taken place. Trace-to-trace connections have become very strong,
  and retrieval has now become independent of the link system.

The four stages portray a process whereby the neural basis of the
memory representations is slowly moved from the link system to the
trace system. At the same time, the neural basis in the link systems
declines in strength, for example, because it is gradually overwritten
by newly stored patterns. This (apparent) movement from link system to trace system is the basis for explaining retrograde amnesia,
which is analogous to that of the models discussed earlier (Alvarez &
Squire, 1994; McClelland et al., 1995). By inactivating the link nodes
(i.e., modeling a hippocampal lesion), all memory representations at
Stage 2 are lost. Stage 3 representations may be preserved if they
have received sufficient consolidation, and Stage 4 representations always remain intact. Lesioning of the link system, therefore, results

in a characteristic gradient of retrograde amnesia first described by Théodule Ribot in 1881. This gradient, often named *Ribot gradient* in his honor, shows a characteristic pattern with disproportional memory loss for recent time periods.

4.3 THE MEMORY CHAIN MODEL

As we illustrate next, the TraceLink is useful for studying in detail the process that may drive consolidation. It allows us to relate aspects of neurobiology to behavior. The model is not very well suited, however, for quantitative studies, e.g., to fit the shape of memory curves from experiments with amnesic patients and healthy controls. Even on modern computers, it takes a long time to run one simulation. Data fitting necessitates a parameter search, that would multiply the total simulation time well beyond feasible limits. Furthermore, because TraceLink was not developed for data fitting, it is not clear how its output should be mapped onto behavioral data and what would constitute the relevant parameters. Learning and consolidation parameters seem likely candidates, but perhaps also the size of the neural network layers, the choice of pattern representation, or the way the answers are evaluated. It is a justified criticism of neural networks that they often contain many hidden parameters in this manner. Their function is to provide a proof of principle—to show that some mechanism can work. Once this has been accomplished, one may either delve deeper into the neural mechanisms involved or abstract the model, extracting its principal characteristics. Such an abstract model, a summary model as it were, can then be compared with behavioral data. This is the approach we take here: to abstract the TraceLink model and derive a new model that incorporates some of the fundamental structures and processes of TraceLink.

The resulting model is called the *Memory Chain Model*. TraceLink has two main structures to represent and store a pattern: the link system and the trace system. We extend this idea to an arbitrary number of neural stores. In TraceLink, a representation is consolidated from the link system to the trace system. We generalize this idea as well, assuming that representations can induce representations in later stores, like the link system can induce representations in the trace system. Thus, we arrive at a chain of neural stores, where a memory representations are cascaded from early to late stores. In TraceLink, memory representations decline over time, with a higher decline rate in the link system than in the trace system. In the Memory Chain Model, memory representations also decline, with higher decline rates in the early stores compared with the later stores.

The neural mechanisms involved in memory are not uniform. On the contrary, they differ vastly depending on the time-scale considered. A memorized stimulus mobilizes a cascade of mechanisms such as firing neurons, activated neural assemblies, synaptic changes, neural recruitment, and axonal growth (e.g., McGaugh, 2000; Milner, Squire & Kandel, 1998). These processes are all able to hold a memory for a certain time period—from ultra-brief to very long. Alhough the mechanisms of memory will differ in the various stores, we propose that they nonetheless share the two fundamental characteristics outlined earlier: (a) a process' memory strength diminishes at a constant rate, and (b) as long as a memory has not been forgotten, it may induce more permanent memory processes in later stores.

In the current version of the Memory Chain Model, we assume an exponential decline. It should be pointed out that the model can also use other decline functions such as power law decline, but we observe that many of the processes that could cause the decline tend to lead to exponential loss processes:

- In most formulations of activation rules, neural firing declines exponentially once the source of external activation has been removed (Rumelhart & McClelland, 1986).

- Neural noise and other autonomous decay processes usually cause exponential loss of information of the synaptic weights.

- Exponential decline of LTP in hippocampus has been observed by Barnes and McNaughton (1980).

- Overwriting of old patterns by new patterns also tends to cause an exponential decline of information.

- The effectiveness of contextual cues also tends to decline exponentially over time (Mensink & Raaijmakers, 1988).

Our model shares the exponential-decline assumption with classic models in memory psychology—for example, the classic two-store model (Atkinson & Shiffrin, 1968) and the Bower-Lockhart attribute models (Murdock, 1974). Recall data obtained from laboratory experiments that intend to measure short-term memory decline through the classical Brown-Peterson learning and distraction task also support an exponential decline (Peterson & Peterson, 1959).

We generalize the induction over all time scales: Each store induces representations in the next store. For example, as long as neural assemblies are firing, synaptic enhancement may take place: One process induces a more permanent process in a later store.

We assume that properties 1 and 2 operate on all time-scales. This explains why, as we believe, forgetting curves can be described by the same function whether measured over seconds, months, or years, despite disparate underlying processes. Because the forgetting curve is a composite, it does not necessarily have a uniform shape. It may even have bumps under certain circumstances depending on the way the underlying processes are influenced by the experimental conditions.

Intuitively, the model assumes that a newly learned memory passes through one or more of the stores. Stores are chained in a feed-forward manner (see Figure 4.4). Each copy in a store generates copies of its representation in the next higher store. This is a chance process, the generation probability being one of the parameters in the model. During initial learning, we assume that the to-be-learned material gradually generates copies in the first store in the chain. It should be pointed out here that the meaning of the stores in the chain depends on the domain of application. The number of the stores in the Memory Chain Model is arbitrary, but throughout this chapter we designate as Store 1 the link system or medial-temporal lobe (MTL) area and as Store 2 the trace system or neocortex. Other applications of the model may include earlier stores as well.

A copy has a probability of being lost, for example, because it is overwritten by different copies or because of neural noise. All copies in a store share the same loss probability. Once a copy is lost, it can no longer generate new copies in higher stores. Higher stores in the chain have lower decline rates, so that the process sketched here is one of rapidly declining stores trying to salvage their representations by generating copies in more slowly declining stores.

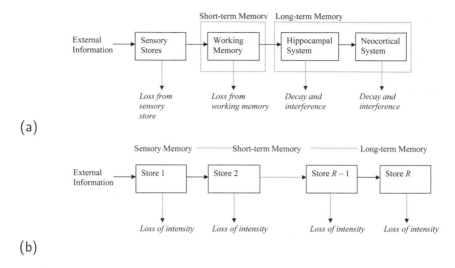

(a)

(b)

Fig. 4.4: Illustration of the memory chain. (a) Memory systems at different time scales, with feed-forward induction of novel memory representations in later stores and decline within stores. (b) Abstract representation used in the Memory Chain Model.

4.4   FORMALIZATION OF THE MEMORY CHAIN MODEL

To be able to generalize the model, we assume that a memory representation consists of one or more copies, any of which suffices to retrieve the memory. It can be either a full copy (cf. *trace replicas* in Nadel, Samsonovich, Ryan & Moscovitch, 2000,) or a *critical feature* (in the sense of feature models, as in Murdock, 1974) that allows retrieval of the entire memory representation. In this chapter, we assume that a single copy in any of the stores suffices for complete recall. The search process initiated by the retrieval cue will typically cover only a small section of a store. This makes memory retrieval a stochastic process: Even if copies are present in the store, it is possible that none will be found if the searched sections happen to not include any of the copies. The expected total number of copies in the sections searched is called the *intensity* of the memory. New learning trials add their contribution to the existing intensity, which may have been partially declined. Longer learning periods and repeated learning trials lead to a proportional increase in intensity by simply adding their contribution, up to a point. After learning, various processes typically lead to a loss of copies, described by the *decline function*, which describes the decline of intensity after learning as a function of time. The size of the searched sections of the stores is determined by the quality of retrieval cues presented to the subject.

In the formal model, the prior effects of learning, storage, and retrieval are multiplied to arrive at the memory intensity, which increases with learning and decreases with forgetting as a function of time:

$$intensity(time) \quad = \quad acquired\ intensity \times intensity\ decline(time)$$
$$\times cue\ quality$$

Acquired intensity represents the contribution of the learning trial, decline represents the effects of time-dependent storage processes, and cue quality represents the effectiveness of the memory search.

All experiments analyzed in this chapter use probability of recall, $p(t)$, as the dependent measure, where t is the time since acquisition of the memory. The relation between memory intensity and recall probability can be described by a simple function (see appendix for details): $p(t) = 1\text{-}e^{-intensity(t)}$.

In accordance with the two main principles described earlier, each store in the chain is characterized by exactly two parameters. The first parameter is the decline rate, which we denote as a_1 and a_2, for the hippocampus and neocortex, respectively. In this chapter, a subscript 1 denotes the hippocampus (MTL) and a subscript 2 denotes the neocortex. The second parameter concerns the rate with which a store fills up with newly generated copies. In particular, μ_1 refers to the intensity acquired during a single learning trial, and μ_2 refers to the rate with which the neocortex is filled during consolidation. Figure 4.5 shows a typical forgetting function, where Store 1 declines rapidly, and Store 2 first builds up intensity, and subsequently declines.

In this chapter, we focus on experiments that compare normal forgetting with the effects of lesions and disruptions of the medial temporal lobe or neocortex. Like with TraceLink, our working hypothesis is that these structures can be identified as two stores of the model. It should be pointed out that this model presents the

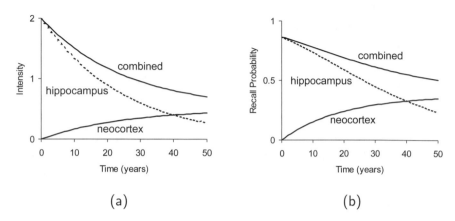

Fig. 4.5: Example of typical forgetting curve with underlying processes in Store 1 and Store 2. (a) Intensity as a function of time. (b) Recall probability as a function of time. The curves in (a) and (b) are based on the same parameters.

minimal model that could be applied to these data. In our recent neural network models (e.g., Meeter, Murre & Talamini, 2002; Talamini, Meeter, Elvevåg, Murre & Goldberg, in press) we have found it worthwhile to include a third, intermediate store (parahippocampal gyrus). The data considered in this chapter, however, are too noisy to allow testing of such higher-order models.

4.5   APPLYING THE MODELS

In this section, we illustrate how the models can be applied to a variety of data. We use the TraceLink model to study a possible mechanism of consolidation. Then, we use the more abstract and concise Memory Chain Model to verify whether the resultant forgetting and amnesia gradients correspond with patient data. We also apply both models to semantic dementia, which can in certain respects be seen as the mirror image of the classic amnesic syndrome.

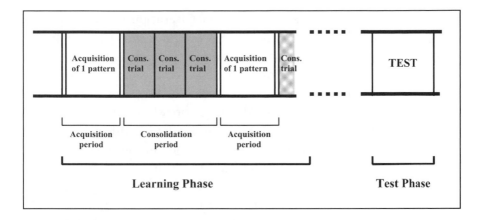

Fig. 4.6: Diagram showing the order of events in most simulations. A simulation was divided into a learning phase and a test phase. The learning phase was subdivided into alternating acquisition periods, in which one pattern was acquired, and consolidation periods. Consolidation periods consisted of three consolidation trials.

4.5.1 Normal Learning and Forgetting

It would hardly suffice if a model would be able to mimic pathological behavior but not that of health controls. In this section, therefore, we first examine the normal behavior of the models.

TraceLink

In basic simulations, the Tracelink model goes through a learning phase and a test phase. The learning phase consists of acquisition of a pattern followed by consolidation (see Figure 4.6). On each simulated day, the model acquires one pattern and then passes through a consolidation phase. In one simulation, the model typically learns a set of 15 or more patterns with interspersed consolidation phases, after which all the patterns are tested.

Patterns consisted of random sets of trace and link nodes. Because patterns are random, they tend to overlap with one another. In a consolidation period, three consolidation trials occur. A single trial proceeds as follows: (a) The model is set to a random pattern, and then allowed to cycle freely for a fixed number of iterations (150); and

(b) whichever pattern is active at the last iteration is consolidated.

The model usually does not settle on the same pattern for all three consolidation trials. More than one pattern is thus typically consolidated in a consolidation period. Also, the model can consolidate noisy patterns, mixtures of patterns, or no pattern at all. For further details, see Meeter and Murre (in pressb).

After learning and consolidation, the model is subjected to a test phase, in which part of each pattern is clamped in the trace layer only (the cue), and the model must activate the remaining trace nodes in the pattern. Figure 4.7 shows the results of a basic simulation of normal memory (the filled circles). Performance is very high for the most recent pattern; the older a pattern was, the lower it scored on the test. The figure shows that, although forgetting was substantial, pattern recall remained well above chance.

These results show the forgetting that occurs in the model when new patterns are learned. When a new pattern overlaps with an old one at a certain node, the old pattern is partly unlearned. There is more overlap in the link system than in the trace system. The link portion of a pattern is therefore lost relatively rapidly and the trace portion more slowly. Because old patterns decay rapidly in the link system, they quickly lose their ability to be activated by a cue in the trace system or to maintain a stable activation of the pattern in the trace system. During the time that the pattern is still strong in the link system, however, it may be consolidated, and its strength will continue to build up in the trace system. This enables retrieval of the older patterns from the trace layer. An old pattern may be activated on the basis of a strong trace representation alone. Overwriting by subsequent memories seems a crude explanation for forgetting as compared with decaying connections or forgetting through contextual cue changes. However, a recent review suggested that overwriting indeed plays an important role in the reversal of long-term potentiation in the hippocampus (Rosenzweig, Barnes & McNaughton, 2002).

Memory Chain Model

We have already tested our model with about 100 forgetting and learning curves (Murre & Chessa, 2002, Submitted) from a variety of experiments, with normal subjects demonstrating that our model

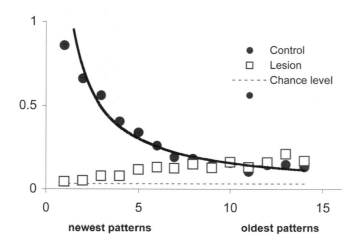

Fig. 4.7: Results of the basic simulation of normal learning and forgetting (filled circles) and the simulation of retrograde amnesia (open squares). Fifteen patterns were learned; the patterns on the left were the most recently learned, and the patterns on the right are the oldest. The first-learned pattern is not shown. Scores are the mean proportion of nodes in the trace portion of the pattern that are active at test and not part of the cue. The continuous line is a power fit of the normal data series ($R^2 = 0.93$).

describes the shape of forgetting and learning with a high degree of accuracy. Two examples of fits to curves with 1,800 and over 4,000 observations per data point are given in Figure 4.8. Because the model can handle simultaneous learning and forgetting, it is also suitable for application to learning and forgetting of advertising as a function of their advertising schedule (Chessa & Murre, 2001). The impact of a prominent single trial and its subsequent decline was studied on the basis of internet hits following a radio interview in which the web site address was mentioned (Chessa & Murre, 2004). For our application advertising, advertisement contacts are viewed as separate learning trials, of which the resulting memory intensities are added. It is even possible to optimize the impact of an advertising campaign on the basis of the model (Chessa & Murre, Submitted). The model has been applied to modeling Ebbinghaus-style savings (Chessa & Murre, Submitted; Ebbinghaus, 1885/1913) and to a study with Galton-Crovitz type data from 2,000 subjects. Such data are a time distribution of dated autobiographical memories elicited through standardized cues (Crovitz & Schiffman, 1974; Galton, 1879; Janssen, Chessa & Murre, in press). The model can also easily be applied to reaction time data.

In all of these applications, we use the model as outlined earlier. The challenge is to derive the different measures of memory with minimal assumptions from the same basic model. We follow the same strategy next, deriving forgetting gradients for amnesic patients and experimental animals with the sole assumptions that the two stores represent the hippocampus (MTL) and neocortex, the structures thought to be implicated in the types of amnesia studied here.

4.5.2   Retrograde Amnesia

Both the Tracelink model and the Memory Chain Model exhibit realistic normal forgetting. In the Tracelink model, this is true only at a qualitative level, whereas the Memory Chain Model can also fit data quantitatively. For both models, this was secondary to the goal of explaining some of the principal characteristics of retrograde amnesia. We first examine TraceLink's behavior with retrograde amnesia. Then we review how the Memory Chain Model has been fitted to several studies with experimental animals and with human patients.

TraceLink

In the TraceLink model, retrograde amnesia is modeled by a lesioning of the link nodes. Recent memories are still at Stage 2, and their representations are dependent on a functioning link system for their retrieval and internal coherence. Remote memories are at Stage 4 and will have developed sufficient supporting trace-to-trace connectivity; their retrieval is independent of the link system. With intermediate memories, successful retrieval after a lesion of the link system will depend on which link nodes are unavailable and what trace-to-trace connections have been formed already.

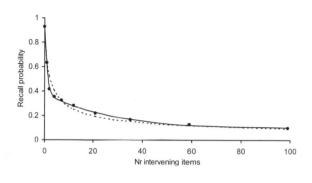

(a)

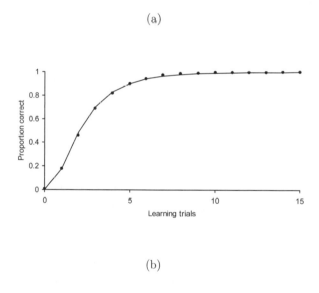

(b)

Fig. 4.8: Example with two fits of the Memory Chain Model to curves with very high numbers of observations per data point. (a) Forgetting curve with fits of a three-store recall probability function (solid curve) and the power-law (dotted curve) to a recall data set concerning word pairs from Rubin, Hinton, and Wenzel (1999). Each data point is based on 1800 observations. The fit was excellent on the chi-square test, which becomes more severe with the number of observations ($\alpha = 0.55$ and $R^2 > 0.999$). The power-law was rejected by the chi-square test. (b) Data and fits for the learning of nouns from Turkish to Dutch. Average learning curve of proportion correct over 141 subjects as a function of learning trials. Each data point is based on 4230 observations. The fit was exceptional ($\alpha = 0.90$, $\chi^2 = 6.29$, and $R^2 = 0.9994$). See Murre and Chessa (submitted) for details.

Thus, to test the TraceLink model for retrograde amnesia, one merely has to deactivate the link system to simulate a lesion in the medial temporal lobe. After having done this, performance was relatively low for all patterns, but the most recent patterns suffered more from the deactivation of the link layer than the oldest patterns. In that condition, the most recent patterns do not score much better than chance (see Figure 4.7). This corresponds to the Ribot gradient found in patients with retrograde amnesia.

One difference between this simulation and a typical retrograde amnesia study deserves mentioning. Our items were all learned with the same strength, and our control condition shows a normal (i.e., quite steep) forgetting curve. Tests of retrograde amnesia, however, are typically constructed so that an equal number of items from various decades are answered correctly by normal controls (Meeter, 2003). Because one can assume that more information from previous decades is forgotten, this equality of performance for normal controls implies that the items selected from the various decades differ in average initial learning strength. For example, items about forty-year-old events ask about very prominent political figures, whereas items about the last decade will ask about much less prominent politicians. The aim is often to have all items reach an average score of 85% with normal controls. To compare data from the simulations with data from retrograde amnesia tests, one might plot the retrograde amnesia scores as a percentage of the normal control scores as is illustrated in Figure 4.12; next we introduce a more rigorous solution to this problem.

In Meeter and Murre (in pressb), we describe eight additional simulations, including anterograde amnesia, the shrinkage of retrograde amnesia (a recovery process that is often observed), and Transient Global Amnesia (a short-lasting form of amnesia).

Memory Chain Model

The approach taken by the Memory Chain Model to explaining retrograde amnesia is the same as in TraceLink. Given the assumption that Store 1 is the damaged hippocampal (MTL) store, the shape of the Ribot gradient can immediately be derived from the Memory Chain Model: It is simply a retention curve lacking the contribution of the hippocampal (MTL) store.

In this chapter, $r_1(t)$ refers to the intensity of the hippocampal store and $r_2(t)$ to the neocortical store. A convenient characteristic of the Memory Chain Model (see appendix) is that the total intensity is simply the sum of the intensities of the individual stores: $r(t) = r_1(t) + r_2(t)$. A full lesion at time t of the hippocampus translates to simply removing the contribution of $r_1(t)$ to the total intensity $r(t)$. What remains is the neocortical intensity, $r_2(t)$. Thus, it immediately follows that the shape of the Ribot gradient with a full hippocampal lesion is identical to the expression for $r_2(t)$. Most tests of retrograde amnesia do not measure intensity directly, but rather they measure recall probability. The predicted shape of the test gradients is, therefore, given by $p_{\text{Ribot}}(t) = 1\text{-}e^{-r_2(t)}$. We often find that neocortical decline, a_2, is close to zero for the material and time periods used in the experiments tested here, for example, because the time period is too short for any neocortical decline to become prominent. This allows us to drop one free parameter and to simplify our equations. Equations for the normal forgetting curve and the Ribot gradient equation are given in **Table 1** for the case of no neocortical forgetting (i.e., $a_2 = 0$) and a full lesion of the hippocampal area. Additional details of the expression are given in the appendix.

In some lesions studies discussed later, we leave the size of the lesion as a free parameter. The lesion parameter is denoted as λ, with $0 \leq \lambda \leq 1$. If the lesion parameter is 0, no lesion is present, and if $\lambda = 1$, we have a 100% lesion. In case of a partial lesion, the Ribot gradient is equal to $1 - \exp(-((1 - \lambda)r_1(t) + r_2(t)))$.

Thus, we have derived a fairly concise, closed-form equation (i.e., one that can be expressed analytically) for the Ribot gradient. Unfortunately, it cannot immediately be applied to most retrograde amnesia studies with human patients. As mentioned earlier, in tests of retrograde amnesia, the difficulty of the questions is manipulated such that scores on remote time period do not show a strong floor effect. In practice, items about remote events are made easier than recent items. This manipulation makes the shape of the individual curves impossible to interpret. The Memory Chain Model offers a straightforward way to still use these data. As we show in the appendix, dividing the intensity of the patient's curve by that of the control's curve results in a new curve from which the acquired intensity parameter μ_1 and the cue specificity parameter q have been elim-

Table 4.1: Overview of the equations and symbols used for the case $a_2 = 0$

Component	Expression/description
Normal forgetting curve	$p(t) = 1 - e^{e\{r_1(t) + r_2(t)\}}$ $= 1 - \exp\left(-\mu_1 e^{-a_1 t} - \frac{\mu_1 \mu_2}{a_1}(1 - e^{-a_1 t})\right)$
Ribot gradient	$p_{\text{Ribot}}(t) = 1 - e^{-r_2(t)}$ $= 1 - \exp\left(\frac{-\mu_1 \mu_2}{a_1}(1 - e^{-a_1 t})\right)$
rr-gradient (data transformation)	$rr(t) = \dfrac{-\log_e(1 - p_{\text{lesioned}}(t))}{-\log_e(1 - p_{\text{control}}(t))}$
Relative retrograde gradient	$rr(t) = \left\{ \dfrac{-a_1(1 - e^{a_1 t}) - 1}{\mu_2} + 1 \right\}^{-1}$

Free Parameters

μ_1	Acquired intensity (contribution of a learning trial) of hippocampal store (not used with rr-gradient)
μ_2	Consolidation rate to the neocortical store
a_1	Decline rate of hippocampal store
λ	Lesion size (0 is no lesion; 1 is full lesion)

Fixed parameters

a_2	Decline rate of neocortical store (assumed to be 0 here)
q	Cue quality (often assumed 1 and suppressed in the equations)

Derived functions

$p(t)$	Recall probability as a function of time t
$r_1(t)$	Intensity of the hippocampal (MTL) store
$r_2(t)$	Intensity of the neocortical store
$rr(t)$	Relative retrograde gradient

inated. These parameters are associated among others with how well the items have been learned and how easily they can be retrieved. Removing their effects, therefore, also removes the distortion. We call the resulting curve the *relative retrograde gradient* or rr-gradient because it expresses the shape of the Ribot gradient *relative* to the normal forgetting curve.

Most tests of retrograde amnesia give us recall probabilities as a function of time elapsed, which is denoted as $p(t)$. The observed recall probability can be transformed into the underlying intensity.[1]

---

[1]This is only true if the retrieval threshold is equal to 1, as is assumed in this

Figure 4.9 illustrates how manipulation of item difficulty leads to distorted forgetting and Ribot gradients, but undistorted rr-gradients. When easy and hard questions in a test are plotted separately, they should have the same rr-gradients because, as we claim, these are not affected by item difficulty. In Figure 4.10, we have done just that, using data from Korsakoff patients and control subjects. For each study, the upper panels 1 and 2 show the recall probabilities, whereas the lower panels 3 and 4 show the empirical rr-gradient (i.e., the transformed data) with a best-fitting curve based on our model. The rr-gradients tend to be smoother than the nontransformed curves. Also, the rr-gradients of easy and hard items of one study are more similar than their nontransformed curves. The rr-gradient allows us to examine the sizable database of human studies in retrograde amnesia in a rigorous, quantitative manner.

It should be pointed out that the Memory Chain Model predicts that simply taking the relative probabilities (see e.g., the approach taken in Brown, 2002) would not completely solve the problem. Suppose, for example, that the underlying intensity for unlesioned (healthy subjects) case is 1.5 and for the lesioned (patients) case 0.75. The rr-transformation would give $0.75/1.5 = 0.5$. Now suppose that the test developer makes this item easier (e.g., by giving more distinct cues), such that the intensities increase to 3 and 1.5, respectively. Then, the rr-value would still be 0.5. The relative p-values, however, would be 0.82 in the difficult case and 0.68 in the easy case: they are not invariant under item difficulty manipulation. This is illustrated in Figure 4.10 for data set b, for which the relative probabilities are also shown (as $b3'$ and $b4'$). The tendency for easy items to be estimated too high is well visible. The Memory Chain Model predicts that as items are made increasingly easier, the relative probabilities, as illustrated in Figure 4.10 $b3' - 4'$, will eventually approach 1.0, whereas the rr-values would remain stable. Although the expected value of rr-values is thus not sensitive to item difficulty, the transformation makes the gradient sensitive to noise when items are either very easy or very difficult. When one of the curves approaches floor or ceiling, the rr-gradient tends to amplify noise.

We fitted our model to studies in which different neuropathologies were investigated, such as Korsakoff's disease and Alzheimer's

chapter. In the more general case, the transformation is more complex.

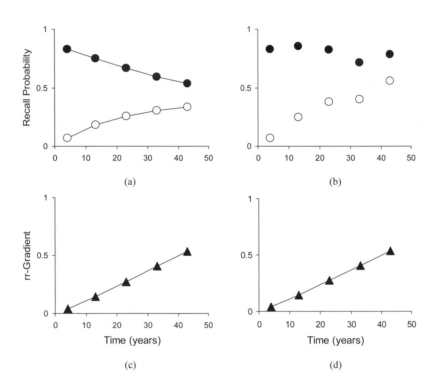

Fig. 4.9: The relative retrograde gradient remains unaffected by manipulation of item difficulty. (a) Example forgetting curve and Ribot gradient (generated with the model using $\mu_1 = 2$, $a_1 = 0.04$, $\mu_2 = 0.01$ and $a_2 = 0$). (b) Distorted curve where μ_1 has been multiplied with (from left to right) 1, 1.4, 1.8, 1.4, and 2. (c) Relative retrograde gradient for the undistorted curves. (d) Relative retrograde gradient for the distorted curves.

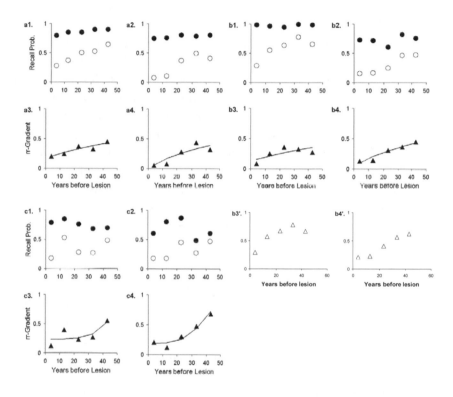

Fig. 4.10: Data from three tests of Korsakoff patients and controls by Albert et al. (1979). In each study, panels 1 and 2 represent easy and hard items, respectively. Open circles represent patient data, solid circles controls. Panels 3 and 4 give the relative retrograde gradient for easy and hard items, respectively. The solid curves are fits by the model, assuming that $a_2 = 0$.

disease. The areas with greatest damage in Korsakoff's disease are ones thought to form one memory system with the hippocampus (Aggleton & Brown, 1999). Therefore, we modeled this disease by partially eliminating the contribution of Store 1. In Alzheimer's disease, hippocampal atrophy is accompanied by diffuse cortical damage. Patients with Alzheimer's disease were therefore fitted by taking into account both hippocampal lesions and making the intensity function of the neocortex equal to $(1 - \lambda_2)r_2(t)$, where λ_2 is the neocortical lesion size. It should perhaps be clarified that these lesion parameters represent only the lesion at the time of testing. (Our approach does not take into consideration the possibly impaired learning that may have hampered acquisition of information in the years before the time of testing; adding such a process would probably improve the fits, but would also add another parameter to the model.) Thus, we expected that Korsakoff patients would show rr-gradients that reflect Ribot gradients because the medial temporal system is partially lesioned. Alzheimer patients' rr-gradients should be similar, but lower because of additional neocortical lesions.

We obtained adequate fits with three free parameters: a_1 (hippocampal decline rate), μ_2 (consolidation), and λ (lesion size; 0 is no lesion, 1 is full lesion). Checks with a_2 left free were performed as well, but rarely gave a significant improvement in fit. We also repeated all fits using a power function instead of an exponential decline, obtaining very similar fits (within a few percentage points of the quoted values), indicating that an exponential decline is not critical for these results. There is analytical evidence that supports these findings: Both the Ribot gradient and the rr-gradient have properties that are independent of the choice of the memory decline function (see appendix).

Some illustrative rr-gradients and fitted curves for memory performance with Alzheimer's dementia are shown in Figure 4.11 . The fits shown in Figure 4.11 explain 97.9% of the variance. Additional results for other pathologies and for animal studies are given in (Murre et al., Submitted).

The advantages and limitations of the empirical rr-gradients can be observed in these figures: Even when the measured curves are quite erratic, the rr-gradients tend to be smooth. When one of the curves approaches floor or ceiling, however, the transformation to the

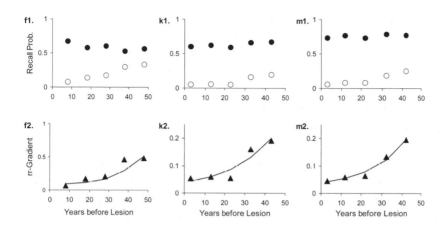

Fig. 4.11: Three studies with Alzheimer patients and matched controls. The ordinate represents percentage correct. The studies are: (f) Kopelman (1989), News Events, cued recall, (k) Beatty et al. (1988), Mean of Famous Faces and Public Events, cued recall, (m) idem, cued recall with extra cues. The panels are presented in pairs, where panel 1 of a pair contains the measured data (solid circles are controls, open circles are patients), and panel 2 is the data transformed to a relative retrograde gradient (always shown as triangles, with the solid line indicating the model fit). For more details on the tests and model fits, see Murre, Chessa, Meeter (submitted).

underlying intensity becomes more sensitive to error.

4.5.3 Semantic Dementia

Semantic dementia is an important disease to model because in many ways it presents as a mirror image of the classic amnesic syndrome. Patients typically show a progressive deterioration in their semantic knowledge, and yet they seem to possess relatively preserved day-to-day (episodic) memory. They are unable to name previously familiar objects, people, and places, and they show poor language comprehension. They show deficits on verbally-based semantic memory tests

such as category fluency and picture naming, but also on non-verbal
tests of semantic memory: They have difficulty matching animal and
object sounds to pictures of the animal or object, and they may have
difficulties handling previously familiar objects.

Its pathology reflects this mirror image as well. Semantic dementia is associated with non-Alzheimer degenerative pathology of
especially the inferolateral temporal neocortex, with relative sparing
(at least in the early stages) of medial temporal regions, although
some damage in the left hippocampus is evident in some patients.

Episodic memory is relatively spared in semantic dementia. Nevertheless, it is not normal. Murre et al. (2001) discussed semantic
dementia in the context of neuroanatomically-based computational
models of long-term memory and suggested several characteristics of
semantic dementia that these models should address. Three salient
ones were related to episodic memory: (a) relative sparing of recent
versus remote memories; (b) preservation of new learning, as measured by recognition memory, early in the disease; and (c) increased
long-term forgetting of newly learned material.

1. Patients with semantic dementia show retrograde amnesia. The
   amnesia is far more pronounced for the distant past than for
   recent periods. This has been demonstrated in both the autobiographical (Graham & Hodges, 1997) and public knowledge
   domains. These results stand in contrast to the Ribot gradient typically found in patients with an amnesic syndrome,
   in which remote memories are preferentially affected and recent memories are relatively spared (e.g., see Figure 4.11). Figure 4.12(a) shows a comparison of a group of semantic dementia patients with normal controls and patients with Alzheimer's
   disease on a test of remote autobiographical memory (Graham
   & Hodges, 1997). Although the Alzheimer's patients, like other
   amnesic groups (Kopelman, 1989), were especially impaired for
   the most recent period, semantic dementia patients showed relatively preserved recent memory and were impaired on remote
   memories.

2. One of the consistent findings in semantic dementia is that patients, even those with severe semantic memory deficits, are
   still able to acquire new episodic memories. The capacity for

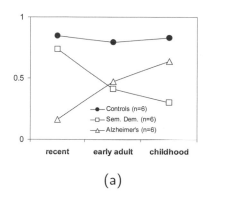 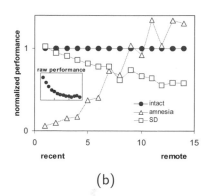

(a)   (b)

Fig. 4.12: (a) Remote memory gradients from a study in which patients with Alzheimer's (AD), semantic dementia patients (SD), and controls (Ctrl) performed a remote memory task, the AMI-autobiographical incidents (adapted from Graham & Hodges, 1997). (b) Results of the remote memory gradient simulation. The x-axis gives the pattern number, listed from the most recent to the left to the first-learned to the right. Performance in the amnesia and semantic dementia (SD) conditions is presented as a fraction of the performance in the control condition with an intact model, which is set to 1.

new learning becomes compromised, however, as the disease progresses.

3. Murre predicted, on the basis of an analytical review of the TraceLink model, that patients with semantic dementia might experience increased forgetting. Some evidence for this prediction came both from a recent semantic dementia case study and from cases of lateral temporal lobe lesions unrelated to semantic dementia. In two case studies, a patient was able to relearn, via repeated training sessions, forgotten exemplars for categories, so as to perform normally on category fluency tests. Once the training sessions ceased, however, the exemplars were quickly forgotten. This is the opposite pattern of that found in amnesic patients who, once they have acquired memories, tend to show forgetting similar to that of normal controls.

Tracelink

In this chapter, we discuss only Tracelink simulations of the first characteristic in some detail. Simulations of other aspects can be found in Meeter and Murre (2004). In Tracelink, the trace system represents cortical memory structures. The natural implementation of semantic dementia is therefore as a loss of trace elements and of trace-trace connections (i.e., cortico-cortical connections). This mimics the atrophy of temporal neocortex seen in semantic dementia. At the onset of the disease, loss of trace-trace connections dominates with sparing of the majority of trace elements. Stage 1 memories (see Figure 4.3) can be transformed into Stage 2 memories, because the link system and modulatory system are still fully operational. The transition to Stages 3 and 4, however, is severely impaired because there are not enough trace-trace connections left to form supporting networks at the trace level. Therefore, the system will show (a) a diffuse but possibly extensive loss of existing well-consolidated memories, (b) preservation of the formation of episodic memories through the link system, and (c) strong interference of new over old episodic memories because of the limited capacity of the link system. This will cause learned episodes to be forgotten faster than in the intact model. If a memory is not rehearsed regularly, it will be lost from the link system. This behavior is very similar to that observed in patients with semantic dementia.

The retention curve was simulated under three conditions: normal memory, retrograde amnesia, and semantic dementia. Training was as described earlier. To simulate a state of progressed semantic dementia, trace nodes and connections within the trace layer were lesioned. Our standard lesion was 80% of all connections within the trace layer and 10% of trace nodes (other lesion sizes are reported in Meeter & Murre, 2004).

As can be seen in Figure 4.12(b), deactivating the link layer in the retrograde amnesia condition generates a Ribot curve: recent patterns are lost, but remote ones were still available after deactivation of the link layer. In the semantic dementia condition, however, exactly the opposite occurs: the most recent patterns are still available, whereas old patterns are severely degraded by the lesion of the trace-trace connections. This amounts to a reverse pattern of retrograde amnesia similar to the one observed in semantic dementia patients (see Figure 4.12(a) for comparison).

4.5.4 Memory Chain Model

A possible (partial) animal model for semantic dementia may be the mice tested in the forgetting study by Frankland et al. (2001). In these genetically manipulated mice, neocortical plasticity is nearly absent as measured by long-term potentiation. Hippocampal plasticity is intact. We modeled this in the Memory Chain Model by simply assuming no consolidation from the hippocampus to the neocortex for the genetically altered mice (i.e., $\mu_2 = 0$ for these mice), but normal consolidation for the wild-type mice (i.e., the unaltered ones).

Frankland et al.'s (2001)'s first experiment used a fear-conditioning paradigm (see their Figure 1). A foot shock was paired with a context; after a retention delay, the animal's fear reaction when placed in the experimental context was evaluated. In Experiment 1a, both experimental and control mice (wild-type) were given three foot shocks and evaluated for freezing after retention delays of 1, 3, 10, 17, and 50 days. In Experiment 1b, eight foot shocks were given. In Experiment 1c, control mice that were given one foot shock were compared with experimental mice that were given eight foot shocks. In Experiment 1d, freezing was measured after daily single-foot shocks for three days.

We fitted the data using four parameters: intensity acquired per learning trial (i.e., per shock) μ_1, hippocampal decline rate a_1, consolidation rate (hippocampus to cortex) μ_2, and the learning saturation limit r_{max}. We assumed that cortical decline rate a_2 was zero for the time course of the experiment. We do not discuss the repeated learning experiment here, but merely show its result (see Murre, Chessa & Meeter, Submitted, for a full description).

Without learning in the neocortex, retention depends solely on hippocampal decline. Like the TraceLink model, the Memory Chain model predicts that the genetically manipulated mice would, therefore, show abnormally steep forgetting. The data and model fits are shown in Figure 4.13a-c. The fit is excellent using only four parameters for all curves. We were able to fit the basic result of the study by Frankland et al (2001), namely, evidence of lack of consolidation

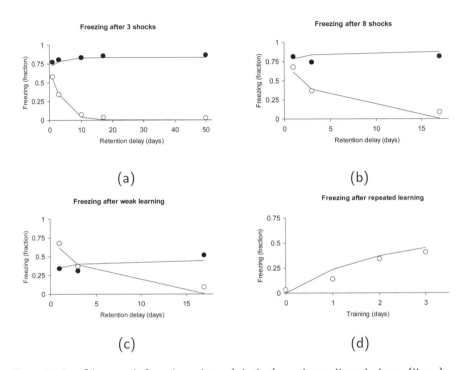

(a)

(b)

(c)

(d)

Fig. 4.13: Observed freezing data (circles) and predicted data (lines) of the study by Frankland et al. (2001) using the assumption of zero consolidation in the experimental condition. Open circles refer to experimental subjects, closed circles to controls. The parameters were $\mu_1 = 0.372$, $a_1 = 0.326$, $\mu_2 = 0.519$, and $r_{\max} = 1.533$. (a) Forgetting curves after learning with three foot shocks. (b) Forgetting curves after learning with eight foot shocks. (c) Forgetting curves after learning with one foot shock (controls) and eight foot shocks (experimental). (d) Repeated learning in experimental animals receiving one foot shock per day. The observed data are averaged over two conditions (see text).

to the cortex (Figure 4.13(a)). In addition, we could also account for the effects of different learning strengths (Figure 4.13[a-c]) and for the effects of repeated learning (Figure 4.13(a)). These results were achieved simultaneously using only four free parameters; with these parameters, the model explained 97.6% of the variance in all four experiments.

It would be interesting to apply the Memory Chain Model to data from semantic dementia patients, but published studies thus far are only based on a few patients, and they do not include a sufficient number of data points to make such a project informative. The same approach as taken with the Frankland data, however, should work with semantic memory patients. In addition, the retrograde amnesia data should be able to fit an extended Frankland experiment, adding a condition with mice that have a lesioned hippocampus. The Memory Chain Model predicts the shape of the Ribot curve with these mice in some detail.

4.6 GENERAL DISCUSSION

The two models described in this chapter illustrate how one might investigate some prevalent ideas. Both models can be seen as implementations of consolidation theory, a theory that when applied to long-term memory states the memories attain a strong neural basis in the course of time. The nature of this elusive long-term consolidation process is hotly debated in the literature but rather then review the various theories and pros and cons here, we refer to Metter and Murre (in pressa), who give a detailed overview of the various theories and models of long-term consolidation.

In contrast to the TraceLink model, the Memory Chain Model was not developed specifically to explain amnesia. Nonetheless, as shown here, without any modifications and with minimal assumptions, it can fit much of the data. This suggests that the structures and mechanisms implemented in TraceLink and generalized in the Memory Chain Model are viable candidates to explain the data. This is an important point because consolidation theories would not be very interesting if they are only invoked to explain amnesia data, but have little to add to normal processes of learning and forgetting.

An adequate fit to the data does not prove a model right; many models might fit the data. The converse, however, would force rejection of a model. Fitting the data is therefore a necessary first step for a quantitative model. Another step would be to see whether the model generalizes to other data sets or whether new predictions could be derived. The advantage of an analytical model is that predictions can be derived analytically. For example, it can be shown that the rr-gradient crosses the ordinate (at $t = 0$) at a value equal to the lesion size. In Study m, for example, in Figure 4.11 the rr-gradient crosses the ordinate around 0.04, suggesting that the medial temporal lobe is still 4% functional for recall of public events. As a test of this, predicted functional lesion parameters could be related to fMRI data to verify the relative level of activity in this structure. More generally, the model predicts that rr-gradients should be invariant under manipulation of item difficulty. Furthermore, it predicts that if the medial temporal lobe is no longer functioning, short-term memory should decline exponentially. Such a condition might be (partially) induced pharmacologically, for example, with scopolamine. Similarly, if consolidation to the cortex is no longer working, as might be the case in semantic dementia, we expect an exponential—but long-term— decline for memories stored in the hippocampus, rather than the decreasing rate of decline usually observed. More predictions along these lines may be derived.

The TraceLink model, although not amenable to analysis in this manner, can nonetheless give rise to novel predictions. One testable prediction that comes out of simulations with mixtures of strongly and weakly patterns is that (a) weak patterns show a stronger long-term forgetting, and (b) strong patterns suffer far less from lesions to the hippocampus. The reason for this is that strong patterns receive a disproportionate number of consolidation trials compared with weak patterns. The MCM does not make this prediction because of its strict feed-forward induction of memories. In TraceLink, the consolidation process is not strictly feed-forward, but also uses recurrent activation. This allows the current strength of a memory in a store to influence its further strengthening (already strong patterns have a higher probability of being selected for further consolidation).

So, although the Memory Chain Model is a summary model, it does not always make the same predictions. The reason of course lies in the fact that it ignores some of the details of the TraceLink model (such as recurrent activations). Although it is possible to include such details, this would only be wise if the discrepancy with the behavioral data was very significant. This in turn also depends on the modeling domain. As a comparison, we may consider Newton's laws that describe the trajectory of a bullet. The basic model for this is simple, but sometimes circumstances demand that we add in other factors such as air turbulence and the rotation of the object. The same is true for models in cognitive neuroscience; details can be added at the expense of complicating the model. Cognitive neuroscience bridges neurobiology and behavior, both exceedingly complex subjects, and so it would be naive to expect models to be simple. This does not necessarily imply that all models should always be geared toward the complexity of the brain. On the contrary, We feel that there is an important role for highly abstract models, in particular when they are abstractions of more complex models at a lower level. Such a multi-level approach makes it possible to address the richness of the brain while still allowing a rigorous analysis of the principal characteristics of behavior with reference to major neuroanatomical systems.

APPENDIX

Forgetting Curve

To derive recall probability, we note that the number of copies in the region searched during retrieval follows a Poisson distribution (Murre & Chessa, Submitted). If we assume that retrieving a single copy suffices for recall, the form of the forgetting function becomes:

$$p(t) = 1 - e^{-\mu(t)} \qquad (4.1)$$

where $p(t)$ is the recall probability at time t and $\mu(t)$ is the intensity of the memory process at t. For higher recall thresholds, additional terms are added to Equation 4.1. The intensity consists of three aspects—namely the effects of (a) encoding and learning conditions, μ_1; (b) memory decline following learning; and (c) the quality of the retrieval cue, q. In particular, we have

$$\mu(t) = \underbrace{\mu_1}_{\text{encoding}} \underbrace{\tilde{r}_1(t)}_{\text{storage}} \underbrace{q}_{\text{retrieval}} . \qquad (4.2)$$

The effects of learning and memory decline are combined in the intensity function $r(t)$:

$$= r(t) = r_1(t) + r_2(t) + \ldots + r_R(t) \tag{4.3}$$

for a multi-store model with R stores.

The intensity function of the first store, which in some variants may be the only store, is expressed as

$$r_1(t) = \mu_1 e^{-a_1 t} \tag{4.4}$$

which expresses a decline in intensity, assuming a constant (proportional) rate a_1. To derive the intensity function of the second store, we hypothesize that there is a rehearsal or consolidation process that generates representations in the second one. The generation rate is assumed to be proportional to $r_1(t)$. Although this generation process is still continuing, the content of the second store starts to decline with constant decline rate a_2. These assumptions give rise to the following expression for $r_2(t)$:

$$r_2(t) = \mu_2 \int_0^t r_1(\tau) e^{-a_2(t-\tau)} d\tau. \tag{4.5}$$

The integral term expresses an interaction (technically, a convolution) of the generation process from the rapidly declining first store to the more gradually declining second store. Straightforward integration and substitution yields:

$$r_{12}(t) = \mu_1 e^{-a_1 t} + \frac{\mu_1 \mu_2}{a_1 - a_2} (e^{-a_2 t} - e^{-a_1 t}), \tag{4.6}$$

where r_{12} denotes the intensity function r for two stores.

Ribot gradient

If Store 1 is used to model the hippocampal store with a partial lesion of size λ, with $0 \leq \lambda \leq 1$, 0 meaning no lesion and 1 meaning a full lesion, the expression for the Ribot gradient is:

$$r_{(1)2}(t) = \gamma \mu_1 e^{-a_1 t} + \frac{\mu_1 \mu_2}{a_1 - a_2} (e^{-a_2 t} - e^{-a_1 t}) \tag{4.7}$$

where $\gamma = 1 - \lambda$ and the round brackets indicate a partial lesion of Store 1. It can be shown that if $a_2 = 0$ and $\gamma = 1 - \lambda = \mu_2/a_1$, the Ribot gradient is flat with constant intensity $\mu_1\mu_2/a_1$. In case of a full hippocampal lesion ($\gamma = 0$) and if $a_2 = 0$, Equation 4.7 has properties that are independent of the choice of memory decline function: $r_{[1]2}(0) = 0$, the derivative for $t \downarrow 0$ is equal to $\mu_1\mu_2$, $r^{[1]2}$ is an increasing function, and it has no flex points if $\mu_1 > 0$.

Relative Retrograde Gradient

The relative retrograde gradient (rr-gradient) with a full lesion (indicated with square brackets around the lesioned store) is defined as $r_{[1]2}/r_{12}$. We obtain a three-parameter curve as follows:

$$rr_{[1]2}(t) \;=\; \frac{r_{[1]2}(t)}{r_{12}(t)}$$

$$= \left[\frac{a_1 - a_2}{\mu_2} \left(e_{(a_1-a_2)t} - 1 \right)^{-1} + 1 \right]^{-1}. \qquad (4.8)$$

For $a_2 = 0$, this expression can be simplified to

$$rr_{[1]2}(t) = \left[\frac{-a_1(1 - e^{a_1 t})^{-1}}{\mu_2} + 1 \right]^{1}. \qquad (4.9)$$

In case of partial lesioning of Store 1, we have

$$rr_{(1)2}(t) \;=\; \frac{r_{(1)2}(t)}{r_{12}(t)}$$

$$= \frac{\gamma r_1(t) + r_2(t)}{r_1(t) + r_2(t)}$$

$$= \gamma rr_{1[2]}(t) + rr_{[1]2}(t) \qquad (4.10)$$

where $\gamma = 1 - \lambda$ as before. For $t = 0$, we have $r_2(0) = 0$, so that $rr_{(1)2}(0) = \lambda$. In other words, in the case of a partial lesion, the rr-gradient intersects the ordinate at λ. The rr-gradient has more properties that are independent of the choice of memory decline function: it tends to 1 as $t \to \infty$. Furthermore, if $a_2 = 0$, then $rr_{(1)2}$ is strictly increasing, its derivative for $t \downarrow 0$ is equal to $\lambda\mu_2$, and it has no flex points if and only if $r_1'(t) + \mu_2 r_1(t) > 0$ for every t—that is, when the induction rate from Store 1 to Store 2 is greater than the decline rate in Store 1.

References

Aggleton, J. P. & Brown, M. W. (1999). Episodic memory, amnesia, and the hippocampal-anterior thalamic axis. *Behavioral and Brain Sciences*, *22*, 425–489.

Alvarez, R. & Squire, L. R. (1994). Memory consolidation and the medial temporal lobe: A simple network model. *Proceedings of National Academy of Sciences*, *91*, 7041–7045.

Atkinson, R. C. & Shiffrin, R. M. (1968). *The psychology of learning and motivation: Advances in research and theory*, Volume 2, chapter Human memory: A proposed system and its control processes. New York: Academic Press.

Barnes, C. A. & McNaughton, B. L. (1980). *The psychobiology of aging: Problems and perspectives*, chapter Spatial memory and hippocampal synaptic plasticity, (pp. 253–272). New York: Elsevier/North Holland.

Beatty, W. M., Salmon, D. P., Butters, N., Heindel, W. C. & Granholm, E. L. (1988). Retrograde amnesia in patients with alzheimer's disease or huntington's disease. *Neuropsychology of Aging*, *9*, 181–186.

Brown, A. S. (2002). Consolidation theory and retrograde amnesia in humans. *Psychonomic Bulletin and Review*, *9*, 403–425.

Chessa, A. G. & Murre, J. M. J. (2001). A new memory model for ad impact and scheduling. *Admap*, *36*, 37–40.

Chessa, A. G. & Murre, J. M. J. (2004). A memory model for internet hits after media exposure. *Physica A*, *333*, 541–552.

Chessa, A. G. & Murre, J. M. J. (Submitted). New insights from ebbinghaus' classic savings data: An analysis with the memory chain model. Submitted.

Crovitz, H. F. & Schiffman, H. (1974). Frequency of episodic memories as a function of age. *Bulletin of the Psychonomic Society*, *5*, 517–518.

Ebbinghaus, H. (1885/1913). *Memory a contribution to experimental psychology (H. A. Ruger & C. E. Bussenius, Trans.)*. New York: Teachers College, Columbia University. Originally published in German in 1885.

Estes, W. K. (1950). Toward a statistical theory of learning. *Psychological-Review, 57*, 94–107.

Felleman, D. J. & van Essen, D. C. (1991). Distributed hierarchical processing in the primate cerebral cortex. *Cerebral Cortex, 1*, 1–47.

Frankland, P. W., O'Brien, C., Ohno, M., Kirkwood, A. & Silva, A. J. (2001). α-CaMKB-dependent plasticity in the cortex is required for permanent memory. *Nature, 411*, 309–313.

Galton, F. (1879). Psychometric experiments. *Brain, 2*, 148–162.

Graham, K. S. & Hodges, J. R. (1997). Differentiating the roles of the hippocampal complex and the neocortex in long-term memory storage: Evidence from the study of semantic dementia and alzheimer's disease. *Neuropsychology,, 11*, 77–89.

Hasselmo, M. E. (1995). Neuromodulation and cortical function: Modeling the physiological basis of behavior. *Behavioral Brain Research, 67*, 1–27.

Hasselmo, M. E. (1999). *Disorders of Brain, Behavior and Cognition: The Neurocomputational Perspective*, chapter Neuromodulation and the hippocampus: Memory function and dysfunction in a network simulation., (pp. 3–18). Amsterdam: Elsevier.

Hebb, D. O. (1949). *The organization of behavior*. New York: Wiley.

Janssen, S. M. J., Chessa, A. G. & Murre, J. M. J. (in press). The reminiscence bump in autobiographical memory: Effects of age, gender, education and culture. *Memory.* in press.

Kopelman, M. D. (1989). Remote and autobiographical memory, temporal context memory, and frontal atrophy in korsakoff and alzheimer patients. *Neuropsychologia, 27*, 437–460.

Leutgeb, S. L., Leutgeb, J. K., Treves, A., Moser, M.-B. & Moser, E. I. (in press). Distinct ensemble codes in hippocampal areas CA3 and CA1. *Science.* in press.

McClelland, J. L., McNaughton, B. L. & O'Reilly, R. C. (1995). Why there are complementary learning systems in the hippocampus and neocortex: Insights from the successes and failures of connectionist models of learning and memory. *Psychological Review, 102*, 419–457.

McGaugh, J. L. (2000). Memory: A century of consolidation. *Science, 287*, 248–251.

Meeter, M. (2003). Long-term memory disorders: Measurement and modelling. Unpublished dissertation.

Meeter, M. & Murre, J. M. J. (2004). Simulating episodic memory deficits in semantic dementia with the TraceLink model. *Memory, 12*, 272–287.

Meeter, M. & Murre, J. M. J. (in pressa). Consolidation of long-term memory: Evidence and alternatives. *Psychological Bulletin.* in press.

Meeter, M. & Murre, J. M. J. (in pressb). TraceLink: A model of consolidation and amnesia. *Cognitive Neuropsychology.* in press.

Meeter, M., Murre, J. M. J. & Talamini, L. M. (2002). A computational approach to memory deficits in schizophrenia. *Neurocomputing, 44*, 929–936.

Meeter, M., Murre, J. M. J. & Talamini, L. M. (in press). Mode shifting between storage and retrieval based on novelty detection in oscillating hippocampal circuits. *Hippocampus.* in press.

Mensink, G. J. & Raaijmakers, J. G. W. (1988). A model for interference and forgetting. *Psychological Review, 95*, 434–455.

Milner, B., Squire, L. R. & Kandel, E. R. (1998). Cognitive neuroscience and the study of memory. *Neuron, 20*, 445–468.

Milner, P. M. (1957). The cell assembly: Mark II. *Psychological Review, 64*, 242–252.

Milner, P. M. (1989). A cell assembly theory of hippocampal amnesia. *Neuropsychologia*, *6*, 215–234.

Mishkin, M. (1982). A memory system in the monkey. *Philosophical Transactions of the Royal Society B*, *298*, 85–95.

Murdock, Jr, B. B. (1974). *Human memory: Theory and data*. Potomac, MD: Lawrence Erlbaum Associates.

Murre, J. M. J. (1994). *Proceedings of the Cognitive Neuroscience Meeting 1994*, chapter A model for categorization and recognition in amnesic patients, (p.38).

Murre, J. M. J. (1996). TraceLink: A model of amnesia and consolidation of memory. *Hippocampus*, *6*, 675–684.

Murre, J. M. J. (1997). Implicit and explicit memory in amnesia: Some explanations and predictions by the TraceLink model. *Memory*, *5*, 213–232.

Murre, J. M. J. & Chessa, A. G. (2002). *Marketing for Sustainability – Towards Transactional Policy-Making*, chapter Learning and forgetting communicative messages, (pp. 191–201). Amsterdam: IOS Press.

Murre, J. M. J. & Chessa, A. G. (Submitted). The memory chain model: A model of learning, forgetting, and retrograde amnesia. Submitted.

Murre, J. M. J., Chessa, A. G. & Meeter, M. (Submitted). Quantitative consolidation theory. Submitted.

Murre, J. M. J., Graham, K. S. & Hodges, J. R. (2001). Semantic dementia: Relevance to connectionist models of long-term memory. *Brain*, *124*, NEED.

Murre, J. M. J. & Raffone, A. (2006). Long-range synaptic self-organization in cortical networks. in press.

Murre, J. M. J. & Sturdy, D. P. F. (1995). The mesostructure of the brain: Analyses of quantitative neuroanatomy. *Biological Cybernetics*, *73*, 529–545.

Nadel, L. & Moscovitch, M. (1997). Memory consolidation, retrograde amnesia and the hippocampal complex. *Current Opinion in Neurobiology, 7*, 217–227.

Nadel, L., Samsonovich, A., Ryan, L. & Moscovitch, M. (2000). Multiple trace theory of human memory: Computational, neuroimaging, and neuropsychological results. *Hippocampus, 10*, 352–368.

Peterson, L. R. & Peterson, M. J. (1959). Short-term retention of individual verbal items. *Journal of Experimental Psychology, 58*, 193–198.

Rosenzweig, E. S., Barnes, C. A. & McNaughton, B. L. (2002). Making room for new memories. *Nature Neuroscience, 5*, 6–8.

Rubin, D. C., Hinton, S. & Wenzel, A. (1999). The precise time course of retention. *Journal of Experimental Psychology: Learning, Memory, and Cognition, 25*, 1161–1176.

Rumelhart, D. E., Hinton, G. E. & Williams, R. (1986). *Parallel distributed processing. Explorations in the microstructure of cognition*, Volume 1, chapter Learning internal representations by error propagation. Cambridge, MA: MIT Press.

Rumelhart, D. E. & McClelland, J. L. (1986). *Parallel distributed processing. Explorations in the microstructure of cognition*, Volume 1. Cambridge, MA: MIT Press.

Squire, L. R. (1992). Memory and the hippocampus: A synthesis from findings with rats, monkeys, and humans. *Psychological Review, 99*, 195–231.

Squire, L. R., Cohen, N. J. & Nadel, L. (1984). *Memory consolidation*, chapter The medial temporal region and memory consolidation: A new hypothesis, (pp. 185–210). Hillsdale, NJ: Lawrence Erlbaum.

Squire, L. R. & Zola-Morgan, S. (1991). The medial temporal lobe memory system. *Science, 253*, 1380–1386.

Stickgold, R., James, L. & Hobson, J. (2000). Visual discrimination learning requires sleep after training. *Nature neuroscience, 3*, 1237 1238.

Talamini, L. M., Meeter, M., Elvevåg, B., Murre, J. M. J. & Goldberg, T. E. (in press). Reduced parahippocampal connectivity produces schizophrenia-like memory deficits in simulated neural circuits. *Archives of General Psychiatry*.

Teyler, T. J. & DiScenna, P. (1986). The hippocampal memory indexing theory. *Behavioral Neuroscience*, *100*, 147–154.

Wickelgren, W. A. (1979). Chunking and consolidation: A theoretical synthesis of semantic networks, configuring in conditioning, S-R versus cognitive learning, normal forgetting, the amnesic syndrome, and the hippocampal arousal system. *Psychological Review*, *86*, 44–60.

Wickelgren, W. A. (1987). *Neuroplasticity, learning, and memory*, chapter Site fragility theory of chunking and consolidation in a distributed associative memory, (pp. 301–325). New York: Alan R. Liss.

Wilson, M. A. & McNaughton, B. L. (1994). Reactivation of hippocampal ensemble memories during sleep. *Science*, *255*, 676–679.

5

Who Does What: Taking Measures

Alon Keinan
Tel-Aviv University

Alon Kaufman
Hebrew University

Claus C. Hilgetag
International University Bremen

Isaac Meilijson and Eytan Ruppin
Tel-Aviv University

How is neural information processing to be understood? One of the principal first challenges is to identify the roles of the network elements, be they single neurons, neuronal assemblies or cortical regions, depending on the scale on which the system is analyzed. Even simple nervous systems are capable of carrying out multiple and unrelated functions. Each function recruits some of the elements of the system, and often the same element participates in several functions. A precise quantification of the elements' contributions to the different functions may provide insights regarding the functioning of the nervous system, raise new hypotheses, and lead the way to further research.

Localization of specific functions in the nervous system is conventionally done by recording the activity of the system elements during cognition and behavior, mainly using electrical recordings and functional neuroimaging techniques. Using the recorded activity, the correlation between elements and different behavioral and functional observables can be inferred. However, this correlation does not necessarily identify causality. For example, it is possible that a region does not contribute to the processing of a function, but its activity is still raised when the function is performed because it is activated by other regions that do play a role in performing the function. Such difficulties and others that arise using a correlation-based analysis have been discussed elsewhere (Kosslyn, 1999). To overcome these inherent shortcomings, lesion studies have been traditionally employed in neuroscience, in which the function performance is measured after lesioning different elements of the system. Lesioning enables, in principle, the correct identification of the elements that are causally responsible for a given function. Grobstein (1990) provided a thorough discussion of what can and cannot be concluded from lesion experiments, giving evidence for their usefulness.

Most of the prospective lesion investigations in neuroscience have been *single-lesion* studies, in which only one element is lesioned at a time (e.g. Farah, 1996; Squire, 1992). Such single lesions are limited in their ability to reveal the significance of interacting elements. One obvious example is provided by two elements that exhibit a high degree of functional overlap, that is, *redundancy*: Lesioning either element alone will not reveal its significance. Another classical example is that of the *paradoxical lesioning effect* (Kapur, 1996; Sprague, 1966). In this paradigmatic case, lesioning an element is harmful, but lesioning it when another specific element is lesioned is beneficial for performing a particular function. In such cases, and more generally in cases of *compound processing*, where the contribution of an element depends on the state of other elements, single-lesion analysis is likely to be misleading, resulting in erroneous conclusions. The caveats of single-lesion analysis have already been widely noted in the neuroscience literature (Farah, 1990; Sitton, Mozer & Farah, 2000; Sprague, 1966; Young, Hilgetag & Scannell, 2000).

Acknowledging that single lesions are insufficient for localizing functions in neural systems, we present the Multiperturbation Shapley-value Analysis (MSA). The MSA analyzes a data set composed of numerous multiple lesions, or other types of perturbations, that are afflicted on a neural system. In each multiple perturbation experiment composing the data set, several elements are perturbed concurrently, and the system's level of performance in a given set of functions is measured. In this framework, we view a set of multiple perturbation experiments as a *coalitional game*, borrowing relevant analyses from the field of game theory. Specifically, we define the set of sought contributions to be the *Shapley value* (Shapley, 1953), which stands for the unique fair division of the game's worth (the network's performance score when all elements are intact) among the different players (the network elements). Although in traditional game theory the Shapley value is a theoretical tool that assumes full knowledge of the behavior of the game at all possible coalitions, we have developed and studied methods to compute it approximately with high accuracy and efficiency from a relatively small set of multiple perturbation experiments. The MSA framework further quantifies the interactions between groups of elements, allowing for higher order descriptions of the network.

The MSA has a wide range of potential applications for the analysis of artificial and biological neural systems. In this chapter, after presenting the MSA, we focus on two applications: (a) analysis of reversible deactivation and lesion experiments in cats for identifying the contributions and interactions of different sites to the brain functions of spatial attention to auditory and visual stimuli; and (b) analysis of artificial neurocontrollers of evolved autonomous agents (EAAs). EAAs are a promising model for studying neural processing and developing methods for its analysis (see Ruppin, 2002, for a detailed discussion of this issue). They are less biased than conventional neural networks used in neuroscience modeling because their architecture is typically emergent, rather than predesigned. Furthermore, numerous EAA studies have yielded networks that manifest interesting biological-like characteristics (Aharonov-Barki, Beker & Ruppin, 2001; Cangelosi & Parisi, 1997; Ijspeert, Hallam & Willshaw, 1999).

5.1 THE MULTI-PERTURBATION SHAPLEY VALUE ANALYSIS

5.1.1 Theoretical Foundations

Given a system (network) consisting of many elements, we wish to ascribe to each element its contribution in carrying out a studied function. The MSA presented in this chapter aims to quantify the contribution of system elements while overcoming the inherent shortcomings of the single-lesion approaches. The starting point of the MSA is a data set of a series of multi-perturbation experiments studying the system's performance in a certain function. In each such experiment, a different subset of the system elements are perturbed concomitantly (denoting a perturbation configuration), and the system's performance following the perturbation in the function studied is measured. Given this data set, our main goal is to assign values that capture the elements' contribution (importance) to the function in a fair and accurate manner. Note that this assignment is nothing but the classical functional localization goal in neuroscience, but now recast in a formal, multi-perturbation framework.

The basic observation underlying the solution presented in this chapter to meet this goal is that the multi-perturbation setup is essentially equivalent to a coalitional game. That is, the system elements can be viewed as players in a game. The set of all elements that are left intact in a perturbation configuration can be viewed as a coalition of players. The performance of the system following the perturbation can then be viewed as the worth of that coalition of players in the game. Within such a framework, an intuitive notion of a player's importance (or contribution) should capture the worth of coalitions containing it (i.e., the system's performance when the corresponding element is intact), relative to the worth of coalitions that do not (i.e., relative to the system's performance when this element, perhaps among others, is perturbed). This intuitive equivalence, presented formally later, enables us to harness the pertaining game theoretical tools to solve the problem of function localization in biological systems.

Using the terminology of game theory, let a *coalitional game* be defined by a pair (N, v), where $N = \{1, \ldots, n\}$ is the set of all *players* and $v(S)$, for every $S \subseteq N$, is a real number associating a worth with the *coalition* S, such that $v(\phi) = 0$.[1] In the context of multi-perturbations, N denotes the set of all elements, and for each $S \subseteq N$, $v(S)$ denotes the performance measured under the perturbation configuration in which all the elements in S are intact and the rest are perturbed.

A *payoff profile* of a coalitional game is the assignment of a payoff to each of the players. A *value* is a function that assigns a unique payoff profile to a coalitional game. It is *efficient* if the sum of the components of the payoff profile assigned is $v(N)$. That is, an ef-

---

[1]This type of game is most commonly referred to as a coalitional game with transferable payoff.

ficient value divides the overall game's worth (the networks' performance when all elements are intact) between the different players (the network elements). A value that captures the importance of the different players may serve as a basis for quantifying, in the context of multi-perturbations, the contributions of the network elements.

The definite value in game theory and economics for this type of coalitional game is the *Shapley value* (Shapley, 1953), defined as follows. Let the *marginal importance* of player i to a coalition S, with $i \notin S$, be

$$\Delta_i(S) = v(S \cup \{i\}) - v(S). \tag{5.1}$$

Then the Shapley value is defined by the payoff

$$\gamma_i(N, v) = \frac{1}{n!} \sum_{R \in \mathcal{R}} \Delta_i(S_i(R)) \tag{5.2}$$

of each player $i \in N$, where $\mathcal{R}$ is the set of all $n!$ orderings of N and $S_i(R)$ is the set of players preceding i in the ordering R. The Shapley value can be interpreted as follows: Suppose that all the players are arranged in some order, all orders being equally likely. Then $\gamma_i(N, v)$ is the expected marginal importance of player i to the set of players who precede him. The Shapley value is efficient because the sum of the marginal importance of all players is $v(N)$ in any ordering.

An alternative view of the Shapley value is based on the notion of balanced contributions. For each coalition S, the *subgame* (S, v^S) of (N, v) is defined to be the game in which $v^S(T) = v(T)$ for any $T \subseteq S$. A value Ψ satisfies the *balanced contributions* property if for every coalitional game (N, v) and for every $i, j \in N$

$$\Psi_i(N, v) - \Psi_i(N \setminus \{j\}, v^{N \setminus \{j\}}) = \Psi_j(N, v) - \Psi_j(N \setminus \{i\}, v^{N \setminus \{i\}}), \tag{5.3}$$

meaning that the change in the value of player i when player j is excluded from the game is equal to the change in the value of player j when player i is excluded. This property implies that *objections* made by any player to any other regarding the division are exactly balanced by the *counterobjections*. The unique efficient value that satisfies the balanced contributions property is the Shapley value (Myerson, 1977, 1980).

The Shapley value also has an axiomatic foundation. Let player i be a *null player* in v if $\Delta_i(S) = 0$ for every coalition S ($i \notin S$).

Players i and j are interchangeable in v if $\Delta_i(S) = \Delta_j(S)$ for every coalition S that contains neither i nor j. Using these basic definitions, *the Shapley value is the only efficient value that satisfies the three following axioms, further pointing to its uniqueness* (Shapley, 1953):

Axiom 1 *(Symmetry) If i and j are interchangeable in game v, then* $\Psi_i(v) = \Psi_j(v)$.

Intuitively, this axiom states that the value should not be affected by a mere change in the players' names.

Axiom 2 *(Null player property) If i is a null player in game v, then* $\Psi_i(v) = 0$.

This axiom sets the baseline of the value to be zero for a player whose marginal importance is always zero.

Axiom 3 *(Additivity) For any two games v and w on a set N of players,* $\Psi_i(v + w) = \Psi_i(v) + \Psi_i(w)$ *for all $i \in N$, where $v + w$ is the game defined by $(v + w)(S) = v(S) + w(S)$.*

This last axiom constrains the value to be consistent in the space of all games.

In the 50 years since its construction, the Shapley value as a unique fair solution has been successfully used in many fields. Probably the most important application is in cost allocation, where the cost of providing a service should be shared among the different receivers of that service. This application was first suggested by Shubik (1962), and the theory was later developed by many authors (e.g., Billera, Heath & Raanan, 1978; Roth, 1979). This use of the Shapley value has received recent attention in the context of sharing the cost of multicast routing (Feigenbaum, Papadimitriou & Shenker, 2001). In epidemiology, the Shapley value has been utilized as a mean to quantify the population impact of exposure factors on a disease load (Gefeller, Land & Eide, 1998). Other fields where the Shapley value has been used include, among others, politics (starting from the strategic voting framework Shapley & Shubik, 1954), international environmental problems, and economic theory (see Shubik, 1985, for discussion and references).

The MSA, given a data set of multi-perturbations, uses the Shapley value as the unique fair division of the network's performance between the different elements, assigning to each element its contribution, as its average importance to the function in question.[2] The higher an element's contribution according to the Shapley value, the larger is the part it causally plays in the successful performance of the function.[3]

In the context of multi-perturbations, Axiom 1 of the Shapley value formulation entails that if two elements have the same importance in all perturbation configurations, their contributions will be identical. Axiom 2 assures that an element which has no effect in any perturbation configuration will be assigned a zero contribution. Axiom 3 indicates that if two separate functions are performed by the network, such that the overall performance of the network in all multi-perturbation configurations is defined to be equal to the sum of the performances in the two functions, then the total contribution assigned to each element for both functions will be equal to the sum of its individual contributions to each of the two functions.

It should be noted that other game-theoretical values can be used instead of the Shapley value within the MSA framework. Specifically, Banzhaf (1965) suggested an analogue of the Shapley value, and Dubey et al. (1981) later generalized the Shapley value to a whole family of semi-values all satisfying the three axioms but without the efficiency property, a natural requirement for describing fair divisions.

Once a game is defined, its Shapley value is uniquely determined. Yet employing different perturbation methods may obviously result in different values of v and, as a consequence, different Shapley values. A range of authors (Aharonov, Segev, Meilijson & Ruppin, 2003; Keinan, Meilijson & Ruppin, 2003; Keinan, Sandbank, Hilgetag, Meilijson & Ruppin, 2004; Saggie, Keinan & Ruppin, 2004) have discussed different perturbation methods and the effects they may have on the elements' contributions found.

---

[2]Because $v(\phi) = 0$ does not necessarily hold in practice, as it depends on the performance measurement definition, Shapley value efficiency transcribes to the property according to which the sum of the contributions assigned to all the elements equals $v(N) - v(\phi)$.

[3]Because no limitations are enforced on the shape of v, a negative contribution is possible, indicating that the element hinders, on the average, the function's performance.

5.1.2   Methods

Full Information Calculation: The Original Shapley Value

In an ideal scenario, in which the full set of 2^n perturbation configurations along with the performance measurement for each is given,
the Shapley value may be straightforwardly calculated using Equation 5.2, where the summation runs over all $n!$ orderings of N. Equivalently, the Shapley value can be computed as a summation over all
2^n configurations, properly weighted by the number of possible orderings of the elements,

$$\gamma_i(N, v) = \frac{1}{n!} \sum_{S \subseteq N \setminus \{i\}} \Delta_i(S) \cdot |S|! \cdot (n - |S| - 1)!. \qquad (5.4)$$

Substituting according to Equation 5.1 results in

$$\gamma_i(N, v) = \frac{1}{n!} \quad \sum_{S \subseteq N, i \in S} v(S) \cdot (|S| - 1)! \cdot (n - |S|)! -$$
$$\frac{1}{n!} \quad \sum_{S \subseteq N, i \notin S} v(S) \cdot (|S|)! \cdot (n - |S| - 1)!, \qquad (5.5)$$

where each configuration S contributes a summand to either one of
the two sums depending on whether element i is perturbed or intact
in S. Thus, the Shapley value calculation consists of going through
all perturbation configurations and calculating for each element the
two sums in the prior equation.

Predicted Shapley Value

Obviously, calculating the performance levels of all perturbation configurations required for the calculation of the Shapley value is often
intractable. In such cases, one may train a predictor, using a given
subset of perturbation configurations, to predict the performance levels of all unseen configurations. Given such a predictor, a *predicted
Shapley value* can be calculated as the Shapley value based on the
predicted performance levels.

*Estimated Shapley Value and Estimated Predicted Shapley
Value*

The predicted Shapley value relieves the MSA of the need for the full
set of 2^n perturbation configurations. Nevertheless, $n \cdot 2^n$ computa-

tions are still required for its calculation (summing over all predicted configurations for each element). When the number of elements is too large for such a method to be tractable, sampling may be used, facilitating the MSA's scalability. Rather than sampling single configurations, the estimated MSA variant samples whole permutations of the n elements. Let $\hat{\mathcal{R}}$ be a randomly sampled set of permutations (with replacement). Then, based on Equation 5.2,

$$\hat{\gamma}_i(N, v) = \frac{1}{|\hat{\mathcal{R}}|} \sum_{R \in \hat{\mathcal{R}}} \Delta_i(S_i(R)) \tag{5.6}$$

is an unbiased estimator of the Shapley value $\gamma_i(N, v)$. To calculate these estimates for every i, for each permutation $a_1, \ldots, a_n$ in $\hat{\mathcal{R}}$, the performance measurements $v(\phi), v(\{a_1\}), v(\{a_1, a_2\}), \ldots,$ $v(\{a_1, a_2, \ldots, a_{n-1}\}), v(N)$ are needed. Notice, however, that a perturbation configuration should be calculated only once while it may appear in different permutations. Thus, the number of new multi-perturbation experiments to be performed for each sampled permutation tends to decrease as more permutations are sampled. The resulting *estimated Shapley value* is an efficient value, because the sum of the marginal importance of all elements in any permutation is $v(N) - v(\phi)$.

The empirical standard deviation of the marginal importance of element i,

$$s_i(N, v) = \sqrt{\frac{1}{|\hat{\mathcal{R}}|} \sum_{R \in \hat{\mathcal{R}}} (\Delta_i(S_i(R)) - \hat{\gamma}_i(N, v))^2}, \tag{5.7}$$

yields an estimator of the standard deviation of the Shapley value estimator $\hat{\gamma}_i(N, v)$

$$\hat{\sigma}(\hat{\gamma}_i(N, v)) = \frac{s_i(N, v)}{\sqrt{|\hat{\mathcal{R}}|}}. \tag{5.8}$$

The standard deviation measures how close the estimated Shapley value is to the true value. Specifically, using the Shapley value estimator and the standard deviation estimator, confidence intervals for the contribution of each of the elements can be constructed. It is further possible to test statistical hypotheses on whether the contribution of a certain element equals a given value (e.g., zero or $1/n$).

Both the confidence intervals and the hypothesis tests are based on the t-distribution. Sampling permutations for constructing the set $\hat{\mathcal{R}}$ can be done with a given sample size or sequentially—for instance, stopping when reaching a fixed maximal limit for the number of perturbation experiments (the number of perturbation configurations) or when all standard deviation estimates are small enough.

The multi-perturbation experiments that should be performed in the estimated Shapley value method are dictated by the sampled permutations. At times, however, one is given an existing data set of performance measures for some set of perturbation configurations, which does not necessarily match a random permutation sample. In this case, the MSA offers an additional estimation variant: A performance predictor is trained using the given set of perturbation configurations and serves as an oracle supplying performance predictions for any perturbation configuration as dictated by the sampled permutations, resulting in an *estimated predicted Shapley value*.

A Two-Phase Procedure for Large Scale Analysis

We suggest another scalable method within the MSA framework for handling systems with a large number of elements. This *two-phase MSA procedure* is motivated by the observation that often only a small fraction of the possibly large number of elements significantly contributes to the specific function tested within the analysis. Hence, the first phase finds those elements with significant contributions. This phase uses a small sample to calculate the estimated Shapley value and the standard deviation estimates. A two-sided t-test is then performed on the contribution of each element, where the null hypothesis indicates that the contribution is zero, thus identifying the significant elements.

The second phase focuses on finding the accurate contributions of the significant elements. This phase may use the same small sample from the first phase, but it focuses on the coalitional game $(N', v^{N'})$, where N' is the set of elements found as significant in the first phase. Given the characteristic function v of the original game consisting of all elements, $v^{N'}$ may be defined such that for $S \subseteq N'$, $v^{N'}(S)$ equals the average of $v(T)$ over all $T \subseteq N$ satisfying $T \cap N' = S$. Thus, using the original sample, some of the $v^{N'}$ are based on an average over many perturbation configurations, whereas others might not be evaluated due to lack of data. In the case where the characteristic function $v^{N'}$ cannot be fully calculated, a predictor is trained using the available data. The predictor is trained on perturbation configurations of size $|N'|$ and not of size $|N|$, allowing for faster training and increased scalability. In the case where the number of significant elements is too large for the explicit calculation of a predicted Shapley value, sampling is also incorporated in this second phase, using the much smaller configuration space. When the two-phase procedure is used for localizing several functions in a large network (i.e., when a multi-perturbation experiment measures several performance values), the two-phase procedure is applied for each and every function separately, as the set of significant elements yielded by the first phase depends on the function analyzed.

Bounded Perturbation Level Analysis

In scenarios where it might not be possible to concomitantly perturb any number of a system elements, as is the case in most types of biological experiments, a more delicate procedure should be carried out. Specifically, suppose that, for some perturbation level k, one is given with all perturbation configurations in which no more than k elements are perturbed. In such a case, let the marginal importance of element i to a coalition S, with $i \notin S$, be

$$\Delta_i^k(S) = \begin{cases} v(S \cup \{i\}) - v(S) & : \quad |S| \geq n - k \\ 0 & : \quad |S| < n - k \end{cases} \tag{5.9}$$

Then the contribution of element i, in the spirit of the Shapley value (Equation 5.2), can be defined as

$$\gamma_i^k(N, v) = \frac{1}{k(n-1)!} \sum_{R \in \mathcal{R}} \Delta_i^k(S_i(R)). \tag{5.10}$$

These MSA k-bounded contributions coincide with the Shapley value for $k = n$ and with single-lesion analysis for $k = 1$. Similarly to the full ($k = n$) case, if the calculation of all perturbation configurations with up to k perturbed elements is intractable, a predictor can be trained to predict the performance levels of all those configurations, and predicted k-bounded contributions can be calculated. Further, when the set of those configurations is too large to even enumerate them, an unbiased estimator for the k-bounded contributions, estimated k-bounded contributions, can be calculated by sampling permutations while ignoring the configurations with more than k perturbed elements in each permutation. Based on these, an estimated predicted variant can also be calculated, and a two-phase procedure can be carried out.

5.1.3 Two-Dimensional MSA

The Shapley value serves as a summary of the game, indicating the average marginal importance of an element over all possible elements' orderings. For complex networks, where the importance of an element strongly depends on the state (perturbed or intact) of other elements, a higher order description may be necessary to capture sets of elements with significant interactions. For example, when two elements exhibit a high degree of functional overlap—that is, *redundancy*—it is necessary to capture this interaction aside from the average importance of each element. Such high-dimensional analysis provides further insights into the network's functional organization.

We focus on the description of two-dimensional interactions. A natural definition of the interaction between a pair of elements is as follows: Let $\gamma_{i,\bar{j}} = \gamma_i(N \setminus \{j\}, v^{N \setminus \{j\}})$ be the Shapley value of element i in the subgame of all elements without element j. Intuitively, this is the average marginal importance of element i when element j is perturbed. Let us now define the coalitional game (M, v^M), where $M = N \setminus \{i, j\} \cup \{(i,j)\}$, (i,j) is a new compound element, and $v^M(S)$, for $S \subseteq M$, is defined by

$$v^M(S) = \begin{cases} v(S) & : & (i,j) \notin S \\ v(S \setminus \{(i,j)\} \cup \{i,j\}) & : & (i,j) \in S \end{cases} \tag{5.11}$$

where v is the characteristic function of the original game with elements N. Then, $\gamma_{i,j} = \gamma_{(i,j)}(M, v^M)$, the Shapley value of element (i,j) in this game, is the average marginal importance of elements i and j when jointly added to a configuration. The two-dimensional interaction between element i and element j, $j \neq i$, is then defined as

$$I_{i,j} = \gamma_{i,j} - \gamma_{i,\bar{j}} - \gamma_{j,\bar{i}} \tag{5.12}$$

which quantifies how much the average marginal importance of the two elements together is larger (or smaller) than the sum of the average marginal importance of each of them when the other one is perturbed. Intuitively, this symmetric definition ($I_{i,j} = I_{j,i}$) states how much "the whole is greater than the sum of its parts" (*synergism*), where the whole is the pair of elements. In cases where the whole is smaller than the sum of its parts—that is, when the two elements exhibit functional overlap—the interaction is negative (antagonism). This two-dimensional interaction definition coincides with the Shapley interaction index, which is a more general measure for the interaction among any group of players (Grabisch & Roubens, 1999).

The MSA can classify the type of interaction between each pair even further: By definition, $\gamma_{i,\bar{j}}$ is the average marginal importance of element i when element j is perturbed. Based on Equation 5.12, $\gamma_{i,j} + I_{i,j}$ is the average marginal importance of element i when element j is intact. When both $\gamma_{i,\bar{j}}$ and $\gamma_{i,\bar{j}} + I_{i,j}$ are positive, element i's contribution is positive irrespective of whether element j is perturbed or intact. When both are negative, element i hinders the performance irrespective of the state of element j. In cases where the two measures have inverted signs, we define the contribution of element i as *j-modulated*. The interaction is defined as *positive modulated* when $\gamma_{i,\bar{j}}$ is negative, whereas $\gamma_{i,\bar{j}} + I_{i,j}$ is positive, causing a paradoxical effect. We define the interaction as *negative modulated* when the former is positive and the latter is negative. The interaction of j with respect to i may be categorized in a similar way, yielding a full description of the type of interaction between the pair. Classical paradoxical lesioning effects—for instance, of the kind reported in the neuroscience literature (Kapur, 1996; Sprague, 1966)—are defined when both elements exhibit positive modulation with respect to one another. As evident, the rigorous definition of the type of interaction presented in this section relies on an average interaction over all perturbation configurations. Thus, it does not necessarily coincide with the type of interaction found by using only single perturbations and a double perturbation of the pair, as conventionally described in the neuroscience literature.

5.2 MSA OF REVERSIBLE DEACTIVATION EXPERIMENTS

To test the applicability of the approach to the analysis of biological "wet-ware" network data, we applied the MSA to data from reversible cooling deactivation experiments in the cat. Specifically, we investigated the brain localization of spatial attention to auditory and visual stimuli. Spatial attention is an essential brain function in many species, including humans, that is underlying several other aspects of sensory perception, cognition, and behavior. Although attentional mechanisms proceed efficiently, automatically and inconspicuously in the intact brain, perturbation of these mechanism can lead to dramatic behavioral impairment. So-called *neglect patients*, for instance, have great difficulties, or even fail, to reorient their attention to spatial locations after suffering specific unilateral brain lesions, with resulting severe deficits of sensory (e.g., visual, auditory) perception and cognition (Vallar, 1998). From the perspective of systems neuroscience, attentional mechanisms are particularly interesting because this function is known to be widely distributed in the brain. Moreover, lesions in the attentional network have resulted in paradoxical effects (Kapur, 1996), in which the deactivation of some elements results in a better-than-normal performance (Hilgetag, Theoret & Pascual-Leone, 2001) or reversed behavioral deficits resulting from earlier lesions (e.g., Sprague, 1966). Such effects challenge traditional approaches for lesion analysis and provide an ideal testbed for novel formal analysis approaches, such as the MSA.

5.2.1 Auditory Spatial Attention

The elements studied in the auditory experiments were left and right Superior Colliculus (SC) and left and right posterior Middle Suprasylvian (pMS) cortex. These structures were further subdivided into superficial and deep laminar compartments, so that altogether there were eight regions in the system's description.

Figure 5.1(a) presents the MSA contributions of the different regions, calculated using prediction based on 33 available lesion experiments. The analysis revealed that only regions SC_L-deep and SC_R-deep play a role in determining auditory attentional performance in

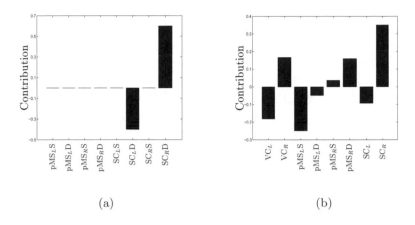

(a)   (b)

Fig. 5.1. MSA contributions of the different regions to auditory (a) and visual (b) spatial attention, in the left hemifield of the cat.

the left hemifield, which is in line with previous functional character-izations of the collicular system (Lomber, Payne & Cornwell, 2001). The contralateral deep layer of the SC has a positive contribution, suggesting that lesioning this region hinders performance. In con-trast, the negative contribution of the ipsilateral SC indicates that lesioning of this region tends to improve the performance. Due to the restricted experimental access to deeper brain structures when a deep layer of the SC was lesioned, the superficial one was lesioned as well. Nevertheless, the MSA framework successfully revealed that only the deep SC regions are the ones of significance.

We further performed a two-dimensional MSA to quantify the in-teractions between each pair of regions, finding only one significant interaction—between SC_L-deep and SC_R-deep. Observing that SC_L-deep has no contribution when SC_R-deep is intact, while it has an average negative contribution when SC_R-deep is lesioned, the MSA concluded that SC_L-deep exhibits a positive modulated interaction with respect to SC_R-deep, uncovering the type of interaction as-sumed to take place in this function (Hilgetag, Lomber & Payne, 2000; Lomber, Payne & Cornwell, 2001). One should emphasize that a single lesioning analysis of the same data would not have revealed this paradoxical effect and would have concluded that SC_R-deep is

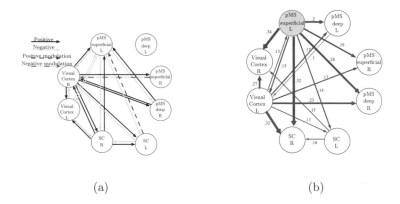

(a)   (b)

Fig. 5.2: Significant interactions in the visual experiments. (a). The type, in both directions, of the twelve most significant two-dimensional interactions. (b). The positive contributions of lesioning a region knowing a specific other region is lesioned $(-\gamma_{i,\bar{j}})$. The figure shows the significant values, arrows representing the contribution of lesioning the arrow's base region (i), given that the arrow's end region (j) is already lesioned.

the only important region in this function.

5.2.2   Visual Spatial Attention

We turn to analyzing data from similar experiments studying the localization of spatial attention to moving visual stimuli. The analyzed data set was collected from various lesion and reversible deactivation experiments of striate and parastriate visual cortex (VC), SC and deep and superficial layers of the pMS cortex in the cat (e.g., Lomber & Payne, 1996; Lomber, Payne & Cornwell, 2001; Lomber, Payne, Hilgetag & Rushmore, 2002; Sprague, 1966). The MSA contributions were calculated using predictions based on 21 available lesion experiments out of the 2^8 multi-lesion space. This small number of lesion experiments is not sufficient to precisely predict the full multiple-lesion set; hence, the results might be inaccurate. However, any additional experimental results, as they become available, can be added in a straightforward manner to refine the prediction. Figure 5.1(b) shows the contributions of the different regions involved in the experiments. The analysis yielded opposite contributions of left- and right-hemispheric structures, with the structures on the ipsilateral side to the tested (left) field having negative contributions and the structures on the contralateral side having positive ones. The largest positive contribution made by SC_R is in line with the presumed central role of the SC in visual spatial attention in cats. Conversely, the largest negative contribution is made by the superficial layers of the ipsilateral pMS due to their powerful role in reversing the impact of contralateral lesions. For example, deactivation of the ipsilateral superficial pMS is sufficient to reverse the impact of a complete deactivation (superficial and deep) of contralateral pMS (Lomber & Payne, 1996) or even a lesion of the entire contralateral VC including the pMS (Lomber, Payne, Hilgetag & Rushmore, 2002). The role of cortical regions in visual spatial attention in the cat has been previously investigated in great detail for pMS. Our analysis also suggests important contributions of other cortical regions (VC). It remains a challenge for future deactivation experiments to test this prediction and identify additional regions within the cat visual cortex that specifically contribute to attentional behavior.

Detailed two-dimensional MSA reveals the functional interactions between the regions. Figure 5.2(a) illustrates the type of the most significant interactions.Figure 5.2(b) quantifies the contributions of lesioning various regions with respect to a given lesion in the network. The contribution of lesioning region i while region j is already lesioned $(-\gamma_{i,\bar{j}})$ is based on the average marginal contribution of such lesioning, taking into consideration other possible unknown lesions to other regions in the network. The figure clearly shows the significant reverse impact of the ipsilateral superficial layers of pMS. This graph is just one example of displaying the causal effects that can be revealed by the MSA, testifying to its usefulness in deducing the functionally important regions as well as their significant interactions.

5.3   ANALYSIS OF EVOLVED AUTONOMOUS AGENTS

The MSA was mainly developed and studied for the analysis of neurocontrollers of EAAs described in the first section to follow. The computations needed to calculate the predicted Shapley value grow exponentially with the number of elements in the analyzed system. This is reasonable for the applications just presented, because they involve networks of only eight elements. However, for larger systems such as EAAs' neurocontrollers containing many elements, these computations become infeasible. Hence, in this section, we utilize the different scalable MSA variants for their analysis.

5.3.1   The EAA Environment

The EAA environment used to study and develop the MSA is described in detail elsewhere (Aharonov-Barki, Beker & Ruppin, 2001). A brief overview is provided herewith. The EAAs live in a virtual discrete two-dimensional grid world surrounded by walls. Poison items are scattered all around the world, while food items are scattered only in a food zone located in one corner. An agent's goal is to find and eat as many food items as possible during its life, while avoiding the poison items. The performance score of an agent is proportional to the number of food items minus the number of poison items it consumes. The agents are equipped with a set of sensors, motors, and a fully recurrent neurocontroller, which is evolved using a genetic algorithm (Aharonov-Barki, Beker & Ruppin, 2001).

Four sensors encode the presence of a wall, a resource (food or poison, without distinction between the two) or a vacancy in the cell the agent occupies and in the three cells directly in front of it (Figure 5.3). A fifth sensor is a smell sensor that can differentiate between food and poison directly underneath the agent, but gives a random reading if the agent is in an empty cell. The four motor neurons dictate movement forward (neuron 1), a turn left (neuron 2) or right (neuron 3), and control the state of the mouth (open or closed, neuron 4). In each step, a sensory reading occurs, network activity is then synchronously updated, and a motor action is taken according to the resulting activity in the motor neurons.

Previous analysis (Aharonov-Barki, Beker & Ruppin, 2001) revealed that successful agents possess one or more command neurons that determine the agent's behavioral strategy. Artificially clamping these command neurons to either constant firing activity or to complete quiescence causes the agent to constantly maintain one of the two behavioral modes it exhibits, regardless of its sensory input.

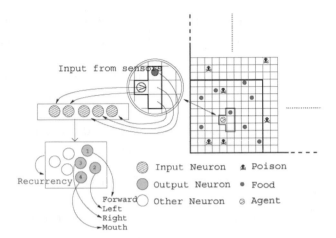

Fig. 5.3: The EAA environment. An outline of the grid world and the agent's neurocontroller. The agent is marked by a small arrow on the grid, whose direction indicates its orientation. The curved lines indicate where in the arena each of the sensory inputs comes from.

These two behavioral modes are *exploration* and *grazing*. Exploration, which normally takes place when the agent is outside of the food zone, consists of moving in straight lines, ignoring resources in the sensory field that are not directly under the agent, and turning at walls. Grazing, which usually takes place when the agent is in the food zone, consists of turning toward resources to examine them, turning at walls, and maintaining the agent's location on the grid in a relatively small region.

Throughout this chapter, we focus on the analysis of four agents, which have been successfully evolved in this environment. All four agents are equipped with sensors and motors, and their neurocontrollers are all fully recurrent, consisting of 10 internal neurons, including the motor neurons (not including the sensors). The differences between the agents follow:

1. The neurocontroller of S10 (Aharonov-Barki, Beker & Ruppin, 2001) is composed of binary McCulloch-Pitts neurons, whose synaptic strengths were evolved.

2. P10 was obtained by a process in which, after the evolution

of a successful agent, its synapses are pruned using an evolutionary network-minimization algorithm (Ganon, Keinan & Ruppin, 2003) that deletes synapses and modifies the weights of the remaining ones so as to produce a similar agent with a smaller neurocontroller. Like S10, P10 is equipped with a neurocontroller composed of binary McCulloch-Pitts neurons, but only 14 recurrent synapses out of the 100 original ones are left after applying the minimization algorithm.

3. To encourage the creation of a fault-tolerant neurocontroller, F10 was evolved using the same network architecture of S10, but while introducing faults to the neurocontroller, resulting in a more robust agent (Keinan, 2004).

4. Last, W10 copes with a more difficult version of the task, which also involves counting, as the agent has to wait and remain still in a grid cell containing food for five steps without moving or turning to eat (Saggie, Keinan & Ruppin, 2004). Eating takes place in this version only if the agent closes its mouth in the last waiting step. The neurocontroller of W10 is composed of discrete-time integrate-and-fire neurons, whose membrane time constants were also evolved, in addition to the synaptic strengths.

5.3.2   Full Information Analysis

We apply the full information MSA to agent P10 to determine the contributions of each of its 14 synapses to its performance. To this end, we measure the agent's performance score under the entire set of 2^{14} synaptic perturbation configurations, where each synaptic perturbation configuration indicates for each of the 14 recurrent synapses in the neurocontroller whether it is perturbed or left intact. The perturbation method used is *stochastic lesioning* (Aharonov, Segev, Meilijson & Ruppin, 2003), which is performed by randomizing the activity of a perturbed element while keeping the mean activity unchanged. Figure 5.4 plots the Shapley value, calculated in a straightforward manner using the full information. The four most important synapses are, by order of importance, the synapse from the right motor to the left one, from the forward motor to the command neuron

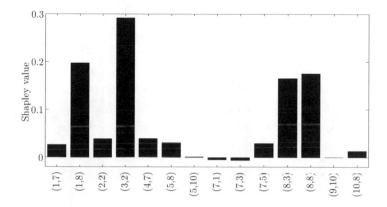

Fig. 5.4: Shapley value contributions of the synapses of P10. The contributions are normalized, as in all the results to follow (except where stated otherwise), such that the sum over all synapses equals 1. The x-axis presents the synapses in the form (presynaptic neuron, postsynaptic neuron).

(neuron number 8), the recurrent synapse from the command neuron to itself, which has been shown to facilitate the short-term memory of the agent (Aharonov-Barki, Beker & Ruppin, 2001), and the synapse from the command neuron to the right motor. The analysis uncovers the main mechanism underlying this minimized neurocontroller's operation while quantifying the part played by each of the mechanism's constituents. The rest of the synapses exhibit minor contributions, with two synapses ([7,1] and [7,3]) having negative contributions, testifying to the fact that, on the average, they hinder the performance.

For W10, the counting agent, the performance score under the entire set of 2^{10} neuronal perturbation configurations was measured using stochastic lesioning and from which the neurons' contributions were calculated (Figure 5.5). Previous analysis (Saggie, Keinan & Ruppin, 2004) revealed neuron number 10 to be the command neuron, neuron numbers 4 and 9 to participate in the temporal counting required for the precise timing of food consumption, and neuron number 1, the forward motor, to count the last two steps before moving

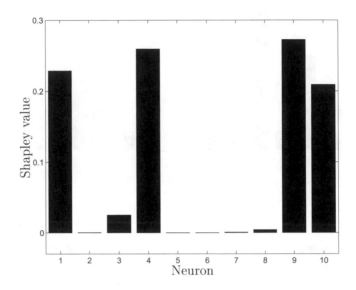

Fig. 5.5: Shapley value contributions of the neurons of W10.

forward. The MSA accurately reveals those neurons to be the most significant ones.

5.3.3   Predicted Shapley Value Analysis

To test the accuracy of the predicted Shapley value, predictors were trained with training sets of randomly chosen synaptic perturbation configurations of P10 of sizes $100, 200, \ldots, 1,000$ (out of $2^{14} = 16,384$ configurations). Figure 5.6 plots the predicted Shapley value contribution of the most important synapse of P10 against the number of configurations in the training set, along with the real Shapley value. The predicted Shapley value is very close to the real one, even for very small numbers of perturbation configurations used for training, and exhibits stability across the different runs, as noted by the small standard deviations. Remarkably, this is true even though the prediction is not very accurate (average test MSE corresponding to explaining less than 60% of the variance when 100 perturbation configurations

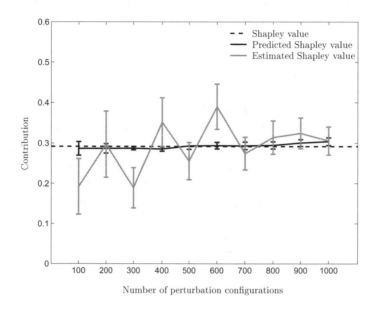

Fig. 5.6: Predicted Shapley value and estimated Shapley value using small perturbation sets. These values for the most important synapse of P10, (3,2), are plotted against the number of perturbation configurations $(100, 200, \ldots, 1000)$. The black line plots the mean and standard deviation of the predicted Shapley value, based on 10 predictors. The gray line plots the estimated Shapley value and the standard deviation estimates. Dashed black line denotes the real Shapley value, calculated using the full set of 2^{14} configurations.

are used for training; the prediction improves as the training set size increases). This might be explained by the fact that the Shapley value is obtained via an averaging of a large number of predictions. Assuming that the prediction is unbiased, prediction errors cancel each other out, resulting in a predicted Shapley value that is similar to the real one.

5.3.4   Estimated Shapley Value and Estimated Predicted Shapley Value Analysis

Figure 5.6 plots the estimated Shapley value, along with its standard deviation estimate, for the most important synapse of P10, against the number of perturbation configurations used.[4] As expected from the theory, the estimated Shapley value appears to be an unbiased estimator for the real Shapley value, and its standard deviation generally decreases with the sample size. Notably, the standard deviation of the estimated Shapley value is much larger than that of the predicted Shapley value, which testifies to the consistent generalization performed by the predictor to the full set of 2^{14} configurations, compared with the consistency of mere random sampling, when both use the same number of lesion configurations with actual performance scores.

We now turn to examine a case where the entire set of 2^n predictions needed for extracting the predicted Shapley value is computationally intractable—the analysis of the full recurrent synaptic neurocontroller of S10, consisting of 100 synapses. An estimated Shapley value is calculated based on a sample of 100 permutations ($9,833$ perturbation configurations), where a more minute perturbation method is employed to capture the long-term contributions (ILM, developed by Keinan et al., 2003, lesioning level of 0.5). Training a predictor with the same sample, the estimated predicted Shapley value is computed by sampling configurations from the predictor using sequential sampling, stopping when the standard deviation estimates of all 100 estimated predicted contributions are below 0.005. Arbitrarily defining an important synapse as one with a normalized contribution above 0.03 (3% of the total performance of the neurocontroller), the same nine synapses are yielded as important by both the estimated Shapley value and the estimated predicted one (Figure 5.7), with similar contributions. These conclusions are rather insensitive to the choice of threshold used for defining an important synapse. By finding the important synapses, the MSA reveals the recurrent backbone of the neurocontroller, containing, in this case, only 9 out of the 100 synapses. Focusing on the backbone may simplify the further

---

[4] Because whole permutations are sampled, the actual number of configurations used for a defined size s is between s and $s + n - 2$, where $n = 14$ in this case.

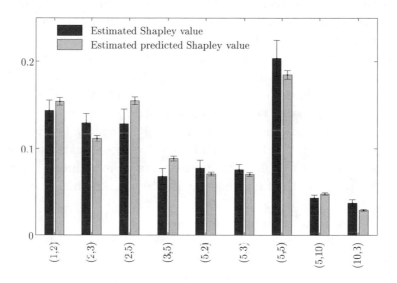

Fig. 5.7: Estimated Shapley value and estimated predicted Shapley value of the important synapses of S10. Error bars of both denote the standard deviation estimates

analysis of such fully recurrent networks (Aharonov, Segev, Meilijson & Ruppin, 2003; Keinan, Sandbank, Hilgetag, Meilijson & Ruppin, 2004).

5.3.5 Two-Phase Analysis

We begin by applying the two-phase MSA procedure to the analysis of a moderate size system to allow for the comparison of the results of the procedure with the real Shapley value. Such a moderate size system is obtained by focusing on part of S10's synaptic network, consisting of 14 synapses out of the 100, after pruning the rest of the synapses. First, we perform a full information MSA to identify the true contributions. Then we perform a two-phase analysis. In the first phase of the latter, a small random sample of 20 permutations (227 perturbation configurations out of the 2^{14}) is used to estimate the Shapley value and the standard deviations. Performing t-tests (two-sided, $\alpha = .05$) using the estimates results in the identification of 11 significant synapses. The second phase focuses on those significant synapses based on the same sample of 227 configurations. A predictor is trained on the sample,[5] and a two-phase predicted Shapley value is calculated using the predictions for the full set of 2^{11} configurations. Figure 5.8 presents the results of this analysis. First, the three synapses with near-vanishing contributions according to the real Shapley value are the ones found as insignificant in the first phase of the procedure. Second, the final two-phase predicted Shapley value is much closer to the true contributions than the estimated Shapley value calculated in the first phase and with a much smaller standard deviation.

To examine the two-phase MSA procedure on a larger scale (thus losing the ability to calculate and compare to the true contributions), we turn to analyze the full recurrent synaptic network of S10, consisting of all 100 synapses. The first phase, using a small random sample consisting of 10 permutations, identifies 20 synapses as significant (two-sided t-tests, $\alpha = .05$). A predictor is trained on the set induced by this sample, and a two-phase predicted Shapley value is calculated from the predictions for the full set of 2^{20} synaptic perturbation configurations. The mean normalized training MSE corresponds to explaining more than 99.8% of the variance, which is five times more accurate than when training on the original sample consisting of configurations of all 100 synapses. Figure 5.9 displays the two-phase predicted Shapley value for the 20 significant synapses, illustrating small standard deviations of the contributions, testifying to their consistency. In this two-phase procedure, the nine synapses with largest contributions are the same ones found in the previous section using the single-phase MSA methods.

5.3.6   Bounded Perturbation Level Analysis

The k-bounded contributions enable one to examine the space between the contributions yielded by single perturbations only (single lesion analysis) and the contributions yielded by a full MSA. For

---

[5]The insignificant synapses are ignored in the perturbation configurations, and the performance scores of identical configurations are averaged, resulting in 164 configurations out of the 2^{11} possible ones.

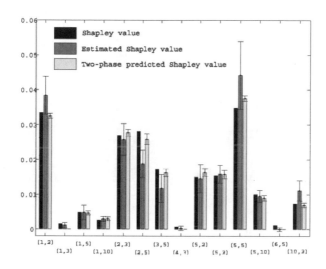

Fig. 5.8: Shapley value, estimated Shapley value (with standard deviation estimates) and two-phase predicted Shapley value (mean and standard deviation across 10 predictors in the second phase) for the 14 synapses network (see main text). Synapses found as insignificant in the first phase ((1,3), (4,3) and (6,5)) are assigned a two-phase predicted contribution of zero. In order for the different values to be comparable, they are not normalized, but rather the sum of the Shapley value and the sum of the estimated one equal $v(N) - v(\phi)$, where N is the group of all 14 synapses, and the sum of the two-phase predicted ones equals $v^{N'}(N') - v^{N'}(\phi)$, where N' is the group of the 11 significant synapses.

each $k = 1, 2, .., 10$, we calculated the k-bounded contributions of the neurons of the fault-tolerant agent F10. Figure 5.10 depicts the distance between the normalized k-bounded contributions vector and the normalized Shapley value vector of contributions as a function of k. The k-bounded contributions gradually approach the Shapley value, starting from the single-perturbation contributions which in this case are as far from the Shapley value as random normalized vectors are. A previous analysis has revealed the distance between the k-bounded contributions and the Shapley value to be larger for fault-tolerant neurocontrollers than for regular ones (Keinan, 2004).

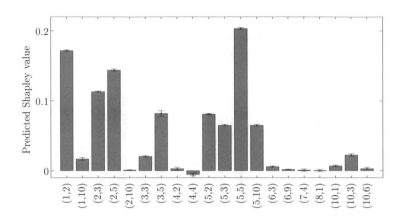

Fig. 5.9: Two-phase predicted Shapley value of the 20 synapses of S10 found as significant in the first phase (mean and standard deviation across 10 predictors).

5.3.7   Two-Dimensional Analysis

Based on the two-dimensional interactions presented earlier, Figure 5.11(a) portrays the results of a two-dimensional analysis performed on the counting agent W10, extending the one-dimensional analysis. Evidently, all pairs of significant neurons found previously in the one-dimensional analysis (1, 4, 9, and 10) exhibit strong synergism, whereas the pairs involving non-significant neurons exhibit weak synergism or weak antagonism. Specifically, neurons 4 and 9, participating in the counting process when waiting in a food cell, exhibit the strongest interaction. Further examining the marginal contributions of each with respect to the other, neuron 9 has a very significant contribution of 0.16 when neuron 4 is intact. When neuron 4 is perturbed, however, neuron 9 has a near-vanishing contribution of 0.005, showing that neuron 9 cannot count by itself without neuron 4. The opposite is also true, because neuron 4 has a significant contribution of 0.15 when neuron 9 is intact and a vanishing contribution when it is perturbed. Interestingly, the multitude of synergistic over antagonistic interactions indicates that there is an evolutionary pressure toward the formation of cooperation between neurons.

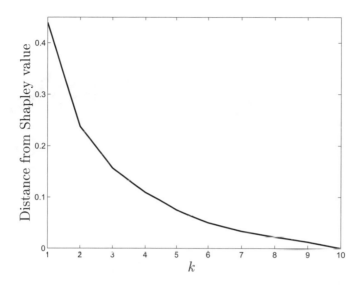

Fig. 5.10: k-bounded contributions versus Shapley value contributions. The Euclidean distance between the normalized MSA k-bounded contributions and the normalized full MSA contributions (the Shapley value) as a function of the perturbation level k, for agent F10.

Observing the interactions among all pairs of neurons of the fault-tolerant agent F10 (Figure 5.11(b)) reveals many negative ones, pointing to pairs of neurons that back up each other's function. These results exemplify the multiplicity of negative interactions in agents evolved while faults are introduced to the neurocontrollers. The necessity of fault-tolerance induces the emergence of functional overlap between the neurons at the expense of the formation of cooperation (Keinan, 2004).

5.4   DISCUSSION

This chapter describes a new framework for quantitative causal function localization via multi-perturbation experiments, the MSA (Keinan, Sandbank, Hilgetag, Meilijson & Ruppin, 2004, 2006). The MSA is

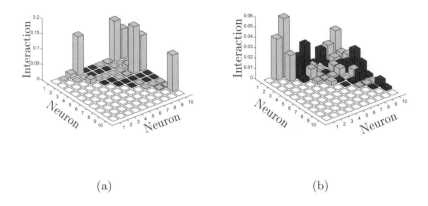

(a)   (b)

Fig. 5.11: Two-dimensional interactions. The symmetric interaction $I_{i,j}$ between each pair of neurons ($i < j$) is portrayed for agent W10 (a) and agent F10 (b). The figures present the absolute values of the interactions, with dark bars denoting the negative (antagonistic) interactions and light bars denoting the positive (synergistic) ones. Note the different scale of the two figures.

based on an axiomatic approach borrowed from Game Theory and yields a unique and fair attribution of contributions among the investigated elements in a system. We demonstrate the applicability of the MSA and its different variants to biological systems as well as artificial neurocontrollers. The more advanced scalable MSA variants, demonstrated in the analysis of the artificial neurocontrollers, are specifically geared toward experimental biological applications, in which only a limited number of multi-perturbation experiments can be performed.

We show that the MSA framework is capable of dealing with behavioral data from experimental deactivation studies of the cat brain, quantitatively identifying the main interaction underlying a paradoxical lesioning phenomenon observed previously in studies of spatial attention (Hilgetag, Kotter & Young, 1999; Hilgetag, Lomber & Payne, 2000; Lomber, Payne & Cornwell, 2001), along with suggesting important contributions of other cortical regions contributing to attention behavior.

As pointed out previously and as evident from effects such as paradoxical lesion phenomena and functional backup, single-perturbation approaches do not suffice to portray the correct function localization in a network. Why, then, has the great majority of perturbation studies in neuroscience until now relied on single perturbations? First, it has been difficult (and, in many systems, practically impossible) to reliably create and test multiple perturbations. Second, single-perturbation studies have been perceived as already being fairly successful in providing insights to the workings of neural systems. Naturally, the lack of a more rigorous multi-perturbation analysis has made the testing and validation of this perception practically impossible, and it may well have been the case that the lack of an analysis method has made such experiments seem futile. We hope that at least this last obstacle has been remedied by the introduction of the MSA.

Addressing the first issue—technical and scalability problems— we attempt to aid by approximating the correct contribution based on small samples of perturbation experiments. We demonstrate the MSA's applicability to large-scale systems by applying it to the analysis of EAAs solving a food-foraging task and guided by fully-recurrent neurocontrollers consisting of up to 100 synapses. The analysis uncovers the important neuronal and synaptic elements in each agent and quantifies their contributions to its performance, as well as their functional interactions.

As to the second concern, because multi-perturbation experiments are technically difficult and costly, an emerging question is whether the multiple-perturbation data will enhance our understanding of the system and, if so, to what extent. Within the MSA framework, this question is dealt in a quantitative manner, measuring the additional insights gained by performing a multi-perturbation analysis over a single-perturbation one. The MSA is currently being applied to quantify how misleading the picture isarising from classical single-perturbation analysis, utilizing an in-silico model of *S. cerevisiae* metabolism (Price, Papin, Schilling & Palsson, 2003) to compare the full information MSA results with those of the k-bounded analysis, gradually increasing k as demonstrated in this chapter for the analysis of a fault-tolerant agent. Such a procedure allows an exact quantification of the extent to which the multi-perturbations clarify the picture, which depends on the system's complexity.

An essential issue in any causal localization analysis is the choice of functions to be analyzed. Applying the MSA to a number of different functions performed by the same system will uncover the contribution of each element to each function separately. A thoughtful specification of these functions may help illuminate different aspects of the system's behavior. Constructing for each function a contribution vector, and describing the contribution of each of the elements to the specific function allow a comparison between functions in an analytical way. We can further assess the degree of localization of each function, as well as the extent to which each element is specialized to a given function. Analyzing the similarities between the functions' contribution patterns can imply which functions are processed in a similar way and suggest grouping elements into similar functional modules.

The MSA is a general function localization framework applicable to a wide variety of systems. Indeed, there are only two requirements for a system to be eligible to such an analysis: (a) an ability to inflict multi-perturbations on its constituent elements, and (b) an ability to measure its performance with respect to the studied functions. Recent technological advances have enabled real biological systems to meet these requirements. In neuroscience, lesioning, reversible deactivations, and Transcranial Magnetic Stimulation (TMS) all allow the collection of multi-perturbation performance data. TMS induces virtual lesions in normal subjects performing various cognitive and perceptual functions (Pascual-Leone, Wasserman, Davey & Rothwell, 2002; Rafal, 2001). The methodology can be utilized to co-deactivate doublets of brain sites (Hilgetag, Kotter, Theoret, Classen, Wolters & Pascual-Leone, 2003) and potentially even triplets. Additionally, recent retrospective lesion studies of stroke patients have reconstructed patients' lesions and analyzed the resulting multi-lesion data using statistical tools (e.g., Adolphs, Damasio, Tranel, Cooper & Damasio, 2000; Bates, Wilson, Saygin, Dick, Sereno, Knight & Dronkers, 2003). Such data may be more rigorously analyzed by the MSA, processing the multi-lesion data to capture the contributions of and the significant high-dimensional interactions between brain regions. Within this scope, we are currently utilizing MSA to analyze spatial attention in Unilateral Spatial Neglect (USN) patients, where the tested functions are the standard clinical tests that denote the severity of USN. The outcome of these studies can determine the long-lasting debate regarding which brain regions, or complexes of regions, damaged during strokes cause USN.

Going beyond the realm of neuroscience to biology in general, the recent discovery of RNA interference (RNAi, Hammond, Caudy & Hannon, 2001; Couzin, 2002) made the possibility of multiple concomitant gene knockouts a reality. Using RNAi, vectors it is now possible to temporarily block the transcription of specified genes for a certain duration and measure the performance of various cellular and metabolic indexes of the cell, including the expression levels of other genes. As with TMS, RNAi is limited at this stage to just a few elements that are knocked out concomitantly, but this is just the beginning. As the biological systems under investigation grow in size, the estimation variants of the MSA will be required for a computationally tractable analysis, with the bounded perturbation-level variant being of particular usefulness for such analyses.

A recent study successfully applied the MSA to analyze genetic systems based on gene multi-knockout experiments (Kaufman, Kupiec & Ruppin, 2004). Within the genetic network analysis setup, a few genes are knocked out together in each perturbation experiment, and the resulting performance level of the investigated UV survival function is recorded. Given these data, the MSA was capable of successfully identifying the importance of genes in the specific DNA repair pathway of the yeast *S. cerevisiae*, quantifying their contributions and characterizing their functional interactions. Incorporating additional biological knowledge, a new functional description of the pathway was provided, predicting the existence of additional genes involved in the pathway.

The MSA is the first framework to make sense out of such multi-perturbation experiments in a formal, axiomatic, and rigorous manner. The discussed variants extend its capabilities by increasing its scalability and allowing for the efficient analysis of large scale systems. Multi-perturbation studies are a necessity, and hence they are bound to take place, starting in the very near future. The MSA framework presented in this chapter is a harbinger of this new kind of studies, offering a way of making sense out of them.

Further MSA papers, as well as a Matlab(R) package implementing the various MSA methods, are available at http://www.cns.tau.ac.il/msa/. The package is freely available for academic use.

References

Adolphs, R., Damasio, H., Tranel, D., Cooper, G. & Damasio, A. R. (2000). A role for somatosensory cortices in the visual recognition of emotion as revealed by three-dimensional lesion mapping. *Journal of Neuroscience, 20(7),* 2683–2690.

Aharonov, R., Segev, L., Meilijson, I. & Ruppin, E. (2003). Localization of function via lesion analysis. *Neural Computation, 15(4),* 885–913.

Aharonov-Barki, R., Beker, T. & Ruppin, E. (2001). Emergence of memory-driven command neurons in evolved artificial agents. *Neural Computation, 13(3),* 691–716.

Banzhaf, J. F. (1965). Weighted voting doesn't work: a mathematical analysis. *Rutgers Law Review, 19,* 317–343.

Bates, E., Wilson, S. M., Saygin, A., Dick, F., Sereno, M. I., Knight, R. T. & Dronkers, N. F. (2003). Voxel-based lesion-symptom mapping. *Nature Neuroscience, 6(5),* 448–450.

Billera, L. J., Heath, D. & Raanan, J. (1978). Internal telephone billing rates—a novel application of non-atomic game theory. *Operations Research, 26,* 956–965.

Cangelosi, A. & Parisi, D. (1997). A neural network model of Caenorhabditis Elegans: The circuit of touch sensitivity. *Neural Processing Letters, 6,* 91–98.

Couzin, J. (2002). Small RNAs make big splash. *Science, 298,* 2296–2297.

Dubey, P., Neyman, A. & Weber, R. J. (1981). Value theory without efficiency. *Mathematics of Operations Research, 6(1),* 122–128.

Farah, M. J. (1990). *Visual agnosia.* Cambridge, MA: MIT Press.

Farah, M. J. (1996). Is face recognition 'special'? evidence from neuropsychology. *Behavioral Brain Research, 76,* 181–189.

Feigenbaum, J., Papadimitriou, C. H. & Shenker, S. (2001). Sharing the cost of multicast transmissions. *Journal of Computer and System Sciences, 63(1),* 21–41.

Ganon, Z., Keinan, A. & Ruppin, E. (2003). Evolutionary network minimization: Adaptive implicit pruning of successful agents. In Banzhaf, W., Christaller, T., Dittrich, P., Kim, J. T. & Ziegler, J. (Eds.), *Advances in Artificial Life - Proceedings of the 7th European Conference on Artificial Life (ECAL),* Volume 2801 of *Lecture Notes in Artificial Intelligence* (pp. 319–327). Springer Verlag Berlin, Heidelberg.

Gefeller, O., Land, M. & Eide, G. E. (1998). Averaging attributable fractions in the multifactorial situation: Assumptions and interpretation. *J Clin Epidemiol, 51(5),* 437–441.

Grabisch, M. & Roubens, M. (1999). An axiomatic approach to the concept of interaction among players in cooperative games. *International Journal of Game Theory, 28,* 547–565.

Grobstein, P. (1990). Strategies for analyzing complex organization in the nervous system: I. lesion experiments. In E. Schwartz (Ed.), *Computational neuroscience.* Cambridge, MA: MIT Press.

Hammond, S. M., Caudy, A. A. & Hannon, G. J. (2001). Post-transcriptional gene silencing by double-stranded RNA. *Nature Rev. Gen., 2(2),* 110–119.

Hilgetag, C. C., Kotter, R., Theoret, H., Classen, J., Wolters, A. & Pascual-Leone, A. (2003). A bilateral competitive network for visual spatial attention in humans. *Neurocomputing, 52–54,* 793–798.

Hilgetag, C. C., Kotter, R. & Young, M. P. (1999). Inter-hemispheric competition of sub-cortical structures is a crucial mechanism in paradoxical lesion effects and spatial neglect. *Prog Brain Res, 121,* 121–141.

Hilgetag, C. C., Lomber, S. G. & Payne, B. R. (2000). Neural mechanisms of spatial attention in the cat. *Neurocomputing, 38*, 1281–1287.

Hilgetag, C. C., Theoret, H. & Pascual-Leone, A. (2001). Enhanced visual spatial attention ipsilateral to rTMS-induced virtual lesions of human parietal cortex. *Nature Neuroscience, 4(9)*, 953–957.

Ijspeert, A. J., Hallam, J. & Willshaw, D. (1999). Evolving swimming controllers for a simulated lamprey with inspiration from neurobiology. *Adaptive Behavior, 7*, 151–172.

Kapur, N. (1996). Paradoxical functional facilitation in brain-behaviour research. A critical review. *Brain, 119*, 1775–1790.

Kaufman, A., Kupiec, M. & Ruppin, E. (2004). Multi-knockout genetic network analysis: The Rad6 example. In *Proceedings of the IEEE Computer Society Conference on Bioinformatics (CSB'04)*, (pp. 332–340).

Keinan, A. (2004). Analyzing evolved fault-tolerant neurocontrollers. In *Proceedings of the Ninth International Conference on the Simulation and Synthesis of Living Systems (ALIFE9)*.

Keinan, A., Meilijson, I. & Ruppin, E. (2003). Controlled analysis of neurocontrollers with informational lesioning. *Philosophical Transactions of the Royal Society of London: Series A, 361(1811)*, 2123–2144.

Keinan, A., Sandbank, B., Hilgetag, C. C., Meilijson, I. & Ruppin, E. (2004). Fair attribution of functional contribution in artificial and biological networks. *Neural Computation, 16(9)*, 1887–1915.

Keinan, A., Sandbank, B., Hilgetag, C. C., Meilijson, I. & Ruppin, E. (2006). Axiomatic scalable neurocontroller analysis via the Shapley value. *Artificial Life, 12(3)*, 333–352.

Kosslyn, S. M. (1999). If neuroimaging is the answer, what is the question? *Philosophical Transactions of the Royal Society of London: Series B, 354*, 1283–1294.

Lomber, S. G. & Payne, B. R. (1996). Removal of two halves restores the whole: Reversal of visual hemineglect during bilateral cortical or collicular inactivation in the cat. *Visual Neuroscience, (13)*, 1143–1156.

Lomber, S. G., Payne, B. R. & Cornwell, P. (2001). Role of the superior colliculus in analyses of space: Superficial and intermediate layer contributions to visual orienting, auditory orienting, and visuospatial discriminations during unilateral and bilateral deactivations. *J Comp Neurol, 441*, 44–57.

Lomber, S. G., Payne, B. R., Hilgetag, C. C. & Rushmore, R. J. (2002). Restoration of visual orienting into a cortically blind hemifield by reversible deactivation of posterior parietal cortex or the superior colliculus. *Exp Brain Res, 142*, 463–474.

Myerson, R. B. (1977). Graphs and cooperation in games. *Mathematics of Operations Research, 2*, 225–229.

Myerson, R. B. (1980). Conference structures and fair allocation rules. *International Journal of Game Theory, 9*, 169–182.

Pascual-Leone, A., Wasserman, E., Davey, N. & Rothwell, J. (2002). *Handbook of Transcranial Magnetic Stimulation*. Oxford University Press.

Price, N. D., Papin, J. A., Schilling, C. H. & Palsson, B. O. (2003). Genome-scale microbial in silico models: the constraints-based approach. *Trends Biotechnol, 21(4)*, 162–169.

Rafal, R. (2001). Virtual neurology. *Nature Neuroscience, 4(9)*, 862–864.

Roth, A. E. (1979). *Axiomatic models of bargaining*. Berlin: Springer Verlag.

Ruppin, E. (2002). Evolutionary autonomous agents: A neuroscience perspective. *Nature Reviews Neuroscience, 3*, 132–141.

Saggie, K., Keinan, A. & Ruppin, E. (2004). Spikes that count: Rethinking spikiness in neurally embedded systems. *Neurocomputing, 58–60C*, 303–311.

Shapley, L. S. (1953). A value for n-person games. In H. W. Kuhn & A. W. Tucker (Eds.), *Contributions to the Theory of Games*, Volume II of *Annals of Mathematics Studies 28* (pp. 307–317). Princeton: Princeton University Press.

Shapley, L. S. & Shubik, M. (1954). A method for evaluating the distribution of power in a committee system. *The American Political Science Review*, *48(3)*, 787–792.

Shubik, M. (1962). Incentives, decentralized control, the assignment of joint costs and internal pricing. *Management Science*, *8*, 325–343.

Shubik, M. (1985). *Game Theory in the Social Sciences*. Cambridge, MA: MIT Press.

Sitton, M., Mozer, M. & Farah, M. J. (2000). Superadditive effects of multiple lesions in a connectionist architecture: Implications for the neuropsychology of Optic aphasia. *Psychological Review*, *107*, 709–734.

Sprague, J. M. (1966). Interaction of cortex and Superior Colliculus in mediation of visually guided behavior in the cat. *Science*, *153*, 1544–1547.

Squire, L. R. (1992). Memory and the Hippocampus: A synthesis of findings with rats, monkeys, and humans. *Psychological Review*, *99*, 195–231.

Vallar, G. (1998). Spatial hemineglect in humans. *Trends in Cognitive Sciences*, *2*, 87–97.

Young, M. P., Hilgetag, C. C. & Scannell, J. W. (2000). On imputing function to structure from the behavioural effects of brain lesions. *Philosophical Transactions of the Royal Society of London: Series B*, *355*, 147–61.

6

Generalized Component Analysis and Blind Source Separation Methods for Analyzing Multichannel Brain Signals

Andrzej Cichocki
Riken, Brain Science Institute
and
Warsaw University of Technology

Blind source separation (BSS) and related methods, e.g., independent component analysis (ICA) are generally based on a wide class of unsupervised learning algorithms and they found potential applications in many areas from engineering to neuroscience. The recent trends in blind source separation and generalized component analysis (GCA) is to consider problems in the framework of matrix factorization or more general signals decomposition with probabilistic generative models and exploit a *priori* knowledge about true nature, morphology or structure of latent (hidden) variables or sources such as sparseness, spatio-temporal decorrelation, statistical independence, non-negativity, smoothness or lowest possible complexity. The goal of BSS can be considered as estimation of true physical sources and parameters of a mixing system, while objective of GCA is finding a new reduced or hierarchical and structured representation for the observed (sensor) data that can be interpreted as physically meaningful coding or blind signal decompositions. The key issue is to find a such transformation or coding which has true physical meaning and interpretation. In this paper we discuss some promising applications of BSS/GCA for analyzing multi-modal, multi-sensory data, especially EEG/MEG data. Moreover, we propose to apply these techniques for early detection of Alzheimer disease (AD) using EEG recordings. Furthermore, we briefly review some efficient unsupervised learning

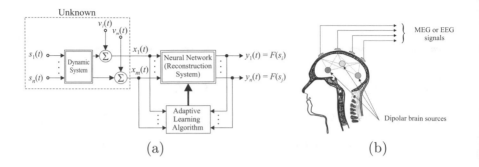

(a)   (b)

Fig. 6.1: (a) General model illustrating blind source separation (BSS).
(b) Such models are exploited in non-invasive multi-sensor recording
of brain activity using EEG (electroencephalography) or MEG (magnetoencephalography). It is assumed that the scalp sensors (electrodes,
SQUIDs) picks up superposition neuronal brain sources and non-brain
sources related, for example, to movements of eyes, muscles, and noise.
Objective is to identify the individual signals coming from different areas
of the brain.

algorithms for linear blind source separation, blind source extraction
and generalized component analysis using various criteria, constraints
and assumptions.

A fairly general blind signal separation (BSS) problem often referred to as blind signal decomposition or blind source extraction
(BSE) can be formulated as follows (see Figure 6.1).

We observe records of sensor signals $\mathbf{x}(t) = [x_1(t), \ldots, x_m(t)]^T$,
where t is time and $(\cdot)^T$ means transpose of a vector, from a MIMO
(multiple-input/multiple-output) dynamical (mixing and filtering) system. These signals are usually superposition of unknown source signals and noises. The objective is to find an inverse system, sometimes
termed a reconstruction system, neural network, or inverse system,
if it exists and is stable, to estimate all the primary source signals
$\mathbf{s}(t) = [s_1(t), \ldots, s_n(t)]^T$ or only some of them with specific properties. This estimation is performed on the basis of only the output
signals $\mathbf{y}(t) = [y_1(t), \ldots, y_n(t)]^T$. Preferably, the inverse (unmixing)
system should be adaptive in such a way that it has some tracking
capability in non-stationary environments. Instead of estimating the
source signals directly, it is sometimes more convenient to identify an

unknown mixing and filtering system first (e.g., when the inverse system does not exist, especially when the system is over-complete; i.e., the number of observations is less than the number of source signals with $m < n$) and then estimate source signals implicitly by exploiting some *a priori* information about the source signals and applying a suitable optimization procedure.

There appears to be something magical about blind source separation; we are estimating the original source signals without knowing the parameters of mixing and/or filtering processes. It is difficult to imagine that one can estimate this at all. In fact, without some *a priori* knowledge, it is not possible to *uniquely* estimate the original source signals. However, one can usually estimate them up to certain indeterminacies. In mathematical terms these indeterminacies and ambiguities can be expressed as arbitrary scaling and permutation of estimated source signals (Tong, Liu, Soon & Huang, 1991). These indeterminacies preserve, however, the waveforms of original sources. Although these indeterminacies seem to be rather severe limitations, in a great number of applications these limitations are not essential, since the most relevant information about the source signals is contained in the temporal waveforms or time-frequency patterns of the source signals and usually not in their amplitudes or order in which they are arranged in the output of the system.[1]

The problems of separating or extracting the source signals from the sensor array, without knowing the transmission channel characteristics and the sources, can be expressed briefly as a number of related BSS or generalized component analysis (GCA) methods such as Independent Component Analysis (ICA) (and its extensions: Topographic ICA, Multidimensional ICA, Kernel ICA, Tree-dependent Component Analysis, Multiresolution Subband Decomposition -ICA) (Hyvärinen, Karhunen & Oja, 2001; Bach & Jordan, 2003; Cichocki & Georgiev, 2003), Sparse Component Analysis (SCA) (Zibulevsky, Kisilev, Zeevi & Pearlmutter, 2002; Li, Cichocki & Amari, 2004; Washizawa & Cichocki, 2005; He & Cichocki, 2006), Sparse Prin-

---

[1] For some dynamical models, however, there is no guarantee that the estimated or extracted signals have exactly the same waveforms as the source signals, and then the requirements must be sometimes further relaxed to the extent that the extracted waveforms are distorted (i.e., time delayed, filtered, or convolved) versions of the primary source signals (see Figure 6.1(a)).

cipal Component Analysis (SPCA) (Chenubhotla, 2004; Zou, Hastie & Tibshirani, 2006), Multichannel Morphological Component Analysis (MMCA) (Bobin, Moudden, J.-L., Starck & Elad, 2006), Nonnegative Matrix Factorization (NMF) (Lee & Seung, 1999; Sajda, Du & Parra, 2003), Smooth Component Analysis (SmoCA) (Cichocki & Amari, 2003), Parallel Factor Analysis (PARAFAC) (Miwakeichi, Martinez-Montes, Valds-Sosa, Nishiyama, Mizuhara & Yamaguchi, 2004), Time-Frequency Component Analyzer (TFCA) (Belouchrani & Amin, 1996) and Multichannel Blind Deconvolution (MBD) (Amari & Cichocki, 1998; Zhang, Cichocki & Amari, 2004; Choi, Cichocki & Amari, 2002a).

The mixing and filtering processes of the unknown input sources s_j may have different mathematical or physical models depending on the specific applications (Hyvärinen, Karhunen & Oja, 2001; Amari & Cichocki, 1998). Most of the linear BSS models in the simplest forms can be expressed algebraically as some specific problems of matrix factorization: Given observation (often called sensor or data matrix) $\mathbf{X} = [\mathbf{x}(1), \ldots, \mathbf{x}(N)] \in \mathbb{R}^{m \times N}$ perform the matrix factorization:

$$\mathbf{X} = \mathbf{AS} + \mathbf{V},$$

where N is the number of available samples, m is the number of observations, n is the number of sources, $\mathbf{A} \in \mathbb{R}^{m \times n}$ represents the unknown basis data matrix or mixing matrix (depending on applications), $\mathbf{V} \in \mathbb{R}^{m \times N}$ is an unknown matrix representing errors or noise and matrix, $\mathbf{S} = [\mathbf{s}(1), \ldots, \mathbf{s}(N)] \in \mathbb{R}^{n \times N}$ contains the corresponding latent (hidden) components that give the contribution of each basis vectors. Usually these latent components represent unknown source signals with specific statistical properties or temporal structures. The matrices usually have clear statistical properties and meanings. For example, the rows of the matrix $\mathbf{S}$ that represent sources or components should be as sparse as possible for SCA or statistically mutually independent as possible for ICA. Often it is required that the estimated components are piecewise smooth (SmoCA) or take only non-negative values (NMF) or values with specific constraints (Lee & Seung, 1999; Cichocki & Georgiev, 2003).

Although some decompositions or matrix factorizations provide an exact reconstruction data (i.e., $\mathbf{X} = \mathbf{AS}$), we shall consider here decompositions which are approximative in nature. In fact, many

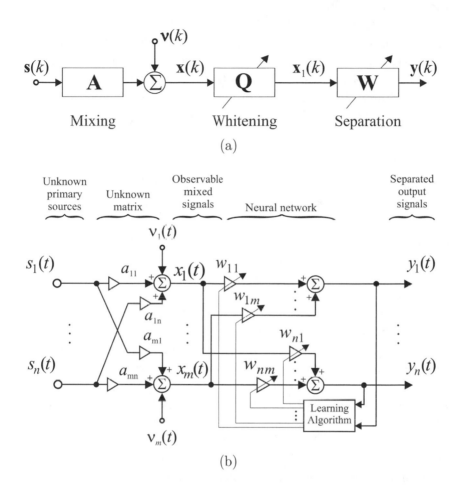

Fig. 6.2: Block diagrams illustrating linear blind source separation or blind identification problem: (a) General schema with optional whitening, (b) detailed model. For the over-complete problem $(m < n)$ the separating matrix $\mathbf{W}$ may not exist; in such cases, we attempt to identify the mixing matrix $\mathbf{A}$ first and next to estimate sources by exploiting some *a priori* knowledge such as sparsity or independence of unknown sources.

problems in signal and image processing can be expressed in such terms of matrix factorization. However, different cost functions and imposed constraints may lead to different types of matrix factorization. In many signal processing applications the data matrix $\mathbf{X} = [\mathbf{x}(1), \mathbf{x}(2) \ldots, \mathbf{x}(N)]$ is represented by vectors $\mathbf{x}(k)$ $(k = 1, 2, \ldots, N)$ for a set of discrete time instants $(k = t)$ as multiple measurements or recordings, thus the compact aggregated matrix equation can be written in a vector form as the system of linear equations (see Figure 6.2):

$$\mathbf{x}(k) = \mathbf{A}\,\mathbf{s}(k) + \mathbf{v}(k), \qquad (k = 1, 2 \ldots, N)$$

where

$$\mathbf{x}(k) = [x_1(k), x_2(k), \ldots, x_m(k)]^T$$

is the vector of the observed signals at the discrete time instant k while

$$\mathbf{s}(k) = [s_1(k), s_2(k), \ldots, s_n(k)]^T$$

is the vector of unknown sources at the same time instant.[2] The above formulated problems are related closely to linear inverse problems or, more generally, to solving a large ill-conditioned system of linear equations (overdetermined or under-determined depending on applications) where it is necessary to estimate reliably vectors $\mathbf{s}(k)$ and in some cases also to identify a matrix $\mathbf{A}$ for noisy data (Kreutz-Delgado, Murray, Rao, Engan, Lee & Sejnowski, 2003; Cichocki & Amari, 2003; Cichocki & Unbehauen, 1994). It is assumed that only the sensor vector $\mathbf{x}(k)$ is available, and it is necessary to design a feed-forward or recurrent neural network and an associated adaptive learning algorithm that enables estimation of sources, identification of the mixing matrix $\mathbf{A}$, and/or separating matrix $\mathbf{W}$ with good tracking abilities. Often BSS/GCA is obtained by finding an $n \times m$, full rank, linear transformation (separating) matrix $\mathbf{W} = \hat{\mathbf{A}}^+$, where $\mathbf{A}^+$ means Moore-Penrose pseudo-inverse of $\mathbf{A}$ such that the output signal vector $\mathbf{y} = [y_1, y_2, \ldots, y_n]^T$, defined by $\mathbf{y} = \mathbf{W}\mathbf{x}$, contains desired components (e.g., sparse, non-negative, independent, spatio-temporally decorrelated).

---

[2]Data are often represented not in the time domain, but in the complex frequency or the time frequency domain, so index k may have a different meaning.

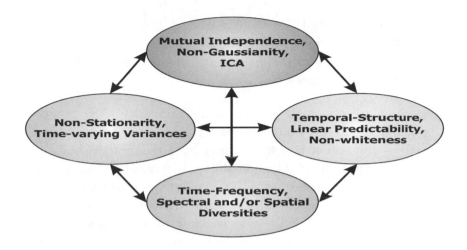

Fig. 6.3: Basic approaches for blind source separation. Each approach exploits some *a priori* knowledge and specific properties of the source signals (Cichocki & Amari, 2003).

Although many different source separation criteria and algorithms are available, their principles can be summarized by the following four fundamental approaches (see Figure 6.3):

- The most popular approach exploits as the cost function some measure of signals statistical independence, non-Gaussianity, or sparseness. When original sources are assumed to be statistically independent, the higher-order statistics (HOS) are essential (implicitly or explicitly) to solve the BSS problem. In such a case, the method does not allow more than one Gaussian source.

- If sources have temporal structures, then each source has non-vanishing temporal correlation, and less restrictive conditions than statistical independence can be used—namely, second-order statistics (SOS) are often sufficient to estimate the mixing matrix and sources. Along this line, several methods have been developed (Molgedey & Schuster, 1994; Belouchrani, Abed-Meraim, Cardoso & Moulines, 1997; Ziehe, Müller, Nolte, Mackert & Curio, 2000; Choi, Cichocki & Belouchrani, 2002c; Tong, Liu, Soon & Huang, 1991; Cichocki &

Belouchrani, 2001; Barros & Cichocki, 2001). Note that these SOS methods do not allow the separation of sources with identical power spectra shapes or i.i.d. (independent and identically distributed) sources.

- The third approach exploits non-stationarity (NS) properties and second-order statistics (SOS). Mainly, we are interested in the second-order non-stationarity in the sense that source variances vary in time. The non-stationarity was first taken into account by Matsuoka et al. (1995), and it was shown that a simple decorrelation technique is able for wide class of source signals to perform the BSS task. In contrast to other approaches, the non-stationarity information-based methods allow the separation of colored Gaussian sources with identical power spectra shapes. However, they do not allow the separation of sources with identical non-stationarity properties. There are some recent works on non-stationary source separation (Barros & Cichocki, 2001; Choi, Cichocki & Belouchrani, 2002c; Choi, Cichocki & Amari, 2002a).

  Methods that exploit either the temporal structure of sources (second-order correlations) and/or the non-stationarity variance of sources, lead in the simplest scenario to the SOS BSS methods. In contrast to BSS methods based on the HOS, all the SOS based methods do not have to infer the probability distributions of sources or nonlinear activation (score) functions (see next sections). This class of methods are referred as spatio-temporal decorrelation (STD) techniques.

- The fourth approach exploits the various diversities[3] of signals, typically, time, frequency, (spectral or "time coherence"), time-frequency diversities, or, more generally, joint space-time-frequency (STF) diversity. Such an approach leads to concept of Time-Frequency Component Analyzer (TFCA) (Cichocki & Amari, 2003). TFCA decomposes the signal into specific components in the time-frequency domain and computes the time-frequency representations (TFRs) of the individual components.

---

[3]By diversities we mean usually different morphology, characteristics or features of the signals.

Usually components are interpreted here as localized, sparse, and structured signals in the time-frequency plain (e.g, spectrogram). In TFCA components are estimated by analyzing the time-frequency distributions of the observed signals and suitable sparsification or decomposition of components. TFCA provides an elegant and promising solution to suppression of some artifacts and interference via masking and/or multi-bandpass filtering of undesired components.

More sophisticated or advanced approaches use combinations or integration of some of the above mentioned approaches: HOS, SOS, NS, and STF (Space-Time-Frequency) diversity in order to separate or extract sources with various morphology, structures or statistical properties and reduce the influence of noise and undesirable interferences.

The above-mentioned BSS methods belong to a wide class of unsupervised learning algorithms. Unsupervised learning algorithms try to discover a structure underlying a data set, extraction of meaningful features, and finding useful representations of the given data. Since data can always be interpreted in many different ways, some knowledge is needed to determine which features or properties represent our true latent (hidden) components. For example, PCA finds a low-dimensional representation of the data that captures most of its variance. On the other hand, SCA tries to explain data as a mixture of sparse components (usually in the time-frequency domain), and NMF seeks to explain data by parts-based localized additive representations (with non-negativity constraints).

Generalized component analysis algorithms (e.g., ICA, SCA, NMF, MMCA, STD, and SPCA) are often considered as pure mathematical formulas, powerful, but rather mechanical procedures: There is the illusion that there not very much left for the user to do after the machinery has been optimally implemented. The successful and efficient use of such tools strongly depends on *a priori* knowledge, common sense, and appropriate use of the preprocessing and postprocessing tools. In other words, it is preprocessing of data and postprocessing of models where an expertise is truly needed in order to extract and identify physiologically significant and meaningful components. Typical preprocessing tools include: Principal Component

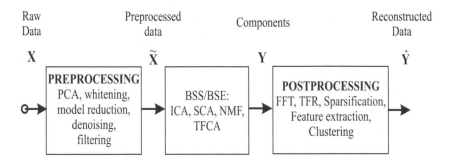

Fig. 6.4: Fundamental three stages implemented and exploited in the BSS/GCA for efficient separation, decomposition, and/or extraction of signals.

Analysis (PCA), Factor Analysis, (FA), whitening, model reduction, filtering, Fast Fourier Transform (FFT), Time Frequency Representation (TFR), and sparsification (Wavelets Package transformation, DCT, Curvelets, Ridgelets) of data (see Figure 6.4). Post-processing tools include: Deflation and reconstruction ("cleaning") of original raw data by removing undesirable components, noise, or artifacts (see Figure 6.5). On the other hand, the assumed linear mixing models must be valid at least approximately, and original source signals should have specified statistical properties (Cichocki & Amari, 2003; Amari & Cichocki, 1998; Cichocki, Amari, Siwek, Tanaka & et al., 2004a).

The main objective of this contribution is to propose extended BSS or GCA approaches which integrate or combine several different criteria to extract physiologically and neuroanatomically meaningful and plausible brain sources and to present their potential applications for analysis EEG/MEG, fMRI data, especially for very early detection of Alzheimer's disease (AD) using EEG recordings.

6.1 EXTENDED BLIND SOURCE SEPARATION AND GENERALIZED COMPONENT ANALYSIS APPROACH TO THE PREPROCESSING OF EEG AND MEG RECORDINGS

A great challenge in neurophysiology is to assess non-invasively the physiological changes occurring in different parts of the brain. These activations can be modeled and measured often as neuronal brain source signals that indicate the function or malfunction of various physiological sub-systems. To extract the relevant information for diagnosis and therapy, expert knowledge is required not only in medicine and neuroscience, but also statistical signal processing. To understand human neurophysiology, we currently rely on several types of non-invasive neuroimaging techniques. These techniques include electroencephalography (EEG) and magnetoencephalography (MEG) (Makeig, Delorme, M., Townsend, Courchense & Sejnowski, 2004b; Jahn, Cichocki, Ioannides & Amari, 1999).

In recent years, there has been great interest in applying high-density EEG systems to analyze patterns and imaging of the human brain, where EEG has the desirable property of excellent time resolution. This property, combined with other systems such as eye tracking and EMG (electromyography) systems with relatively low cost of instrumentation, makes it attractive for investigating the higher cognitive mechanisms in the brain and opens a unique window to investigate the dynamics of human brain functions as they are able to follow changes in neural activity on a millisecond time-scale. In comparison, the other functional imaging modalities, (e.g., positrontomography [PET] and functional magnetic resonance imaging [fMRI]), are limited in temporal resolution to time scales on the order of, at best, one second by physiological and signal-to-noise considerations.

Brain sources are extremely weak, nonstationary signals and usually distorted by large noise, interference, and ongoing activity of the brain. Moreover, they are mutually superimposed and low-passed filtered by EEG recording systems (see Figure 6.1 (b)). Besides classical signal analysis tools (such as adaptive supervised filtering, parametric or non-parametric spectral estimation, time-frequency analysis, and higher-order statistics), intelligent blind source separation techniques (IBSS) and generalized component analysis (GCA) can be used for analyzing brain data, especially for noise and artifact reduction, enhancement, detection, and estimation of neuronal brain source signals.

Determining active regions of the brain, given EEG/MEG measurements on the scalp is an important problem. A more accurate and reliable solution to such a problem can give information about higher brain functions and patient-specific cortical activity. However, estimating the location and distribution of electric current sources within the brain from EEG/MEG recording is an ill-posed problem since there is no unique solution and the solution does not depend continuously on the data. The ill-posedness of the problem and distortion of sensor signals by large noise sources make finding a correct solution a challenging analytic and computational problem.

If one knows the positions and orientations of the sources in the brain, one can calculate the patterns of electric potentials or magnetic fields on the surface of the head. This is called the forward problem. Otherwise, if one only has the patterns of electric potential or magnetic fields on the scalp level, one needs to calculate the locations and orientations of the sources. This is called the inverse problem. Inverse problems are notoriously more difficult to solve than forward problems. In this case, given only the electric potentials and magnetic fields on the scalp, there is no unique solution to the problem. The only hope is that there is some additional information available that can be used to constrain the infinite set of possible solutions to a single unique solution. This is where intelligent blind source separation can be used.

Every EEG electrode montage acts as a kind of spatial filter of cortical brain activity, and the BSS procedure can also be considered as a spatial filter which attempts to cancel the effect of superposition of various brain activities and possibly to estimate components that represent physiologically different processes (Makeig et al., 2004b,a; Delorme & Makeig, 2004).

BSS/GCA is a flexible and powerful approach for the elimination of artifacts and noise from EEG/MEG data and enhancement of neuronal brain sources. In fact, for these applications, ICA/BSS techniques have been successfully applied to remove artifacts and noise, including background brain activity, electrical activity of the

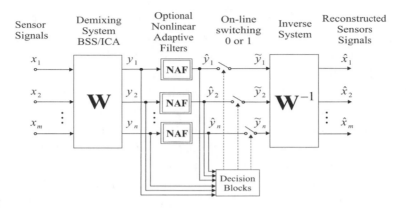

Fig. 6.5: Basic model of deflation for removing undesirable components like noise and artifacts and enhancing multi-sensory (e.g., EEG/MEG) data. Often the estimated components are first filtered, normalized, ranked, ordered, and clustered to identify significant and physiologically meaningful sources or artifacts.

heart, eye-blink and other muscle activity, and environmental noise efficiently (Jung, Makeig, Humphries, Lee, McKeown, Iragui & Sejnowski, 2000; Vorobyov & Cichocki, 2002; Jahn, Cichocki, Ioannides & Amari, 1999; Miwakeichi, Martinez-Montes, Valds-Sosa, Nishiyama, Mizuhara & Yamaguchi, 2004). However, most of the methods require manual detection, classification of interference components, and estimation of the cross-correlation between independent components and the reference signals corresponding to specific artifacts (Jung, Makeig, Humphries, Lee, McKeown, Iragui & Sejnowski, 2000; Makeig, Debener, Onton & Delorme, 2004a).

A conceptual model for the elimination of noise and other undesirable components from multi-sensory data is depicted in Figure 6.5. First, BSS is performed using a suitably chosen robust algorithm with respect to noise by a linear transformation of sensory data as $\mathbf{y}(k) = \mathbf{W}\mathbf{x}(k)$, where the vector $\mathbf{y}(k)$ represents the specific components (e.g., sparse, smooth, spatio-temporally decorrelated or statistically independent components). Then, the projection of interesting or useful components (e.g., independent activation maps) $\tilde{y}_j(k)$ back onto the sensors (electrodes). The corrected or "cleaned" sensor signals are obtained by linear transformation[4] $\hat{\mathbf{x}}(k) = \mathbf{W}^{-1}\tilde{\mathbf{y}}(k)$, where $\mathbf{W}^{-1}$ is the inverse or pseudo-inverse of the unmixing matrix $\mathbf{W}$ and $\tilde{\mathbf{y}}(k)$ is the vector obtained from the vector $\mathbf{y}(k)$ after removal of all the undesirable components (i.e., by replacing them with zeros). The entries of estimated attenuation (mixing) matrix $\hat{\mathbf{A}} = \mathbf{W}^{-1}$ indicate how strongly each electrode picks up each individual component. Back projection of some significant components $\hat{\mathbf{x}}(k) = \mathbf{W}^{-1}\tilde{\mathbf{y}}(k)$ allows us not only to remove some artifacts and noise but also to enhance EEG data.

In many cases, the estimated components must first be filtered or smoothed to identify all significant components. Moreover, the EEG/MEG data can be first decomposed into useful signal and noise subspaces using standard techniques such as PCA or Factor Analysis (FA) (see next sections). Next, we can apply BSS algorithms to decompose the observed signals (signal subspace) into specific components.

In addition to the denoising and artifacts removal, BSS/GCA techniques can be used to decompose EEG/MEG data into individual components, each representing possibly a physiologically distinct process or brain source. The main idea here is to apply localization and imaging methods to each of these components in turn. The decomposition is usually based on the underlying assumption of sparsity and/or statistical independence between the activation of different cell assemblies involved. Alternative criteria for the decomposition are: non-negativity, spatio-temporal decorrelation, temporal predictability, or smoothness of extracted components. The BSS approaches enable us to project each component (localized "brain source") onto an activation map at the skull level. For each activation map, we can apply an EEG/MEG source localization procedure, looking only for a single dipole (or brain source) per map. To localize a single component (say, a source $\hat{s}_j = \hat{y}_j$) we compute the sensor space projection (on the scalp level) for the source j

$$\hat{\mathbf{x}}_j(k) = \hat{\mathbf{A}}\mathbf{D}_j\mathbf{W}\mathbf{x}(k) = \hat{\mathbf{A}}\mathbf{D}_j\tilde{\mathbf{y}}(k) = \hat{\mathbf{a}}_j\hat{s}_j(k), \qquad (6.1)$$

where $\mathbf{D}_j$ is a diagonal matrix with all entries zero except for ones

---

[4]For simplicity, we assumed that $m = n$. In the more general case, for $m > n$ instead of the inverse matrix $\mathbf{W}^{-1}$, we use the Moore-Penrose pseudo-inverse generalized matrix $\mathbf{W}^{+}$.

on the j-th row and the j-th column $(j = 1, 2, \ldots, n)$ and $\hat{\mathbf{a}}_j$ is the j-th column of the estimated mixing matrix $\hat{\mathbf{A}} = \mathbf{W}^{-1}$. It is worth noting that $\hat{\mathbf{x}}_j(k)$ at each time instant k is uniquely represented by the fixed vector $\hat{\mathbf{a}}_j$, which is scaled by $\hat{s}_j(k)$, so dipole-fitting algorithms will localize j-th source to the some location independent on time instant (under the assumption that $\hat{\mathbf{A}}$ is fixed). The sensor space back projection of each component can be used as input data to any localization algorithm for source modeling (e.g., BESA). By localizing multiple sources independently one by one, we can dramatically increase the likelihood of efficiently converging to the correct and reliable solutions for the electromagnetic inverse problems.

One of the biggest strengths of the BSS/GCA approach is that it offers a variety of powerful and efficient algorithms that are able to estimate various kind of sources (sparse, non-negative, statistically independent, spatio-temporally decorrelated, smooth etc.). Some of the algorithms (e.g., AMUSE or TICA Cichocki & Amari, 2003; Cruces, Cichocki & Amari, 2004; Cruces & Cichocki, 2003) are able to automatically rank and order the components according to their complexity or sparseness measures. Some algorithms are quite robust with respect to noise (e.g., SOBI or SONS) (Belouchrani, Abed-Meraim, Cardoso & Moulines, 1997; Choi, Cichocki & Amari, 2002a; Choi, Cichocki & Belouchrani, 2002c; Choi, Cichocki & Amari, 1998).

In real world scenarios, latent (hidden) components (e.g., brain sources) have various complex properties and features. In other words, true unknown involved sources are seldom all sparse or only all statistically independent or all spatio-temporally decorrelated , etc.. Therefore, if we apply only one single technique like ICA, SCA, or STD, we usually fail to extract all interesting components. We need rather to apply fusion strategy by employing several suitably chosen criteria and associated algorithms to extract all desired sources. For this reason, we recommend using algorithms in cascade (multiple) or parallel mode to extract components with various features and statistical properties (Cichocki & Amari, 2003). In other words, we may apply two possible approaches. The most promising approach is a sequential blind extraction (see Figure 6.6), in which we extract components one by one in each stage applying different criterion (e.g., statistical independence, sparseness. smoothness, etc). In this way, we can sequentially extract different components with various statis-

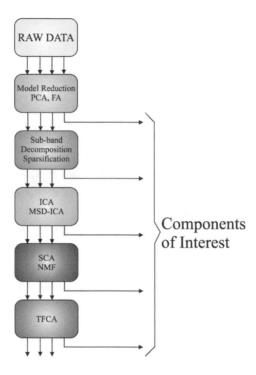

Fig. 6.6: Conceptual model of sequential blind sources extraction. In each stage, different criteria can be used.

tical properties.

In an alternative approach, after suitable preprocessing, we perform simultaneously (in parallel) several GCA (ICA, SCA, MMCA, STD, TFCA). Next the estimated components are normalized, ranked, clustered, and compared to each other using some similarity measures (see Figure 6.7). Furthermore, the components are back-projected to scalp level, and hypothetic brain sources are localized on the basis of clusters of subcomponents. In this way, on the basis of statistics and *a priori* knowledge (e.g., information about external stimuli for event-related brain sources), we can identify sources with electrophysiological meaning and specific anatomic localizations.

In summary, blind source separation and generalized component analysis (BSS/GCA) algorithms allow investigators to accomplish the following:

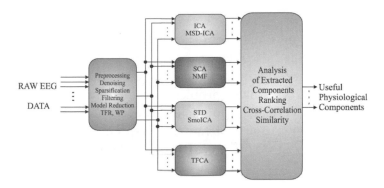

Fig. 6.7: Parallel model of GCA employing fusion strategy with various component analysis algorithms for estimation of physiologically and neuroanatomically meaningful event-related brain sources. The reliability of estimated sources or components should be analyzed by investigating the spread of the obtained components for many trials and possibly many subjects. Usually, the reliable and significant components correspond to small and well-separated clusters from the rest of the components, whereas unreliable components usually do not belong to any cluster.

1. Extract and remove artifacts and noise from raw EEG/MEG data.

2. Recover neuronal brain sources activated in cortex (especially in auditory, visual, somatosensory, motoric, and olfactory cortex).

3. Improve the signal-to-noise ratio (SNR) of evoked potentials (EPs), especially AEP, VEP and SEP.

4. Improve spatial resolution of EEG and reduce the level of subjectivity involved in the brain source localization.

Above mentioned applications of BSS/GCA show special promise in the areas of non-invasive human brain imaging techniques to delineate the neural processes that underlie human cognition and sensorimotor functions. These techniques lead to interesting and exciting new ways of investigating and analyzing brain data and develop new hypotheses about how the neural assemblies communicate and process information. The fundamental problems here are: What are the system's real properties and how can we get information about them? What is valuable information in the observed data and what is only noise or interference? How can the observed (sensor) data be transformed into features or components characterizing the brain sources in a reasonable way? These problems are actually an extensive research area, and presented approaches still remain to be validated at least experimentally to obtain full gain, especially for multi-sensory and multi-modal (EEG, MEG fMRI, PET) data.

6.2   EARLY DETECTION OF ALZHEIMER DISEASE US-ING BLIND SOURCE SEPARATION AND GENER-ALIZED COMPONENT ANALYSIS OF EEG DATA

Finding electrophysiological and other markers of different diseases and psychiatric disorders is generating increasing interest (Jeong, 2004; Petersen, Stevens, Ganguli, Tangalos, Cummings & DeKosky, 2001). The series of studies we have undertaken has been an attempt to find such markers for differential diagnosis of aging, especially for mild cognitive impairment (MCI) and Alzheimer's disease (AD) through BSS/GCA of EEG recordings (Cichocki, Shishkin, Musha, Leonowicz, Asada & Kurachi, 2005; Vialatte, Cichocki, Dreyfus, Musha, Shishkin & Gervais, 2005).

Alzheimer's disease (AD) is characterized by the degeneration of cortical neurons and the presence amyloid plaques and neurofibrillary tangles. These pathological changes, which begin in the entorhinal cortex, gradually spread across the brain, destroying the hippocampus and neocortex. Recent advances in drug treatment for dementia, particularly the acetylcholinesterase inhibitors for AD, are most effective in early stages, which are difficult to accurately diagnose. Recent studies demonstrated that AD has a pre-symptomatic phase, likely lasting years, during which neuronal degeneration is occurring, but clinical symptoms are not clearly observable (Jeong, 2004; DeKosky & Marek, 2003; Petersen, 2003). Since early diagnosis of AD may alter the outcome of the disease, the development of a practical diagnostic test that can detect the presence of the disease well before clinical symptoms is of increasing importance (Musha, Asada, Yamashita, T., Chen, Matsuda, Uno & Shankle, 2002; Jelic, Johansson,

Almkvist, Shigeta, Julin, Nordberg, Winblad & Wahlund, 2000; Petersen, 2003). A diagnostic device should be inexpensive, to make possible screening of many individuals who are at risk of developing this dangerous disease. The electroencephalogram (EEG) is one of the most promising candidates for such a device, since it is cheap and portable; in addition, noninvasive recording of EEG data is safe and simple. However, while many signal processing techniques have already been applied for revealing pathological changes in EEG associated with AD (see Jeong, 2004; Petersen, 2003; Cichocki, Shishkin, Musha, Leonowicz, Asada & Kurachi, 2005; Vialatte, Cichocki, Dreyfus, Musha, Shishkin & Gervais, 2005, for reviews), EEG-based detection of AD at its most early stages is still not sufficiently reliable, and further improvements are necessary. Moreover, the efficiency of early detection of AD is lower for standard EEG compared with modern neuroimaging techniques (fMRI, PET, SPECT), and it is considered only as an additional diagnostic tool (Wagner, 2000; DeKosky & Marek, 2003). This is why a number of more sophisticated or advanced multistage data analysis and signal processing approaches with optimization should be applied to this problem.

6.2.1   Methods for Blind Recovery of Electrophysiological Markers of Alzheimer's Disease

To our best knowledge, no study until now has been reported about the application of BSS and GCA methods as preprocessing tools in AD diagnosis (Cichocki, Shishkin, Musha, Leonowicz, Asada & Kurachi, 2005). Generally speaking, in our novel approach, we first decompose EEG data into suitable components (especially spatio-temporal decorrelated, independent, and/or sparse). Next we rank them according to some measures (such as linear predictability, increasing complexity, or sparseness), and then we project to the scalp level only some significant and specific components, possibly of physiological origin, that could be apparently the brain signal markers for dementia and, more specifically, for Alzheimer's disease (see Figure 6.8).

We believe that BSS/GCA are promising methods for discrimination dementia due the following reasons:

1. GCA and BSS algorithms allow us to extract and eliminate

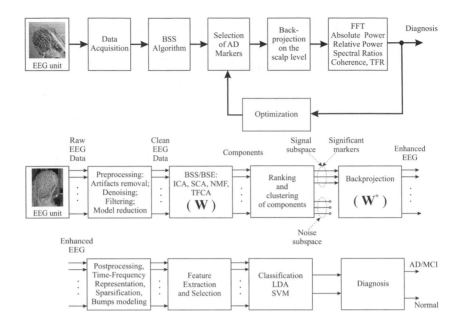

Fig. 6.8: Conceptual block diagrams of the proposed preprocessing (enhancement and filtering) method for early diagnosis of AD; the main novelty lies in suitable ordering of components and selection of only a few significant AD markers (components) and back-projecting (deflation) of these components on the scalp level for further analysis and processing in the frequency or the time-frequency domain using sparsification, bump modeling, and feature extraction. The components are selected via an optimization procedure.

various artifacts and high-frequency noise and interference. In this way, we can improve the signal-to-noise ratio and enhance some significant brain source signals.

2. BSS/GCA algorithms, especially those with equivariant and nonholonomic properties, allow us to extract extremely weak brain sources (Cichocki, Unbehauen & Rummert, 1994; Cichocki & Amari, 2003), probably corresponding to the sources located deep in the brain, e.g., in the entorhinal cortex and hippocampus.

One of the hallmarks of EEG abnormalities in AD patients is a shift of the power spectrum to lower frequencies. There is general agreement in literature that the earliest changes in the EEG abnormalities are observed in increasing theta activity and decreasing beta activity, which are followed by a decrease of alpha activity (Jeong, 2004; Musha, Asada, Yamashita, T., Chen, Matsuda, Uno & Shankle, 2002; Jelic, Johansson, Almkvist, Shigeta, Julin, Nordberg, Winblad & Wahlund, 2000). Delta activity typically increases later during the progression of the disease. This suggests that an increase of theta power and a decrease in beta and alpha powers are markers for the subsequent rate of a cognitive and functional decline in early and mild stages of AD. However, these changes in the early stage of AD can be very small and distorted by many factors, thus detection of them directly from raw EEG data is rather difficult . Therefore, we exploit these properties for suitably filtered or enhanced data, rather than for raw EEG data. This filtering is performed using BSS techniques described in the next sections. The basic idea can be formulated as filtering based on BSS/GCA via selection of most relevant or significant components and project them back to scalp level (Cichocki, Shishkin, Musha, Leonowicz, Asada & Kurachi, 2005; Vialatte, Cichocki, Dreyfus, Musha, Shishkin & Gervais, 2005).

In a strict sense, BSS means estimation of true (original) neuronal brain sources, whereas GCA means decomposition of EEG data to meaningful components, although exactly the same procedure can be used for separation of two or more subspaces of the signal without estimation of true sources (see the next section). One procedure currently becoming popular in EEG analysis is removing artifact-related independent components and back projection of independent components originating from the brain (Jung, Makeig, Humphries, Lee, McKeown, Iragui & Sejnowski, 2000; Vorobyov & Cichocki, 2002). In this procedure, components of brain origin are not required to be separated from each other exactly because they are mixed again by back projection after removing artifact-related components. By the similar procedure, we can filter off the ongoing "brain noise" also in a wider sense, improving the signal-to-noise ratio (SNR).

In a recently-developed and very simple procedure, we do not attempt to identify individual brain sources or physiologically meaningful components but rather identify the whole group or cluster of significant AD components (Cichocki, Shishkin, Musha, Leonowicz, Asada

& Kurachi, 2005). In other words, we divide the available EEG data into two subspaces: brain signal subspace and "brain noise" subspace. Finding a fundamental mechanism or principle for identification of significant and non-significant components is critical in our approach and, in general, may require more extensive studies. We attempt here to differentiate clusters or subspaces of components with similar properties or features. In this simple approach, the estimation of all individual components corresponding to separate and physiologically meaningful brain sources is not required, unlike in other applications of BSS to EEG processing discussed in the previous section. The use of clusters of components could be especially beneficial when the data from different subjects are compared: Similarities among individual components for different subjects are usually low, whereas subspaces formed by similar components are more likely to be sufficiently consistent. Differentiation of signal and noise subspaces with high and low amounts of diagnostically useful information can be made easier if components are separated and sorted according to some criterion which, at least to some extent, correlate with the diagnostic value of components. For this reason, we have applied the AMUSE BSS algorithm, which provides automatic ordering of components according to decreasing variance and simultaneously decreasing their linear predictability (see Figure 6.9). The main advantage of AMUSE over other BSS algorithms was highly reproducible components with respect to their ranking or ordering and also across subjects belonging to the same of group of patients. This allows us to identify significant components and optimize their number.

The proposed AMUSE BSS algorithm (see the next sections for details) performs linear decomposition of EEG signals into precisely ordered spatio-temporal decorrelated components that have the lowest possible complexity (in the sense of best linear predictability) (Stone, 2001; Cichocki & Amari, 2003). In other words, in the frequency domain, the power spectra of components have possibly distinct shapes.

Artifact-free 20-second intervals of raw resting EEG recordings from 23 early stage AD patients and 38 age-matched healthy controls were decomposed into spatio-temporally decorrelated components using BSS algorithm AMUSE. AD patients had, at the time of EEG recording, only memory impairment, but no apparent loss in general

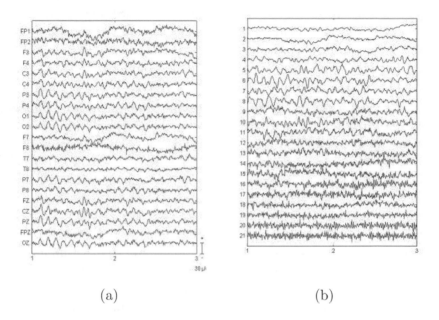

(a)   (b)

Fig. 6.9: Example of raw EEG (a) and its components separated with AMUSE STD algorithm, and (b) for a patient with early stage AD (EarlyAD15). AMUSE was applied to 20 s artifact-free interval of EEG, but only 2 s are shown here. The scale for the components is arbitrary, but linear. Note that the components are automatically ordered according to decreasing linear predictability (increasing complexity).

cognitive, behavioral, or functional status. The MMSE (Mini-Mental Status Exam) score was 24 or higher at the time of recording, and diagnosis was made during follow-up clinical evaluation within the next 12-18 months. Recording was made with eyes closed in an awake resting condition (with vigilance control) using 21 electrodes according to the 10-20 international system, with a sampling frequency of 200 Hz (Musha, Asada, Yamashita, T., Chen, Matsuda, Uno & Shankle, 2002).

We found by extensive experiments that filtering and enhancement of EEG data are the best if we reject components with lowest variance and back project only the first 5-7 spatio-temporally decorrelated components with highest linear predictability and largest variance. Automatic sorting of components by AMUSE algorithm makes it possible to perform this simply and consistently for all subjects by removing components with an index higher than some chosen threshold (in our case, we projected the first six components for 10-20 international EEG system).

After back-projecting the six significant components to scalp level, we performed a standard spectral analysis based on FFT of reconstructed or filtered EEG data and applied linear discriminant analysis (LDA) (Cichocki, Shishkin, Musha, Leonowicz, Asada & Kurachi, 2005) to combine relative power in various frequency bands. Relative spectral powers were computed by dividing the power in six standard frequency bands: delta (1 - 4 Hz), theta (4-8 Hz), alpha 1 (8-10 Hz), alpha 2 (10-13 Hz), beta 1 (13-18 Hz), and beta 2 (18-22 Hz) by the power in 1-22 Hz band. To reduce the number of variables used for classification, we averaged band power values over all 21 channels. Relative power of filtered data in the six bands was processed with the LDA. We found that the filtering or enhancement method based on the BSS AMUSE approach increases differentiability between early stage AD patients and age-matched healthy controls, and considerably improves sensitivity and specificity (from 12% to 18% in comparison to the standard approach without BSS filtering), and gives 86% overall correct classification accuracy.

In particular, our computer simulations indicate that several specific spatio-temporal decorrelated components in the lower frequency range (theta waves 4-8 Hz) and also in the higher frequency range (beta waves 13-22 Hz) have substantially different magnitudes of relative power for early and mild-stage AD patients than for age-matched healthy subjects. In fact, the components in the theta band have higher magnitude of relative power for AD patients, while the components in the beta band have lower magnitude of the relative power in comparison to normal age-matching healthy subjects (see Figure 6.10).

There is obviously room for improvement and extension of the proposed method both, in ranking and selection of optimal (significant) components, apparatus, and post-processing to perform the classification task. In particular, we can apply a variety of BSS/GCA methods discussed in this chapter. We are actually investigating sev-

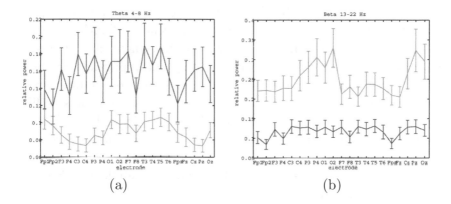

(a)   (b)

Fig. 6.10: Plots of average distribution of relative power for all 21 electrodes for 23 AD patients (blue (dark) lines) and 38 age-matched healthy subjects (green (light) lines) for: (a) theta band, (b) beta band. Error bars indicate the standard deviation fluctuation around the average values of the relative power. These plots indicate that several specific spatio-temporally decorrelated components (back projected to the scalp level) in low-frequency bands (theta waves 4-8 Hz, Figure (a)) and high-frequency band (beta waves 13-22 Hz, Figure (b)) show different magnitudes of relative power for AD patients (blue (dark) lines) and controls (green (light) lines). These components in the case of theta waves have higher relative power for AD patients whereas the same components for beta waves have lower relative power in comparison with normal age-matched healthy subjects. For delta waves (1-4 Hz) and alpha waves (8-13 Hz), we have observed (not shown) also some (but much smaller) differences in the magnitude of relative power between AD patients and the healthy subjects.

eral alternative, more sophisticated, and even more promising approaches, in which we employ a family of BSS algorithms (rather than one single AMUSE BSS algorithm), as explained in the previous section, to extract from raw EEG data significant components whose time courses and electrode projections corresponded to neurophysiologically and neuroanatomically meaningful activations of separate brain regions. We believe that such an approach will enable us to extract not only various noise and artifacts from neuronal signals, but also, under favorable circumstances, to estimate physiologically and functionally distinct neuronal brain sources. Some of them may represent local field activities of the human brain and could be significant markers for early stage AD. To confirm these hypotheses, we need more experimental and simulation works. Nevertheless, by virtue of separating various neuronal and noise/artifacts sources, BSS/GCA techniques offer at least a way of improving the effective SNR and enhancing some brain patterns.

Furthermore, instead of standard linear discriminant analysis (LDA), we can use neural networks or support vector machine (SVM) classifiers. We expect to obtain even better discrimination and sensitivity if we apply these methods. Moreover, classification can be further improved by supplementing the set of spectral power measures which we used with much different indices, such as coherence (Jelic, Johansson, Almkvist, Shigeta, Julin, Nordberg, Winblad & Wahlund, 2000) or alpha dipolarity, a new index depending on prevalence local vs. distributed sources of EEG alpha activity, which was shown to be very sensitive to mild AD (Musha, Asada, Yamashita, T., Chen, Matsuda, Uno & Shankle, 2002).

An additional attractive but still open issue is that, using the proposed BSS/GCA approach, we can detect and measure in a consistent way the progression of AD and influence of medications. Another important open issue is to establish relations of the extracted AD-sensitive EEG components to currently existing neuroimaging, genetic, and biochemical markers (Jelic, Johansson, Almkvist, Shigeta, Julin, Nordberg, Winblad & Wahlund, 2000). The proposed method can also be a potentially useful and effective tool for differential diagnosis of AD from other types of dementia, and possibly for diagnosis of other mental diseases. Particularly, the possibility of differential diagnosis of AD from vascular dementia (VaD) will be very important. For these purposes, more studies would be needed to assess the usefulness and efficiency of the available and future blind source separation and generalized component analysis methods for enhancement/filtering and extraction of the EEG/MEG, fMRI, PET latent components.

6.3 PRINCIPAL COMPONENT ANALYSIS—SIGNAL AND NOISE SUBSPACES

Principal component analysis (PCA) is perhaps one of the oldest and best-known techniques in multivariate analysis and data mining. It was introduced by Pearson, who used it in a biological context, and further developed by Hotelling in works done on psychometry. PCA was also developed independently by Karhunen in the context of probability theory and was subsequently generalized by Loève (see, e.g., Cichocki, Kasprzak & Skarbek, 1996; Rosipal, Girolami, Trejo & Cichocki, 2001; Wang, Lee, Fiori, Leung & Zhu, 2003, and references therein). The purpose of PCA is to derive a relatively small number of uncorrelated linear combinations (principal components) of a set of random zero-mean variables while retaining as much of the information from the original variables as possible. Often the principal components (PCs) (i.e., directions on which the input data have the largest variances) are usually regarded as important or significant, whereas those components with the smallest variances, called minor components (MCs), are usually regarded as unimportant or associated with noise. However, in some applications, the MCs are of the same importance as the PCs—for example, in curve- and surface-fitting or total least squares (TLS) problems (Cichocki & Unbehauen, 1994).

PCA can be converted to the eigenvalue problem of the covariance matrix of $\mathbf{x}(k)$ and it is essentially equivalent to the Karhunen-Loève transform used in image and signal processing. In other words, PCA is a technique for computation of eigenvectors and eigenvalues for the estimated covariance matrix

$$\mathbf{R_{xx}} = E\{\mathbf{x}(k)\,\mathbf{x}^T(k)\} = \mathbf{V}\,\mathbf{\Lambda}\,\mathbf{V}^T \in \mathbb{R}^{m \times m}, \qquad (6.2)$$

where $\mathbf{\Lambda} = \mathrm{diag}\,\{\lambda_1, \lambda_2, ..., \lambda_m\}$ is a diagonal matrix containing the m eigenvalues and $\mathbf{V} = [\mathbf{v}_1, \mathbf{v}_2, \ldots, \mathbf{v}_m] \in \mathbb{R}^{m \times m}$ is the corresponding orthogonal or unitary matrix consisting of the unit length eigenvectors referred to as principal eigenvectors. PCA can be also done via the singular value decomposition (SVD) of the batch data matrix $\mathbf{X} = [\mathbf{x}(1), \mathbf{x}(2), \ldots, \mathbf{x}(N)]$.

The Karhunen-Loéve transform determines a linear transformation of an input vector $\mathbf{x}$ as

$$\mathbf{y}_P = \mathbf{V}_S^T \mathbf{x}, \tag{6.3}$$

where $\mathbf{x} = [x_1(k), x_2(k), \ldots, x_m(k)]^T$ is the zero-mean input vector, $\mathbf{y}_P = [y_1(k), y_2(k), \ldots, y_n(k)]^T$ $(n < m)$ is the output vector called the vector of principal components (PCs), and $\mathbf{V}_S = [\mathbf{v}_1, \mathbf{v}_2, \ldots, \mathbf{v}_n]$ $\in \mathbb{R}^{m \times n}$ is the set of signal subspace eigenvectors, with the orthonormal vectors $\mathbf{v}_i = [v_{i1}, v_{i2}, \ldots, v_{im}]^T$ (i.e., $(\mathbf{v}_i^T \mathbf{v}_j = \delta_{ij})$ for $j \leq i$, where δ_{ij} is the Kronecker delta equals to 1 for $i = j$, otherwise zero. The vectors $\mathbf{v}_i$ $(i = 1, 2, \ldots, n)$ are eigenvectors of the covariance matrix, while the variances of the PCs $y_i(k) = \mathbf{v}_i^T \mathbf{x}(k)$ are the corresponding principal eigenvalues. On the other hand, the $(m - n)$ minor components are given by

$$\mathbf{y}_M = \mathbf{V}_N^T \mathbf{x}, \tag{6.4}$$

where $\mathbf{V}_N = [\mathbf{v}_m, \mathbf{v}_{m-1}, \ldots, \mathbf{v}_{m-n+1}]$ consists of the $(m - n)$ eigenvectors associated with the smallest eigenvalues.

An important problem arising in many application areas is determination of the dimension of the signal and noise subspaces. In other words, a central issue in PCA is choosing the number of principal components to be retained. To solve this problem, we usually exploit a fundamental property of PCA: It projects the input data $\mathbf{x}(k)$ from their original m-dimensional space onto an n-dimensional output subspace $\mathbf{y}(k)$ (typically, with $n \ll m$), thus performing a dimensionality reduction which retains most of the intrinsic information in the input data vectors. In other words, the principal components $y_i(k) = \mathbf{v}_i^T \mathbf{x}(k)$ are estimated in such a way that, for $n < m$, although the dimensionality of data is strongly reduced, the most relevant information is retained in the sense that the original input data $\mathbf{x}$ can be reconstructed from the output data (signals) $\mathbf{y}$ by using the transformation $\hat{\mathbf{x}} = \mathbf{V}_S \mathbf{y}$, that minimizes a suitable cost function. A commonly used criterion is the minimization of mean squared error $\|\mathbf{x} - \mathbf{V}_S^T \mathbf{V}_S \mathbf{x}\|_2^2$.

PCA enables us to divide observed (measured) sensor signals: $\mathbf{x}(k) = \mathbf{x}_s(k) + \boldsymbol{\nu}(k)$ into two subspaces: the *signal subspace* corresponding to principal components associated with the largest eigenvalues called principal eigenvalues: $\lambda_1, \lambda_2, ..., \lambda_n$, $(m > n)$ and associated eigenvectors $\mathbf{V}_s = [\mathbf{v}_1, \mathbf{v}_2, \ldots, \mathbf{v}_n]$ called the principal eigenvectors and the *noise subspace* corresponding to the minor components associated with the eigenvalues $\lambda_{n+1}, ..., \lambda_m$. The subspace spanned by the n first eigenvectors $\mathbf{v}_i$ can be considered as an approximation of the noiseless signal subspace. One important advantage of this approach is that it enables not only a reduction in the noise level, but also allows us to estimate the number of sources on the basis of the distribution of eigenvalues. However, a problem arising from this approach is how to correctly set or estimate the threshold which divides eigenvalues into the two subspaces, especially when the noise is large (i.e., the SNR is low).

6.3.1   Probabilistic PCA—Expectation Maximization Algorithm

Let us assume that we model the vector $\mathbf{x}(k) \subset \mathbb{R}^m$ as

$$\mathbf{x}(k) = \mathbf{A}\,\mathbf{s}(k) + \boldsymbol{\nu}(k), \tag{6.5}$$

where $\mathbf{A} \in \mathbb{R}^{m \times n}$ is a full column rank mixing matrix, with $m > n$ representing factor loading, $\mathbf{s}(k) \in \mathbb{R}^n$ is a vector of zero-mean Gaussian sources with the nonsingular covariance matrix $\mathbf{R_{ss}} = E\{\mathbf{s}(k)\mathbf{s}^T(k)\}$ and $\boldsymbol{\nu}(k) \in \mathbb{R}^m$ is a vector of Gaussian zero-mean i.i.d. noise modeled by the covariance matrix $\mathbf{R}_{\boldsymbol{\nu}\boldsymbol{\nu}} = \sigma_\nu^2 \mathbf{I}_m$, furthermore, random vectors $\{\mathbf{s}(k)\}$ and $\{\boldsymbol{\nu}(k)\}$ are uncorrelated.

The model given by Equation 6.5 is often referred to as probabilistic PCA (PPCA) and has been introduced in the machine learning context. Moreover, such a model can also be considered as a special form of Factor Analysis (FA) with isotropic noise. The only difference is that, in FA, the noise covariance matrix can be, in general, an arbitrary positive definite diagonal matrix. Under the above assumptions, the maximum likelihood estimator of matrix $\mathbf{A}$ in the linear generative model (6.5) is given by

$$\hat{\mathbf{A}}_{ML} = \mathbf{V}_{\mathcal{S}} \left[\boldsymbol{\Lambda}_{\mathcal{S}} - \sigma_\nu^2 \mathbf{I}_n \right]^{1/2} \mathbf{R}, \tag{6.6}$$

where $\mathbf{R} \in \mathbb{R}^{n \times n}$ is arbitrary orthogonal rotation matrix, so $\hat{\mathbf{A}}_{ML}$ estimate only rotated version of principal eigenvectors.[5]

To estimate $\mathbf{A}$ and $\mathbf{S} = [\mathbf{s}(1), \ldots, \mathbf{s}(N)]$, we can formulate the following cost function:

$$J(\hat{\mathbf{A}}, \ \hat{\mathbf{S}}) = \|\mathbf{X} - \mathbf{A}\mathbf{S}\|_F^2. \tag{6.7}$$

By minimizing this cost function using alternating least squares (ALS) or Expectation Maximization (EM) principle, we obtain EM-PCA algorithm for noiseless model ($\sigma_\nu^2 = 0$):

$$\text{E-step} \qquad \hat{\mathbf{S}} = (\hat{\mathbf{A}}^T \hat{\mathbf{A}})^{-1} \hat{\mathbf{A}}^T \mathbf{X}, \tag{6.8}$$

$$\text{M-step} \qquad \hat{\mathbf{A}} = \mathbf{X} \hat{\mathbf{S}}^T (\hat{\mathbf{S}} \hat{\mathbf{S}}^T)^{-1}. \tag{6.9}$$

For noisy data the EM-PCA algorithm can take following form:

$$\hat{\mathbf{M}} = (\hat{\mathbf{A}}^T \hat{\mathbf{A}} + \hat{\sigma}_\nu^2 \mathbf{I}_n)^{-1}, \tag{6.10}$$

$$\hat{\mathbf{S}} = \hat{\mathbf{M}} \hat{\mathbf{A}}^T \mathbf{X}, \tag{6.11}$$

$$\hat{\mathbf{A}} = \mathbf{X} \hat{\mathbf{S}}^T (\hat{\mathbf{S}} \hat{\mathbf{S}}^T + m \hat{\sigma}_\nu^2 \hat{\mathbf{M}})^{-1}, \tag{6.12}$$

$$\hat{\sigma}_\nu^2 = \frac{1}{Nm} \operatorname{tr}(\mathbf{X} \mathbf{X}^T - \hat{\mathbf{A}} \hat{\mathbf{S}} \hat{\mathbf{X}}). \tag{6.13}$$

For noisy data, the EM-PCA algorithm allows us not only to estimates matrices $\{\hat{\mathbf{A}}, \ \hat{\mathbf{S}}\}$, but also the variance $\hat{\sigma}_\nu^2$ of additive Gaussian noise.

6.3.2   Sequential Method for PCA

One of the simplest and intuitively understandable approaches to the derivation of adaptive algorithms for extraction of true principal components is based on self-association (also called self-supervising or the replicator principle) (Cichocki & Unbehauen, 1993, 1994). According to this approach, we first compress the data vector $\mathbf{x}(k)$ to one variable $y_1(k) = \mathbf{v}_1^T \mathbf{x}(k)$. Next we attempt to reconstruct the original data from $y_1(k)$ by using the transformation $\hat{\mathbf{x}}(k) = \mathbf{v}_1 y_1(k)$. Let us assume that we wish to extract principal components (PCs) sequentially by employing the self-supervising principle (replicator)

---

[5]The true principal eigenvectors can be recovered when the columns of $\mathbf{R}^T$ are equal to the eigenvectors of the matrix $\mathbf{A}\mathbf{A}^T$.

and a cascade (hierarchical) neural network architecture (Cichocki & Unbehauen, 1994).

Let us consider a simple processing unit (see Fig.6.11)

$$y_1(k) = \mathbf{v}_1^T \mathbf{x}(k) = \sum_{j=1}^{m} v_{1j} x_j(k), \qquad (6.14)$$

which extracts the first principal component, with $\lambda_1 = E\{y_1^2(k)\}$. Strictly speaking, the factor $y_1(k)$ is called the first principal component of $\mathbf{x}(k)$ if the variance of $y_1(k)$ is maximally large under the constraint that the principal vector $\mathbf{v}_1$ has unit length.

The vector $\mathbf{v}_1 = [v_{11}, v_{12}, \ldots, v_{1m}]^T$ should be determined in such a way so that the reconstruction vector $\hat{\mathbf{x}}(k) = \mathbf{v}_1 y_1(k)$ will reproduce (reconstruct) the input training vectors $\mathbf{x}(k)$ as correctly as possible, according to the following cost function:

$$J(\mathbf{v}_1) = E\{\|\mathbf{e}_1(k)\|_2^2 \approx \sum_{k=1}^{N} \|\mathbf{e}_1(k)\|_2^2,$$

where $\mathbf{e}_1(k) = \mathbf{x}(k) - \mathbf{v}_1 \, y_1(k)$. In general, the loss (cost) function is expressed as

$$J_i(\mathbf{v}_i) = \sum_{k=1}^{N} \|\mathbf{e}_i(k)\|_2^2 \qquad (6.15)$$

where

$$\mathbf{e}_i = \mathbf{x}_{i+1} = \mathbf{x}_i - \mathbf{v}_i y_i, \quad y_i = \mathbf{v}_i^T \mathbf{x}_i, \quad \mathbf{x}_1(k) = \mathbf{x}(k).$$

To increase convergence speed, we can minimize the cost function (6.15) by employing the recursive least-squares (RLS) approach for optimal updating of the learning rate η_i (Cichocki & Unbehauen, 1993; Cichocki, Kasprzak & Skarbek, 1996; Wang, Lee, Fiori, Leung

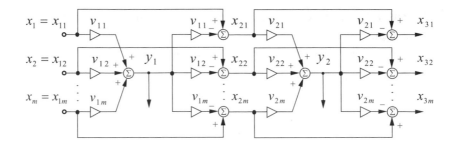

Fig. 6.11: Sequential extraction of principal components (Cichocki & Amari, 2003).

& Zhu, 2003):

$$\mathbf{x}_1(k) = \mathbf{x}(k), \qquad (6.16)$$

$$y_i(k) = \mathbf{v}_i^T(k)\mathbf{x}_i(k) \quad (i = 1, 2, \ldots, n), \qquad (6.17)$$

$$\mathbf{v}_i(k+1) = \mathbf{v}_i(k) + \frac{y_i(k)}{\eta_i(k)}[\mathbf{x}_i(k) - y_i(k)\mathbf{v}_i(k)], \qquad (6.18)$$

$$\eta_i(k+1) = \eta_i(k) + |y_i(k)|^2, \qquad (6.19)$$

$$\mathbf{x}_{i+1}(k) = \mathbf{x}_i(k) - y_i(k)\mathbf{v}_{i*}, \qquad (6.20)$$

$$\eta_i(0) = 2\max\{\|\mathbf{x}_i(k)\|_2^2\} = 2\,\mathbf{x}_{i,max}, \qquad (6.21)$$

$$\mathbf{v}_{i+1}(0) = \mathbf{v}_{i*} - [\mathbf{v}_{1*}, \ldots, \mathbf{v}_{i*}]^T[\mathbf{v}_{1*}, \ldots, \mathbf{v}_{i*}]\mathbf{v}_{i*}, \qquad (6.22)$$

where $\mathbf{v}_{i*}$ means vector $\mathbf{v}_i(k)$ after achieving convergence. The above algorithm is fast and accurate for extracting sequentially arbitrary number of eigenvectors in PCA.

6.3.3 Sparse PCA

The importance of PCA is mainly due to the following three important properties:

1. Principal components sequentially capture the maximum variability (variance) among data matrix $\mathbf{X}$, thus guaranteeing minimal information loss in the sense of mean squared errors.

2. Principal components are uncorrelated (i.e., $E\{y_i y_j\} = \delta_{ij}\lambda_j$, $(i, j = 1, 2, \ldots, n)$).

3. Principal components are hierarchically organized with respect to decreasing values of their variances (eigenvalues of the covariance matrix).

On the other hand, the standard PCA has several disadvantages. A particular disadvantage that is our focus here is that standard principal components $y_i(k) = \mathbf{v}_i^T \mathbf{x} = \sum_{j=1}^{m} v_{ij} x_i(k)$ are usually a linear combination of all variables $x_i(k)$. In other words, all weights v_{ij} (referred as loadings) are not zero. This means that principal vectors $\mathbf{v}_i$ are dense (not sparse), making physical interpretation of the principal components difficult in some applications (Zou, Hastie & Tibshirani, 2006). For example, in many applications (from biology to image understanding), the coordinate axes have physical interpretations (each axis might correspond to specific feature), but only if the components are sparsely represented (i.e., by a very few variables with non zero loadings [coordinates]). Recently several, modifications of PCA have been proposed which impose some sparseness for principal (basis) vectors, and corresponding components are called sparse principal components (SPCA, Chenubhotla, 2004; Zou, Hastie & Tibshirani, 2006). The main idea in SPCA is to force the basis vectors to be sparse. However, the sparsity profile should be adjustable or well controlled via some parameter to discover specific features in the observed data. In other words, our objective is to estimate sparse principal components—the sets of sparse vectors $\mathbf{v}_i$ spanning a low-dimensional space that represent most of the variance present in the data $\mathbf{X}$.

The cost functions (Equation 6.15) for standard PCA can be easily modified to perform the SPCA (using, e.g., the concept of a Laplace prior) as follows:

$$J_i(\mathbf{v}_i) = \sum_{k=1}^{N} \|\mathbf{x}_i(k) - \mathbf{v}_i\, y_i(k)\|_2^2 + \alpha \|\mathbf{v}_i\|_1, \qquad (6.23)$$

where $\mathbf{x}_{i+1} = \mathbf{x}_i - \mathbf{v}_i y_i$, $y_i = \mathbf{v}_i^T \mathbf{x}_i$, $\mathbf{x}_1(k) = \mathbf{x}(k)$, and $\alpha \geq 0$ is a parameter which controls sparsity. The first term in the above cost function is designed by the PC eigenvectors, while the second penalty term promotes sparsity. As α is increased, the sparsity of the SPCA basis vectors is also increased at cost of slight decreasing of variance captured by SPCA and small correlation between the components.

The presence of correlation implies that the reconstruction errors $\mathbf{e}_i = \mathbf{x}_{i+1}$ of the SPCA will not be optimal (in the sense of mean squared error). However, typically for achieving 50-70% sparsity in the basis vectors, the error increases by less than 2%.

An alternative approach is to apply regression type minimization with Lasso constraints (Zou, Hastie & Tibshirani, 2006):

$$J(\mathbf{V}, \mathbf{W}) = \sum_{k=1}^{N} \|\mathbf{x}(k) - \mathbf{W}\mathbf{V}^T\mathbf{x}(k)\|_2^2 + \alpha \sum_{i=1}^{n} \|\mathbf{v}_i\|_1, \quad (6.24)$$

$$\text{subject to} \quad \mathbf{W}^T\mathbf{W} = \mathbf{I}_n,$$

where $\mathbf{V} = [\mathbf{v}_1, \mathbf{v}_2, \ldots, \mathbf{v}_n] \in \mathbb{R}^{n \times m}$ and $\mathbf{W} \in \mathbb{R}^{n \times m}$. The above optimization problem can be solved using the standard procedure— for example, semidefinite programming (SDP).

SPCA, in contrast to standard PCA, often reveals multi-scale hierarchical structures in data (Zou, Hastie & Tibshirani, 2006; Chenubhotla, 2004). For example, for EEG/MEG data, the SPCA generates spatially localized, narrow bandpass functions as basis vectors, thereby achieving a joint space and frequency representation what is impossible using standard PCA.

6.4   BLIND SOURCE SEPARATION BASED ON SPATIO-TEMPORAL DECORRELATION

Temporal, spatial, and spatio-temporal[6] decorrelations play important roles in EEG/MEG data analysis. These techniques are based on second-order statistics (SOS). They are the basis for modern subspace methods of spectrum analysis and array processing and are often used in a preprocessing stage to improve convergence properties of adaptive systems, eliminate redundancy or reduce noise. Spatial decorrelation or prewhitening is often considered a necessary (but not sufficient) condition for stronger stochastic independence criteria. After prewhitening, the BSS or ICA tasks usually become somewhat easier and well-posed (less ill-conditioned) because the subsequent separating (unmixing) system is described by an orthogonal matrix

---

[6]Literally, space and time. Spatio-temporal data has both a spatial (i.e. location) and a temporal (i.e. time related) components.

for real-valued signals and a unitary matrix for complex-valued signals and weights. Furthermore, spatio-temporal and time-delayed decorrelation can be used to identify the mixing matrix and perform blind source separation of colored sources under certain weak conditions (Cichocki & Amari, 2003).

6.4.1   AMUSE Algorithm and its Properties

AMUSE algorithm belongs to the group of the second-order statistics spatio-temporal decorrelation (SOS-STD) algorithms. It provides identical or at least very similar decomposition of raw data as the well-known and popular SOBI and TDSEP algorithms (Belouchrani, Abed-Meraim, Cardoso & Moulines, 1997; Ziehe, Müller, Nolte, Mackert & Curio, 2000). This class of algorithms is sometimes classified or referred to as ICA algorithms. However, these algorithms do not exploit implicitly or explicitly statistical independence. Moreover, in contrast to the standard higher order statistics ICA algorithms, they are able to estimate colored Gaussian distributed sources, and their performance in estimation of original sources is usually better if the sources have temporal structure.

AMUSE algorithms have some similarities with standard PCA algorithms. The main difference is that AMUSE employs PCA two times (in cascade) in two separate steps. In the first step, standard PCA can be applied for whitening (sphering) data, and in the second step SVD/PCA, is applied to the time-delayed covariance matrix of the pre-whitened data. Mathematically, the AMUSE algorithm is the following two-stage procedure. In the first step, we apply a standard or robust prewhitening (sphering) as linear transformation $\mathbf{x}_1(k) = \mathbf{Q}\mathbf{x}(k)$, where $\mathbf{Q} = \mathbf{R}_x^{-1/2} = (\mathbf{V}\mathbf{\Lambda}\mathbf{V}^T)^{-1/2} = \mathbf{V}\mathbf{\Lambda}^{-1/2}\mathbf{V}^T$ of the standard covariance matrix $\mathbf{R}_{xx} = E\{\mathbf{x}(k)\mathbf{x}^T(k)\}$ and $\mathbf{x}(k)$ is a vector of observed data for time instant k. In the next step (for pre-whitened data), the SVD is applied for time-delayed covariance matrix $\mathbf{R}_{x1x1} = E\{\mathbf{x}_1(k)\mathbf{x}_1^T(k-1)\} = \mathbf{U}\mathbf{\Sigma}\mathbf{V}^T$, where $\mathbf{\Sigma}$ is diagonal matrix with decreasing singular values and $\mathbf{U}$, $\mathbf{V}$ are orthogonal matrices of left and right singular vectors. Then, an unmixing (separating) matrix is estimated as $\mathbf{W} = \mathbf{U}^T\mathbf{Q}$ (Cichocki & Amari, 2003).

The main advantage of the AMUSE algorithm in comparison to other BSS/ICA algorithms is that it allows us to automatically order components due to application of SVD (singular value decomposition). In fact, the components are ordered according to decreasing values of singular values of the time-delayed covariance matrix. In other words, the AMUSE algorithm exploits a simple principle that the estimated components tend to be less complex or, more precisely, have better linear predictability than any mixture of those sources. It should be emphasized that all components estimated by AMUSE are uniquely defined and consistently ranked. The consistent ranking is due to the fact that singular values are always ordered in decreasing order.

The main disadvantage of AMUSE algorithm is that its performance is relatively sensitive to additive noise since the algorithm exploits only one time delayed covariance matrix. To alleviate this problem, we can alternatively use SOBI algorithm which allows hundreds of the time delayed covariance matrices with various time delays to be approximately jointly diagonalized simultaneously (Belouchrani, Abed-Meraim, Cardoso & Moulines, 1997; Belouchrani & Cichocki, 2000).

6.5 BLIND SOURCE EXTRACTION USING LINEAR PREDICTABILITY AND ADAPTIVE BAND PASS FILTERS

There are two main approaches to solve the problem of blind source separation. The first approach, which was mentioned briefly in the previous section, is to simultaneously separate all sources. In the second one, we extract sources sequentially in a blind fashion, one by one, rather than separating them all simultaneously. In many applications, a large number of sensors (electrodes, sensors, microphones, or transducers) are available, but only a very few source signals are subjects of interest. For example, in the modern high density array EEG or MEG devices, we typically record more than 100 sensor signals, but only a few source signals are interesting; the rest can be considered as interfering noise. In another example, the cocktail party problem, it is usually essential to extract the voices of specific persons rather than separate all the source signals of all speakers available (in mixing form) from an array of microphones. For such applications, it is essential to develop and apply reliable, robust, and effective learning algorithms which enable us to extract only a small number of source signals that are potentially interesting and contain useful information.

We can use here several different models and criteria. The most frequently used criterion is based on higher order statistics (HOS), which assumes that the sources are mutually statistically independent and non-Gaussian (at most only one can be Gaussian). For independence criteria, we can use some measures of non-Gaussianity (Cichocki & Amari, 2003).

An alternative criterion, based on the concept of linear predictability, assumes that source signals have some temporal structure (i.e., the sources are colored with different autocorrelation functions or equivalently have different spectra shapes). In this approach, we exploit the temporal structure of signals rather than their statistical independence (Cichocki & Thawonmas, 2000; Stone, 2001; Barros & Cichocki, 2001). Intuitively speaking, source signals with temporal structures s_j have less complexity than the mixed sensor signals x_j. In other words, the degree of temporal predictability of any source signal is higher than (or equal to) that of any mixture. For example, waveforms of a mixture of two sine waves with different frequencies are more complex or less predictable than either of the original sine waves. This means that by applying the standard linear predictor model and minimizing the mean squared error, which is a measure of predictability, we can separate or extract signals with different temporal structures. More precisely, by minimizing the error, we maximize a measure of temporal predictability for each recovered signal (Cichocki, Thawonmas & Amari, 1997b; Cichocki, Rutkowski & Siwek, 2002).

It is worth noting that two basic criteria used in BSE—temporal linear predictability and non-Gaussianity based on kurtosis—may lead to different results. Temporal predictability forces the extracted signal to be smooth and possibly of the lowest complexity, whereas the non-Gaussianity measure forces the extracted signals to be as independent as possible with sparse representation for sources that have positive kurtosis.

Let us assume that temporally correlated source signals are mod-

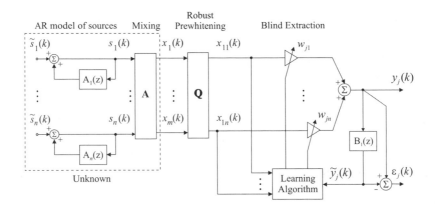

Fig. 6.12: Block diagram illustrating implementation of learning algorithm for blind extraction of a temporally correlated source (Cichocki & Amari, 2003).

eled by autoregressive processes (AR) (see Figure 6.12) as

$$s_j(k) = \widetilde{s}_j(k) + \sum_{p=1}^{L} \widetilde{a}_{jp} s_j(k-p) \tag{6.25}$$

$$= \widetilde{s}_j(k) + A_j(z) s_j(k), \tag{6.26}$$

where $A_j(z) = \sum_{p=1}^{L} \widetilde{a}_{jp} z^{-p}$, $z^{-p} s(k) = s(k-p)$ and $\widetilde{s}_j(k)$ are i.i.d. unknown innovative processes. In practice, the AR model can be extended to more general models such as the Auto Regressive Moving Average (ARMA) model or the Hidden Markov Model (HMM) (Cichocki & Amari, 2003; Hyvärinen, Karhunen & Oja, 2001; Amari, Hyvärinem, Lee, Lee & Sanchez, 2002).

For ill-conditioned problems (when a mixing matrix is ill-conditioned and/or source signals have different amplitudes), we can apply optional preprocessing (prewhitening) to the sensor signals $\mathbf{x}$ in the form

$$\mathbf{x}_1 = \mathbf{Q}\mathbf{x},$$

where $\mathbf{Q} \in \mathbb{R}^{n \times m}$ is a decorrelation matrix ensuring that the autocorrelation matrix $\mathbf{R}_{\mathbf{x}_1 \mathbf{x}_1} = E\{\mathbf{x}_1 \mathbf{x}_1^T\} = \mathbf{I}_n$ is an identity matrix. To model temporal structures of source signals, we consider a linear processing unit with an adaptive filter with the transfer function $B_1(z)$ (which estimates one $A_j(z)$) as illustrated in Figure 6.12.

Let us assume for simplicity that we want to extract only one source signal (e.g. $s_j(k)$) from the available sensor vector $\mathbf{x}(k)$. For this purpose, we employ a single processing unit described as (see Figure 6.13):

$$y_1(k) = \mathbf{w}_1^T \mathbf{x}(k) = \sum_{j=1}^{m} w_{1j}\, x_j(k), \qquad (6.27)$$

$$\varepsilon_1(k) = y_1(k) - \sum_{p=1}^{L} b_{1p}\, y_1(k-p) \qquad (6.28)$$

$$= \mathbf{w}_1^T \mathbf{x}(k) - \mathbf{b}_1^T \bar{\mathbf{y}}_1(k), \qquad (6.29)$$

where

$$\mathbf{w}_1 = [w_{11}, w_{12}, \ldots, w_{1m}]^T, \qquad (6.30)$$
$$\bar{\mathbf{y}}_1(k) = [y_1(k-1), y_1(k-2), \ldots, y_1(k-L)]^T, \qquad (6.31)$$
$$\mathbf{b}_1 = [b_{11}, b_{12}, \ldots, b_{1L}]^T, \qquad (6.32)$$
$$(6.33)$$

and

$$B_1(z) = \sum_{p=1}^{L} b_{1p} z^{-p} \qquad (6.34)$$

is the transfer function of the corresponding FIR filter. It should be noted that the FIR filter can have a sparse representation. In particular, only one single processing unit (e.g.,with delay p and $b_{1p} \neq 0$) can be used instead of L parameters. The processing unit has two outputs: $y_1(k)$, which estimates the extracted source signals, and $\varepsilon_1(k)$, which represents a linear prediction error or estimator of an innovation after passing the output signal $y_1(k)$ through FIR filter.

Our objective is to estimate optimal values of vectors $\mathbf{w}_1$ and $\mathbf{b}_1$, in such a way that the processing unit successfully extracts one of the sources. This is achieved if the global vector defined as $\mathbf{g}_1 = \mathbf{A}^T \mathbf{w}_1 = (\mathbf{w}_1^T \mathbf{A})^T = c_j \mathbf{e}_j$ contains only one nonzero element (e.g. in the j-th row), such that $y_1(k) = c_j s_j$, where c_j is an arbitrary

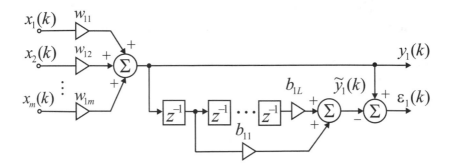

Fig. 6.13: The neural network structure of single extraction unit using a linear predictor.

nonzero scaling factor. For this purpose, we reformulate the problem as a minimization of the cost function

$$\mathcal{J}(\mathbf{w}_1, \mathbf{b}_1) = E\left\{\varepsilon_1^2\right\}. \tag{6.35}$$

The main motivation for applying such a cost function is the assumption that primary source signals (signals of interest) have temporal structures and can be modeled, for example, by an autoregressive model (Cichocki & Amari, 2003; Barros & Cichocki, 2001; Jung & Lee, 2000).

According to the AR model of source signals, the filter output can be represented as $\varepsilon_1(k) = y_1(k) - \tilde{y}_1(k)$, where $\tilde{y}_1(k) = \sum_{p=1}^{L} b_{1p} y_1(k - p)$ is defined as an error or estimator of the innovation source $\tilde{s}_j(k)$. The mean squared error $E\{\varepsilon_1^2(k)\}$ achieves a minimum $c_1^2 E\{\tilde{s}_j^2(k)\}$, where c_1 is a positive scaling constant, if and only if $y_1 = \pm c_1 s_j$ for any $j \in \{1, 2, \ldots, m\}$ or $y_1 = 0$ holds.

Let us consider the processing unit shown in Figure 6.13. The associated cost function (6.35) can be evaluated as follows:

$$E\left\{\varepsilon_1^2\right\} = \mathbf{w}_1^T \widehat{\mathbf{R}}_{\mathbf{x}_1\mathbf{x}_1} \mathbf{w}_1 - 2\mathbf{w}_1^T \widehat{\mathbf{R}}_{\mathbf{x}_1\bar{\mathbf{y}}_1} \mathbf{b}_1 + \mathbf{b}_1^T \widehat{\mathbf{R}}_{\bar{\mathbf{y}}_1\bar{\mathbf{y}}_1} \mathbf{b}_1, \tag{6.36}$$

where $\widehat{\mathbf{R}}_{\mathbf{x}_1\mathbf{x}_1} \approx E\{\mathbf{x}_1\mathbf{x}_1^T\}$, $\widehat{\mathbf{R}}_{\mathbf{x}_1\bar{\mathbf{y}}_1} \approx E\{\mathbf{x}_1\bar{\mathbf{y}}_1^T\}$ and $\widehat{\mathbf{R}}_{\bar{\mathbf{y}}_1\bar{\mathbf{y}}_1} \approx E\{\bar{\mathbf{y}}_1\bar{\mathbf{y}}_1^T\}$, are estimators of the true values of the correlation and cross-correlation matrices: $\mathbf{R}_{\mathbf{x}_1\mathbf{x}_1}, \mathbf{R}_{\mathbf{x}_1\bar{\mathbf{y}}_1}, \mathbf{R}_{\bar{\mathbf{y}}_1\bar{\mathbf{y}}_1}$, respectively. To estimate vectors $\mathbf{w}_1$ and $\mathbf{b}_1$, we evaluate gradients of the cost function and equalize them to zero as follows:

$$\frac{\partial \mathcal{J}_1\left(\mathbf{w}_1, \mathbf{b}_1\right)}{\partial \mathbf{w}_1} = 2\widehat{\mathbf{R}}_{\mathbf{x}_1 \mathbf{x}_1}\mathbf{w}_1 - 2\widehat{\mathbf{R}}_{\mathbf{x}_1 \bar{\mathbf{y}}_1}\mathbf{b}_1 = \mathbf{0}, \qquad (6.37)$$

$$\frac{\partial \mathcal{J}_1\left(\mathbf{w}_1, \mathbf{b}_1\right)}{\partial \mathbf{b}_1} = 2\widehat{\mathbf{R}}_{\bar{\mathbf{y}}_1 \bar{\mathbf{y}}_1}\mathbf{b}_1 - 2\widehat{\mathbf{R}}_{\bar{\mathbf{y}}_1 \mathbf{x}_1}\mathbf{w}_1 = \mathbf{0}. \qquad (6.38)$$

Solving these matrix equations, we obtain a simple iterative algorithm:

$$\tilde{\mathbf{w}}_1 = \widehat{\mathbf{R}}_{\mathbf{x}_1 \mathbf{x}_1}^{-1}\widehat{\mathbf{R}}_{\mathbf{x}_1 \bar{\mathbf{y}}_1}\mathbf{b}_1, \quad \mathbf{w}_1 = \frac{\tilde{\mathbf{w}}_1}{\|\tilde{\mathbf{w}}_1\|_2}, \qquad (6.39)$$

$$\mathbf{b}_1 = \widehat{\mathbf{R}}_{\bar{\mathbf{y}}_1 \bar{\mathbf{y}}_1}^{-1}\widehat{\mathbf{R}}_{\bar{\mathbf{y}}_1 \mathbf{x}_1}\mathbf{w}_1 = \widehat{\mathbf{R}}_{\bar{\mathbf{y}}_1 \bar{\mathbf{y}}_1}^{-1}\widehat{\mathbf{R}}_{\bar{\mathbf{y}}_1 y_1}, \qquad (6.40)$$

where the matrices $\widehat{\mathbf{R}}_{\bar{\mathbf{y}}_1 \bar{\mathbf{y}}_1}$ and $\widehat{\mathbf{R}}_{\bar{\mathbf{y}}_1 y_1}$ are estimated based on the parameters $\mathbf{w}_1$ obtained in the previous iteration step. To avoid the trivial solution $\mathbf{w}_1 = \mathbf{0}$, we normalize the vector $\mathbf{w}_1$ to unit length in each iteration step as $\mathbf{w}_1(l+1) = \tilde{\mathbf{w}}_1(l+1)/\|\tilde{\mathbf{w}}_1(l+1)\|_2$ (which ensures that $E\{y_1^2\} = 1$).

It is worth noting here that in our derivation, matrices $\widehat{\mathbf{R}}_{\bar{\mathbf{y}}_1 \bar{\mathbf{y}}_1}$ and $\widehat{\mathbf{R}}_{\mathbf{y}_1 y_1}$ are assumed to be independent of the vector $\mathbf{w}_1(l+1)$ (i.e., they are estimated based on $\mathbf{w}_1(l)$ in the previous iteration step). This two-phase procedure is similar to the expectation maximization (EM) scheme: (a) Freeze the correlation and cross-correlation matrices and learn the parameters of the processing unit $(\mathbf{w}_1, \mathbf{b}_1)$; (b) freeze $\mathbf{w}_1$ and $\mathbf{b}_1$ and learn new statistics (i.e., matrices $\widehat{\mathbf{R}}_{\bar{\mathbf{y}}_1 y_1}$ and $\mathbf{R}_{\bar{\mathbf{y}}_1 \bar{\mathbf{y}}_1}$) of the estimated source signal, then go back to (a) and repeat. Hence, in (a) our algorithm extracts a source signal, whereas in (b) it learns the statistics of the source (Cichocki & Belouchrani, 2001; Cichocki, Rutkowski & Siwek, 2002; Gharieb & Cichocki, 2003).

6.6 INDEPENDENT COMPONENT ANALYSIS (ICA)

ICA can be defined as follows: The ICA of a random vector $\mathbf{x}(k) \in \mathbb{R}^m$ is obtained by finding an $n \times m$ (with $m \geq n$) full rank separating (transformation) matrix $\mathbf{W}$, such that the output signal vector $\mathbf{y}(k) = [y_1(k), y_2(k), \ldots, y_n(k)]^T$ (independent components) estimated by

$$\mathbf{y}(k) = \mathbf{W}\,\mathbf{x}(k) \qquad (6.41)$$

are as independent as possible, when evaluated by an information-theoretic cost function such as minima of Kullback-Leibler divergence (Hyvärinen, Karhunen & Oja, 2001).

Compared with PCA, which removes second-order correlations from observed signals, ICA further removes higher-order dependencies. Independence of random variables is a more general concept than decorrelation. Roughly speaking, we say that random variables y_i and y_j are statistically independent if knowledge of the values of y_i provides no information about the values of y_j. Mathematically, the independence of y_i and y_j can be expressed by the relationship

$$p(y_i, y_j) = p(y_i)p(y_j), \qquad (6.42)$$

where $p(y)$ denotes the probability density function (pdf) of the random variable y. In other words, signals are independent if their joint pdf can be factorized.

If independent signals are zero-mean, the generalized covariance matrix of $f(y_i)$ and $g(y_j)$, where $f(y)$ and $g(y)$ are different, odd, nonlinear activation functions (e.g., $f(y) = \tanh(y)$ and $g(y) = y$ for super-Gaussian sources), is a non-singular diagonal matrix:

$$
\begin{aligned}
\mathbf{R_{fg}} &= E\{\mathbf{f}(\mathbf{y})\mathbf{g}^T(\mathbf{y})\} \qquad\qquad (6.43)\\
&= \begin{bmatrix} E\{f(y_1)g(y_1)\} & & 0 \\ & \ddots & \\ 0 & & E\{f(y_n)g(y_n)\} \end{bmatrix},
\end{aligned}
$$

that is, the covariances $E\{f(y_i)g(y_j)\}$ are all zero for $i \neq j$. It should be noted that for odd $f(y)$ and $g(y)$, if the probability density function of each zero-mean source signal is even, then the terms of the form $E\{f(y_i)\}E\{g(y_i)\}$ equal zero. The true general condition for statistical independence of signals is the vanishing of high-order cross-cumulants (Cichocki, Unbehauen & Rummert, 1994; Cichocki & Unbehauen, 1996; Amari & J.-F.Cardoso, 1997; Cichocki, Bogner, Moszczyński & Pope, 1997a).

The above diagonalization principle can be expressed as (Fiori, 2003; Nishimori, 1999)

$$\mathbf{R}_{fg}^{-1} = \mathbf{\Lambda}^{-1}, \qquad (6.44)$$

where Λ is any diagonal positive definite matrix (typically, $\Lambda = \mathbf{I}$ or $\Lambda = \text{diag}\{\mathbf{R}_{fg}\}$). By pre-multiplying the earlier equation by separating matrix $\mathbf{W}$ and Λ, we obtain:

$$\Lambda \mathbf{R}_{fg}^{-1} \mathbf{W} = \mathbf{W}, \tag{6.45}$$

which suggests the following iterative multiplicative learning algorithm:

$$\tilde{\mathbf{W}}(l+1) = \Lambda \mathbf{R}_{fg}^{-1} \mathbf{W}(l), \tag{6.46}$$

$$\mathbf{W}(l+1) = \tilde{\mathbf{W}}(l+1) \left[\tilde{\mathbf{W}}^T(l+1) \tilde{\mathbf{W}}(l+1) \right]^{-1/2}, \tag{6.47}$$

where the last equation represents the symmetric orthogonalization to keep the algorithm stable. This algorithm is simple and fast but does require prewhitening the data.

In fact, a wide class of ICA algorithms can be expressed in general form as (see Table 1) (Cichocki & Amari, 2003)

$$\nabla \mathbf{W}(l) = \mathbf{W}(l+1) - \mathbf{W}(l) = \eta \mathbf{F}(\mathbf{y}) \mathbf{W}(l), \tag{6.48}$$

where $\mathbf{y}(k) = \mathbf{W}(l)\mathbf{x}(k)$ and the matrix $\mathbf{F}(\mathbf{y})$ can take different forms—for example, $\mathbf{F}(\mathbf{y}) = \Lambda_n - \mathbf{f}(\mathbf{y})\mathbf{g}^T(\mathbf{y})$ with suitably chosen nonlinearities $\mathbf{f}(\mathbf{y}) = [f(y_1), ..., f(y_n)]$ and $\mathbf{g}(\mathbf{y}) = [g(y_1), ..., g(y_n)]$ (Cichocki, Unbehauen & Rummert, 1994; Cruces, Castedo & Cichocki, 2002; Cruces, Cichocki & Castedo, 2000; Cruces & Cichocki, 2003; Cichocki & Amari, 2003; Hyärinen & Oja, 2000).

Assuming prior knowledge of the source distributions $p_i(y_i)$, we can estimate $\mathbf{W}$ using maximum likelihood (ML):

$$J(\mathbf{W}, \mathbf{y}) = -\frac{1}{2} \log |\det(\mathbf{W}\mathbf{W}^T)| - \sum_{i=1}^{n} \log(p_i(y_i)) \tag{6.49}$$

Using natural gradient descent to increase likelihood, we get

$$\mathbf{W}(l+1) = \eta \left[\mathbf{I} - \mathbf{f}(\mathbf{y})\mathbf{y}^T \right] \mathbf{W}(l), \tag{6.50}$$

where $\mathbf{f}(\mathbf{y}) = [f_1(y_1), f_2(y_2), \ldots, f_n(y_n)]^T$ is an entry-wise nonlinear score function defined by

$$f_i(y_i) = -\frac{p_i'(y_i)}{p_i(y_i)} = -\frac{d \log(p_i(y_i))}{d(y_i)}. \tag{6.51}$$

It should be noted that ICA can perform blind source separation (i.e., enable estimation of true sources only if they are all statistically independent and non-Gaussian, Cichocki & Amari, 2003; Bell & Sejnowski, 1995; Cardoso & Laheld, 1996; Karhunen & Pajunen, 1997).

Table 6.1: Basic equivariant adaptive learning algorithms for ICA. Some of these algorithms require pre-whitening.

	Learning rule	References
1	$\Delta \mathbf{W} = \eta \left[\mathbf{\Lambda} - \langle \mathbf{f}(\mathbf{y})\, \mathbf{g}^T(\mathbf{y}) \rangle \right] \mathbf{W}$ $\mathbf{\Lambda}$ is a diagonal matrix with nonnegative elements λ_{ii}	Cichocki et al. (1994)
	$\mathbf{W}(l+1) = \left[\mathbf{I} + \eta \left[\mathbf{I} - \langle \mathbf{f}(\mathbf{y})\, \mathbf{g}^T(\mathbf{y}) \rangle \right]^{\mp 1} \right] \mathbf{W}(l)$	Cruces et al. (2000)
2	$\Delta \mathbf{W} = \eta \left[\mathbf{\Lambda} - \langle \mathbf{f}(\mathbf{y})\, \mathbf{y}^T \rangle \right] \mathbf{W}, \quad f'(y_i) = -p'(y_i)/p(y_i)$ $\lambda_{ii} = \langle f(y_i(k)) y_i(k) \rangle \quad$ or $\quad \lambda_{ii} = 1, \; \forall i$	Bell & Sejnowski (1995) Amari et al., (1996); Choi et al. (1998)
3	$\Delta \mathbf{W} = \eta \left[\mathbf{I} - \langle \mathbf{y}\,\mathbf{y}^T \rangle - \langle \mathbf{f}(\mathbf{y})\, \mathbf{y}^T \rangle + \langle \mathbf{y}\, \mathbf{f}^T(\mathbf{y}) \rangle \right] \mathbf{W}$	Cardoso & Laheld (1996)
4	$\Delta \mathbf{W} = \eta \left[\mathbf{I} - \langle \mathbf{y}\,\mathbf{y}^T \rangle - \langle \mathbf{f}(\mathbf{y})\, \mathbf{y}^T \rangle + \langle \mathbf{f}(\mathbf{y})\, \mathbf{f}^T(\mathbf{y}) \rangle \right] \mathbf{W}$	Karhunen & Pajunen (1997)
5	$\tilde{\mathbf{W}} = \mathbf{W} + \eta \left[\mathbf{\Lambda} - \langle \mathbf{f}(\mathbf{y})\, \mathbf{y}^T \rangle \right] \mathbf{W}, \; \lambda_{ii} = \langle f(y_i)\, y_i \rangle$ $\mathbf{W} = \tilde{\mathbf{W}} (\tilde{\mathbf{W}}^T \tilde{\mathbf{W}})^{-1/2}$ $\eta_{ii} = [\lambda_{ii} + \langle f'(y_i) \rangle]^{-1};$	Hyvärinen & Oja (1999)
6	$\Delta \mathbf{W} = \eta \left[\mathbf{I} - \mathbf{\Lambda}^{-1} \langle \mathbf{y}\,\mathbf{y}^T \rangle \right] \mathbf{W}$	Amari & Cichocki (1998)

Table 6.1, continued

Learning rule	References
$\lambda_{ii}(k) = \langle y_i^2(k) \rangle$	Choi et al. (2002)
7 $\quad \Delta \mathbf{W} = \eta \Big[\mathbf{I} - \mathbf{C}_{1,q}(\mathbf{y}, \mathbf{y})\, \mathbf{S}_{q+1}(\mathbf{y}) \Big] \mathbf{W}$	Cruces et al. (2002)
$C_{1,q}(y_i, y_j) = Cum(y_i, \underbrace{y_j, \ldots, y_j}_{q})$	
8 $\quad \mathbf{W}(l+1) = \exp(\eta\, \mathbf{F}[\mathbf{y}])\, \mathbf{W}(l)$	Nishimori (1999); Fiori (2003)
$\mathbf{F}(\mathbf{y}) = \mathbf{\Lambda} - \langle \mathbf{y}\,\mathbf{y}^T \rangle - \langle \mathbf{f}(\mathbf{y})\,\mathbf{y}^T \rangle + \langle \mathbf{y}\,\mathbf{f}^T(\mathbf{y}) \rangle$	Cichocki & Georgiev (2002)
9 $\quad \widetilde{\mathbf{W}} = \mathbf{\Lambda}\, \mathbf{R}_{fg}^{-1} \mathbf{W}$	Fiori (2003)
$\mathbf{W} = \widetilde{\mathbf{W}}(\widetilde{\mathbf{W}}^T \widetilde{\mathbf{W}})^{-1/2}$	

6.6.1 Multiresolution Subband Decomposition: Independent Component Analysis (MSD-ICA)

Despite the success of using standard ICA in many applications, the basic assumptions of ICA may not hold for some kinds of signals, hence some caution should be taken when using standard ICA to analyze real-world problems, especially in analysis of EEG/MEG data. In fact, by definition, the standard ICA algorithms are not able to estimate statistically dependent original sources—that is, when the independence assumption is violated. In this section, we present a natural extension and generalization of ICA called Multiresolution Subband Decomposition ICA (MSD-ICA), which relaxes considerably the assumption regarding mutual independence of primarily sources (Cichocki & Georgiev, 2003; Cichocki & Amari, 2003; Tanaka & Cichocki, 2004; Cichocki, Li, Georgiev & Amari, 2004b). The key idea in this approach is the assumption that the unknown wide-band source signals can be dependent. However, some of their narrow-band or sparse linearly transformed subcomponents are independent. In other words, we assume that each unknown source can be modeled or represented as a sum (or linear combinations) of narrow-band sub-signals (sub-components):

$$s_i(k) = s_{i1}(k) + s_{i2}(k) + \cdots + s_{iK}(k). \tag{6.52}$$

For example, in the simplest case, source signals can be modeled or decomposed into their low- and high-frequency sub-components:

$$s_i(k) = s_{iL}(k) + s_{iH}(k) \qquad (i = 1, 2, \ldots, n). \tag{6.53}$$

In practice, the high-frequency sub-components $s_{iH}(k)$ are often found to be mutually independent, whereas the low-frequency sub-components are weakly dependent. In such a case, we can use a High Pass Filter (HPF) to extract mixture of the high-frequency sub-components and then apply any standard ICA algorithm to such preprocessed sensor (observed) signals.

The basic concept in Subband Decomposition ICA is to divide the sensor signal spectra into their subspectra or subbands and then treat those subspectra individually for the purpose at hand. The subband signals can be ranked and processed independently. Let us assume that only a certain set of sub-components are independent.

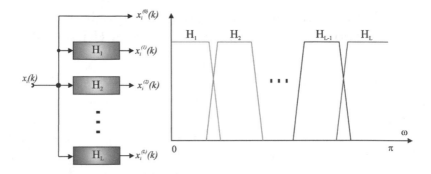

Fig. 6.14: Bank of filters employed in preprocessing stage for MSD-ICA with typical frequency bands. For each sensor signal, we employ the identical set of filters. The sub-bands can be overlapped or not and have more complex sub-bands forms. Instead of subband filters we can use various alternative transforms to sparsify data.

Provided that for some of the frequency subbands (at least one) all sub-components, say $\{s_{ij}(k)\}_{i=1}^n$, are mutually independent or temporally decorrelated, we can easily estimate the mixing or separating system under condition that these subbands can be identified by some *a priori* knowledge or detected by some self-adaptive process. For this purpose, we simply apply any standard ICA algorithm—however, not for all available raw sensor data, but only for suitably pre-processed (e.g., subband filtered or more generally in a transform domain) sensor signals.

By applying any standard ICA/BSS algorithm for specific sub-bands and raw sensor data, we obtain sequence of separating matrices $\mathbf{W}_0, \mathbf{W}_1, \ldots, \mathbf{W}_L$, where $\mathbf{W}_0$ is the separating matrix from the original data $\mathbf{x}$ and $\mathbf{W}_j$ is the separating matrix from preprocessing sensor data $\mathbf{x}_j$ in the j-th sub-band. To identify for which sub-bands corresponding source subcomponents are independent, we propose to compute the global (mixing-separating) matrices $\mathbf{G}_{jq} = \mathbf{W}_j \mathbf{W}_q^{-1}$, $\forall j \neq q$ and $m = n$, where $\mathbf{W}_q$ is estimating separating matrix for q-th sub-band. If subcomponents are mutually independent for at least two sub-bands, say for the sub-band j and sub-band q, then the global matrix $\mathbf{W}_j \mathbf{W}_q^{-1} = \mathbf{P}_{jq}$ will be a generalized permutation matrix with only one nonzero (or dominated) element in each row and each column. This follows from the simple observation that, in such a case, both matrices $\mathbf{W}_j$ and $\mathbf{W}_q$ represent inverses (for $m = n$) of the same mixing matrix $\mathbf{A}$ (neglecting nonessential scaling and permutation ambiguities). In this way, we can blindly identify essential information for which frequency sub-bands the source subcomponents are independent, and we can easily identify correctly the mixing matrix. Furthermore, the same concept can be used to estimate blindly the performance index and compare performance of various ICA algorithms, especially for large-scale problems.

In the preprocessing stage, we can use any linear transforms, especially more sophisticated methods such as block transforms, multirate sub-band filter bank, or wavelets, ridgelets, and curvelets transforms, can be applied in order to sparsify data and extract signals with specific structures or morphological properties. We can extend and generalize further this concept by performing the decomposition of sensor signals in a composite time-frequency domain, rather than in frequency sub-bands as such. This naturally leads to the concept of wavelets packets (sub-band hierarchical trees) and to block transform packets (Cichocki & Amari, 2003; Zibulevsky, Kisilev, Zeevi & Pearlmutter, 2002; Bach & Jordan, 2003; Bobin, Moudden, J.-L., Starck & Elad, 2006). Such preprocessing techniques have been extensively tested and implemented in our ICALAB (Cichocki, Amari, Siwek, Tanaka & et al., 2004a).

Such explanation can be summarized as follows. The MSD-ICA (Multiresolution Subband Decomposition ICA) can be formulated as a task of estimation of the separating matrix $\mathbf{W}$ and/or the estimating mixing matrix $\hat{\mathbf{A}}$ on the basis of suitable wavelet package or subband decomposition of sensor signals and by applying a classical ICA (instead for raw sensor data) for one or several preselected subbands for which source sub-components are independent.

6.7 VALIDITY OF ICA, BSS ALGORITHMS FOR REAL WORLD DATA

One of the fundamental questions in BSS is whether the obtained results of the specific BSS/ICA algorithm are reliable and represent inherent properties of the model and data, or whether they are just random, synthetic or purely mathematical, decompositions of data without any physical meaning. In fact, since most of BSS algorithms are stochastic in nature, their results could be somewhat different in different runs even for the same algorithm. Thus, the results obtained in a single run or for a single set of data of any BSS algorithm should be interpreted with reserve and reliability of estimated sources should be analyzed by investigating the spread of the obtained estimates for many runs (Himberg, Hyvärinen & Esposito, 2004). Such an analysis can be performed, for example, by using resampling or bootstrapping method in which the available data are randomly changed by producing surrogate data sets from the original data (Mainecke, Ziehe, Kawanabe & Müller, 2002). The specific ICA/BSS algorithm is then run many times with bootstrapped samples that are somewhat different from each other. An alternative approach called ICASSO has been developed by Himberg et al. (2004), which is based on running the specific BSS algorithm many times for various different initial conditions and parameters and by visualizing the clustering structure of the estimated sources (components) in the signal subspace. In other words, to estimate algorithmic reliability, it was suggested to run the BSS algorithm many times using different initial conditions and assessing which of the components are found in almost all runs. For this purpose, the estimated components are clustered and classified. The reliable components correspond to small and well-separated clusters from the rest of components, while unreliable components usually do not belong to any cluster (Himberg et al., 2004; Mainecke et al., 2002).

It is worth noting that the concept of MSD-ICA described in the previous section can be easily extended to more general and flexible multidimensional models for checking validity and reliability of ICA (or more generally BSS) algorithms (see Figure 6.14). In this model, we can use a bank of stable filters with transfer functions $H_i(z)$, for example, a set of FIR (finite impulse response) filters. The parameters (coefficients) of such FIR filters can be suitably designed or even randomly generated. In this case, the proposed method has some similarity with resampling or bootstrap approaches proposed by Mainecke et al. (2002). Similarly, as in MSD-ICA, we run any BSS algorithm for sufficiently large number L of filters and generate a set of separating matrices: $\{\mathbf{W}_0, \mathbf{W}_1, \ldots, \mathbf{W}_L\}$ or alternatively set of estimated mixing matrices: $\{\hat{\mathbf{A}}_0, \hat{\mathbf{A}}_1, \ldots, \hat{\mathbf{A}}_L\}$.[7] In the next step, we estimate the global mixing-separating matrices $\mathbf{G}_{pq} = \mathbf{W}_p \mathbf{W}_q^+$ for any $p \neq q$.

The performance of blind separation can be characterized by one single performance index (sometimes referred to as Amari's performance index), which we refer to as blind performance index (since we do not know a true mixing matrix):

$$BPI_i = \frac{1}{n} \sum_{j=1}^{n} \left(\frac{\sum_{i=1}^{n} |g_{ij}|^2}{max_i \, |g_{ij}|^2} - 1 \right) + \frac{1}{n} \sum_{i=1}^{n} \left(\frac{\sum_{j=1}^{n} |g_{ij}|^2}{max_j \, |g_{ij}|^2} - 1 \right) \quad (6.54)$$

where g_{ij} is the ij-th element of the matrix $\mathbf{G}_{pq}$. In many cases, we are not able to achieve perfect separation for some sources or we are able to extract only some sources (not of all them). In such cases, instead of using one global performance index, we can define local performance index as

$$BPI_i = \left(\frac{\sum_{j=1}^{n} |g_{ij}|^2}{max_j \, |g_{ij}|^2} - 1 \right). \quad (6.55)$$

If the performance index BPI_i for specific index i and filters p, q is close to zero, this means that with high probability this component is successfully extracted. To assess significant components, all of the estimated components should be clustered according to their mutual similarities. These similarities can be searched in the time or frequency domain. The natural measure of similarity between the estimated components can be absolute value of their mutual correlation coefficients $|r_{ij}|$ for $i \neq j$, which are elements of the similarity matrix (Himberg, Hyvärinen & Esposito, 2004)

$$\mathbf{R} = \overline{\mathbf{W}} \, \mathbf{R}_{xx} \, \overline{\mathbf{W}}^T, \quad (6.56)$$

where $\overline{\mathbf{W}} = [\mathbf{W}_0, \mathbf{W}_1, \ldots, \mathbf{W}_L]$ and $\mathbf{R}_{xx} = E\{\mathbf{xx}^T\} = \mathbf{A}\mathbf{R}_{ss}\mathbf{A}^T$ is covariance matrix of observations under assumption that the covariance matrix of sources $\mathbf{R}_{ss} = E\{\mathbf{ss}^T\}$ is a diagonal matrix and separating matrices $\mathbf{W}_p$ are normalized (e.g., to unit length vectors).

---

[7]The set of matrices can be further extended if data will be bootstrapped and/or initial conditions will be changed for each run.

6.8 SPARSE COMPONENT ANALYSIS AND SPARSE SIGNAL REPRESENTATIONS

Sparse component analysis (SCA) and sparse signals representations (SSR) arise in many scientific problems, especially where we wish to represent signals of interest by using a small (or sparse) number of basis signals from a much larger set of signals, often called dictionary (Donoho & Elad, 2004). Such problems also arise in many applications such as electromagnetic and biomagnetic inverse problems (EEG/MEG), feature extraction, filtering, wavelet denoising, time-frequency representation, neural and speech coding, spectral estimation, direction of arrival estimation, failure diagnosis, and speed-up processing (Cichocki & Amari, 2003; Li, Cichocki & Amari, 2006).

In contrast to ICA, where the mixing matrix and source signals are estimated simultaneously, the SCA is usually a multi-stage procedure (Zibulevsky, Kisilev, Zeevi & Pearlmutter, 2002; Li, Cichocki, Amari, Shishkin, Cao & Gu, 2003; Li, Cichocki & Amari, 2004; Georgiev & Cichocki, 2004). In the first stage, we need to find a suitable linear transformation which guarantee that sources in the transformed domain are sufficiently sparse. Typically, we represent the observed data in the time-frequency domain using a wavelets package (Li, Cichocki & Amari, 2004). In the next step, we estimate the columns $\mathbf{a}_i$ of the mixing matrix $\mathbf{A}$ using an advanced hierarchical clustering technique. This step is the most difficult and challenging task since it requires identifying precisely intersections of all hyperplanes on which observed data are located (Li, Cichocki, Amari, Shishkin, Cao & Gu, 2003; Theis, Georgiev & Cichocki, 2004). In the last step, we estimate sparse sources using for example a modified robust linear programming (LP), quadratic programming (QP), or semi-definite programming (SDP) optimization. The big advantage of SCA is its ability to reconstruct original sources and also their numbers even if the number of observations (sensors) is smaller than the number of sources under certain weak conditions (Li, Cichocki & Amari, 2004; Cichocki, Li, Georgiev & Amari, 2004b; Georgiev & Cichocki, 2004). Moreover, the system can be highly nonstationary (i.e., the number of active sources can change dramatically in time) and sources can be statistically dependent.

We can state the subset selection sub-problem as follows: Find an optimal subset of $r << n$ columns from the matrix $\mathbf{A}$, which we denote by $\mathbf{A}_r \in \mathbb{R}^{m \times r}$ such that $\mathbf{A}_r \mathbf{s}_{r*} \cong \mathbf{x}$, or equivalently, $\mathbf{A}\mathbf{s}_* + \mathbf{e}_r = \mathbf{x}$, where $\mathbf{e}_r$ represents some residual error vector which norm should below some threshold. The problem consists often not only in estimating the sparse vector $\mathbf{s}_*$, but also correct or optimal sparsity profile that is the sparsity index r, that is detection of the number of sources.

Usually, we have interest in the sparsest and most unique representation (i.e., it is necessary to find solution having the smallest possible number of non-zero-components). The problem can be reformulated as the following robust optimization problem (Cichocki, Li, Georgiev & Amari, 2004b):

$$(P_\rho) \quad J_\rho(\mathbf{s}) = \|\mathbf{s}\|_\rho = \sum_{j=1}^{n} \rho(s_j) \quad \text{s. t.} \quad \mathbf{A}\mathbf{s} = \mathbf{x}, \quad (6.57)$$

where $\mathbf{A} \in \mathbb{R}^{m \times n}$ (usually with $n >> m$), and $\|\mathbf{s}\|_\rho$ is a suitably chosen function which measures the sparsity of the vector $\mathbf{s}$. It should be noted that the sparsity measure does not need to be necessarily a norm, although we use such notation. For example, we can apply Shannon, Gauss, or Renyi entropy or normalized kurtosis as a measure of the sparsity (Cichocki & Amari, 2003; Kreutz-Delgado, Murray, Rao, Engan, Lee & Sejnowski, 2003; Zibulevsky, Kisilev, Zeevi & Pearlmutter, 2002). In the standard form, we use l_p-norm with $0 \leq p \leq 1$. Especially, l_0 quasi-norm has attracted a lot of attention since it ensures sparsest representation (Donoho & Elad, 2004; Li, Cichocki, Amari, Shishkin, Cao & Gu, 2003; Li, Cichocki & Amari, 2004). Unfortunately, such a formulated problem (Equation 6.57) for l_p-norm with $p < 1$ is rather difficult to solve, especially for $p = 0$ it is NP-hard, so for a large-scale problem it is numerically untractable. For this reason, we often use Basis Pursuit (BP) or standard Linear Programming (LP) for $\|\mathbf{s}\|_\rho = \|\mathbf{s}\|_1$, with $\rho = p = 1$.

In practice, due to noise and other uncertainty (e.g., measurement errors), the system of linear underdetermined equations should not be satisfied precisely, but with some prescribed tolerance (i.e., $\mathbf{A}\mathbf{s} \cong \mathbf{x}$ in the sense that $\|\mathbf{x} - \mathbf{A}\mathbf{s}\|_q \leq \varepsilon$). From the practical as well as statistical point of view, it is convenient and quite natural to replace the exact constraints $\mathbf{x} = \mathbf{A}\mathbf{s}$ by the constraint $\|\mathbf{x} - \mathbf{A}\mathbf{s}\|_q \leq \varepsilon$, where choice of l_q-norm depends on the distribution of noise and specific applications. For noisy and uncertain data, we should to use a more flexible and robust cost function (in comparison to the standard (P_ρ) problem) which is referred to as Extended Basis Pursuit Denoising $(EBPD)$(Cichocki, Li, Georgiev & Amari, 2004b):

$$(EBPD) \qquad J_{q,\rho}(\mathbf{s}) = \|\mathbf{x} - \mathbf{A}\,\mathbf{s}\|_q^q + \alpha\,\|\mathbf{s}\|_\rho, \qquad (6.58)$$

There are several possible basic choices for l_q and sparsity criteria $(\|\mathbf{s}\|_\rho = \|\mathbf{s}\|_p)$. For example, for the uniform (Laplacian) distributed noise, we should choose l_∞-Chebyshev norm (l_1-norm). Some basic choices of ρ (for $l_q = 2$) are $\rho = 0$ (minimum l_0 quasi norm or atomic decomposition related with the matching pursuit (MP) and FOCUSS algorithm), $\rho = 1$ (basis pursuit denoising) and $\rho = 2$ (ridge regression) (Kreutz-Delgado, Murray, Rao, Engan, Lee & Sejnowski, 2003; Zibulevsky, Kisilev, Zeevi & Pearlmutter, 2002; Donoho & Elad, 2004). The optimal choice of ρ norms depends on distribution of noise in sparse components. For example, for noisy components, we can use robust norms such as Huber function defined as $\|\mathbf{s}\|_{\rho_H} = \sum_i \rho_H(s_i)$, where $\rho_H(s_i) = s_i^2/2$ if $|s_i| \le \beta$ and $\rho_H(s_i) = \beta\,|s_i| - \beta^2/2$ if $|s_i| > \beta$, and/or epsilon norm defined as $\|\mathbf{s}\|_{+\varepsilon} = \sum_j |s_j|_{+\varepsilon}$ where $|s_j|_{+\varepsilon} = \max\{0,\ (|s_j| - \varepsilon)\}$.

The practical importance of the $EBPD$ approach in comparison to the standard LP or BP approach is that the $EPBD$ allows for treating the presence of noise or errors due to mismodeling. Moreover, using the $EBPD$ approach, we can adjust the sparsity profile (i.e., adjust the number of non-zero components) by tuning the parameter α. In contrast, by using the LP approach, we do not have such an option. Furthermore, the method can be applied both for undercomplete and/or overcomplete models (i.e., when the number of sources is larger or less than the number of sensors).

The practical importance of the extended quadratic programming approach in contrast to the linear programming or standard Basis Pursuit approach is that the (QP) allows for treating the presence of noise or errors due to mismodeling. In practice, in the presence of noise the true model is: $\mathbf{x}(k) = \mathbf{A}\,\mathbf{s}(k) + \mathbf{v}(k)$.

6.9 NONNEGATIVE MATRIX FACTORIZATION AND SPARSE CODING WITH NONNEGATIVITY CONSTRAINTS

The NMF (Nonnegative Matrix Factorization) introduced by Lee and Seung (Lee & Seung, 1999), sometimes called also PMF (Positive Matrix Factorization) which was first proposed by Paatero does not assume explicitly or implicitly sparseness or the mutual statistical independence of components, however, usually provides sparse decomposition. The NMF method is designed to capture alternative structures inherent in the data and, possibly to provide more biological insight. Lee and Seung (1999) introduced NMF in its modern formulation as a method to decompose images. For example, in this context, NMF yielded a decomposition of human faces into parts reminiscent of features such as lips, eyes, nose, etc.. By contrast to other factorization methods, such as ICA or PCA, image data often yielded non-negative components with obvious visual interpretation.

The NMF has found wide applications in spectroscopy, chemometrics and environmental science where the matrices have some physical meanings. The NMF also has potential application in analysis of EEG/MEG data by extracting hidden interesting sparse and localized components from spectra and/or spectrograms of the data. Whereas the original application of NMF focused on grouping elements of images into parts (using the matrix $\mathbf{A}$), we take the dual viewpoint by focusing primarily on grouping samples into components represented by the matrix $\mathbf{S}$.

NMF decomposes the data matrix $\mathbf{X}$ as a product of two matrices $\mathbf{A}$ and $\mathbf{S}$ having only non-negative elements. This results in reduced representation of the original data. In the reduced data set, each feature is a linear combination of the original attribute set. NMF does not allow negative entries in the matrix factors $\mathbf{A}$ and $\mathbf{S}$ in the model $\mathbf{X} = \mathbf{AS} + \mathbf{V}$. Unlike the other matrix factorization, these non-negativity constraints permit the combination of multiple basis signals to represent original signals or images. But only additive combinations are allowed because the non-zero elements of $\mathbf{A}$ and $\mathbf{S}$ are all positive. Thus, in such decomposition, no subtractions can occur. For these reasons, the non-negativity constraints are compatible with the intuitive notion of combining components to form a whole signal or image, which is how NMF learns a parts-based representation (Lee & Seung, 1999).

Let us consider as an illustrative example beta divergence as cost function (Kompass, 2005; Minami & Eguchi, 2002; Cichocki, Zdunek & Amari, 2006b):

$$
D_K^{(\beta)}(\mathbf{X}||\mathbf{AS}) = \sum_{ik} \left(x_{ik} \frac{x_{ik}^{\beta} - [\mathbf{AS}]_{ik}^{\beta}}{\beta(\beta+1)} + [\mathbf{AS}]_{ik}^{\beta} \frac{[\mathbf{AS}]_{ik} - x_{ik}}{\beta+1} \right)
$$
$$
+ \alpha_S ||\mathbf{S}||_1 + \alpha_A ||\mathbf{A}||_1, \tag{6.59}
$$

where α_S and α_A are small positive regularization parameters which control the degree of smoothing or sparseness of the matrices $\mathbf{A}$ and $\mathbf{S}$, respectively and l_1 norms $||\mathbf{A}||_1$ and $||\mathbf{S}||_1$ are introduced to enforce sparse representation of solutions. The choice of the β parameter depends on statistical distribution of data and the beta divergence corresponds to Tweedie models (Minami & Eguchi, 2002). On the basis of such cost function we can derive various kinds of NMF algorithms: Multiplicative based on the gradient descent or the exponentiated gradient (EG)algorithms, additive algorithms using projected gradient (PG) or interior projected gradient (IPG) approaches and fixed point (FP) algorithms.

In order to derive a flexible NMF learning algorithm, we compute the gradient of (6.59) with respect to elements of matrices $s_{jk} = s_j(k) = [\mathbf{S}]_{jk}$ and $a_{ij} = [\mathbf{A}]_{ij}$ as follows

$$
\frac{\partial D_K^{(\beta)}}{\partial s_{jk}} = \sum_{i=1}^{m} a_{ij} \left([\mathbf{AS}]_{ik}^{\beta} - x_{ik} [\mathbf{AS}]_{ik}^{\beta-1} \right) + \alpha_S, \tag{6.60}
$$

$$
\frac{\partial D_K^{(\beta)}}{\partial a_{ij}} = \sum_{k=1}^{N} \left([\mathbf{AS}]_{ik}^{\beta} - x_{ik} [\mathbf{AS}]_{ik}^{\beta-1} \right) s_{jk} + \alpha_A. \tag{6.61}
$$

The simplest approach to design multiplicative algorithm is to apply the exponentiated gradient (EG) method (Cichocki, Amari, Zdunek, He & Kompass, 2006a):

$$
s_{jk} \leftarrow s_{jk} \exp \left(-\eta_{jk} \frac{\partial D_K^{(\beta)}}{\partial s_{jk}} \right), \tag{6.62}
$$

$$
a_{ij} \leftarrow a_{ij} \exp \left(-\tilde{\eta}_{ij} \frac{\partial D_K^{(\beta)}}{\partial a_{ij}} \right), \tag{6.63}
$$

where the positive learning rates η_{jk} and $\tilde{\eta}_{ij}$ can take different forms. Typically, in order to guarantee stability of the algorithm we assume that $\eta_{jk} = \eta_j = \omega \left(\sum_{i=1}^{m} a_{ij} \right)^{-1}$, $\tilde{\eta}_{ij} = \tilde{\eta}_j = \omega \left(\sum_{k=1}^{N} x_{jk} \right)^{-1}$, where $\omega \in (0, 2)$ is an over-relaxation parameter.

Alternatively, similar to the Lee and Seung approach, by choosing suitable learning rates:

$$\eta_{jk} = \frac{s_{jk}}{\sum_{i=1}^{m} a_{ij} [\mathbf{AS}]_{ik}^{\beta}}, \quad \tilde{\eta}_{ij} = \frac{a_{ij}}{\sum_{k=1}^{N} [\mathbf{AS}]_{ik}^{\beta} s_{jk}}, \tag{6.64}$$

we obtain multiplicative update rules (Kompass, 2005; Cichocki, Zdunek & Amari, 2006b):

$$s_{jk} \leftarrow s_{jk} \frac{\left[\sum_{i=1}^{m} a_{ij} \left(x_{ik} / [\mathbf{AS}]_{ik}^{1-\beta} \right) - \alpha_S \right]_{\varepsilon}}{\sum_{i=1}^{m} a_{ij} [\mathbf{AS}]_{ik}^{\beta}}, \tag{6.65}$$

$$a_{ij} \leftarrow a_{ij} \frac{\left[\sum_{k=1}^{N} \left(x_{ik} / [\mathbf{AS}]_{ik}^{1-\beta} \right) s_{jk} - \alpha_A \right]_{\varepsilon}}{\sum_{k=1}^{N} [\mathbf{AS}]_{ik}^{\beta} s_{jk}}, \tag{6.66}$$

where the additional nonlinear operator is introduced in practice, defined as $[x]_{\varepsilon} = \max\{\varepsilon, x\}$ with a small ε in order to avoid zero and negative values.

The projected gradient (PG) NMF algorithm with additive updates can be written in a general form as (Lin, 2005)

$$s_{jk} \leftarrow P_{\Omega} \left[s_{jk} - \eta_{jk} \left(\frac{\partial D_K}{\partial s_{jk}} \right) \right], \tag{6.67}$$

$$a_{ij} \leftarrow P_{\Omega} \left[a_{ij} - \tilde{\eta}_{ij} \left(\frac{\partial D_K}{\partial a_{ij}} \right) \right], \tag{6.68}$$

where the learning rates are not fixed but adjusted in each iteration step in a such way that they keep update nonnegative and/or $P_{\Omega}(x)$ ensures projection of x onto feasible (nonnegative) set Ω.

Using the Interior Projected Gradient (IPG) technique the additive algorithm can take the following form (using MATLAB notation):

$$\mathbf{A} \leftarrow \mathbf{A} - \eta_A \, \mathbf{A} \, ./ \, (\mathbf{ASS}^T) \, . * \, (\mathbf{AS} - \mathbf{X}) \mathbf{S}^T, \tag{6.69}$$

$$\mathbf{S} \leftarrow \mathbf{S} - \eta_S \, \mathbf{X} ./ (\mathbf{A}^T \mathbf{AS}) \, . * \, \mathbf{A}^T (\mathbf{AS} - \mathbf{X}), \tag{6.70}$$

where η_A and η_S are diagonal matrices with positive entries representing suitably chosen learning rates (Merritt & Zhang, 2004).

Finally, the family of fixed point NMF algorithms can be derived for by equalizing the gradients (for $\beta = 1$) to zero (Cichocki & Zdunek, 2006) (compare with EM-PCA algorithm):

$$\nabla_X D_F(\mathbf{X}\|\mathbf{AS}) = \mathbf{A}^T\mathbf{AS} - \mathbf{A}^T\mathbf{X} + \alpha_S = \mathbf{0}, \qquad (6.71)$$
$$\nabla_A D_F(\mathbf{X}\|\mathbf{AS}) = \mathbf{ASS}^T - \mathbf{XS}^T + \alpha_A = \mathbf{0}. \qquad (6.72)$$

These equations suggest the following fixed point updates rules:

$$\mathbf{S} \leftarrow \max\{\varepsilon, [(\mathbf{A}^T\mathbf{A})^+(\mathbf{A}^T\mathbf{X} - \alpha_S)]\} = [(\mathbf{A}^T\mathbf{A})^+(\mathbf{A}^T\mathbf{X} - \alpha_S)]_\varepsilon,$$
$$\mathbf{A} \leftarrow \max\{\varepsilon, [(\mathbf{XS}^T - \alpha_A)(\mathbf{SS}^T)^+]\} = [(\mathbf{XS}^T - \alpha_A)(\mathbf{SS}^T)^+]_\varepsilon.$$

where $[\mathbf{A}]^+$ means Moore Penrose pseudo-inverse and max function is componentwise.

During the above updates, we should update the matrices $\mathbf{A}$ and $\mathbf{S}$ alternatively. Due to some physical constraints and also in order to achieve a unique solution it is necessary usually to normalize in each iteration the columns of $\mathbf{A}$ or rows of $\mathbf{S}$ to unity or fixed norm.

Useful NMF learning algorithms for various flexible and generalized cost functions are presented in Table 6.2 (Cichocki, Zdunek & Amari, 2006c; Cichocki, Amari, Zdunek, He & Kompass, 2006a; Zdunek & Cichocki, 2006; Cichocki & Zdunek, 2006; Dhillon & Sra, 2005). Algorithms are described in the matrix form using MATLAB notation. The operators .*, ./, and .$^\beta$ mean component-wise multiplication, division and rising to the power β each element of a matrix or a vector, respectively. In practice, in order to avoid division by zero and $\log(0)$ a small positive value ε is added when necessary. Furthermore, in order to avoid negative values we use operator $[x]_\varepsilon = \max\{x, \varepsilon\}$, where ε is the small positive number, typically 10^{-16}.

Table 6.2: NMF algorithms and corresponding cost functions (MATLAB notation is used).

Minimization of cost function subject to $a_{ij} \geq 0$ and $s_{ik} \geq 0$	Iterative learning algorithm
Amari alpha divergence $\sum_{ik} x_{ik} \dfrac{(x_{ik}/[\mathbf{AS}]_{ik})^{\alpha-1} - 1}{(\alpha-1)\alpha} + \dfrac{[\mathbf{AS}]_{ik} - x_{ik}}{\alpha}$	$\mathbf{S} \leftarrow \mathbf{S} .* (\mathbf{A}^T(\mathbf{X}./(\mathbf{AS}+\varepsilon)).^{\alpha}) .^{1/\alpha}$ $\mathbf{A} \leftarrow \mathbf{A} .* (((\mathbf{X}./(\mathbf{AS}+\varepsilon)).^{\alpha})\,\mathbf{S}^T) .^{1/\alpha}$ $\mathbf{A} \leftarrow \mathbf{A}\,\mathrm{diag}(1./sum(\mathbf{A},1)),\ \alpha \neq 0$
Shannon entropy $\sum_{ik}(s_{ik} \log s_{ik})$ s.t. $\mathbf{X} = \mathbf{AS}$ $\sum_{ij}(a_{ij} \log a_{ij})$ s.t. $\mathbf{X}^T = \mathbf{S}^T \mathbf{A}^T$	$\mathbf{S} \leftarrow \mathbf{S} .* \exp\left(\eta_S\, \mathbf{A}^T \ln(\mathbf{X}./(\mathbf{AS}+\epsilon))\right)$ $\mathbf{A} \leftarrow \mathbf{A} .* \exp\left(\ln(\mathbf{X}./(\mathbf{AS}+\epsilon))\,\mathbf{S}^T \eta_A\right)$ $\mathbf{A} \leftarrow \mathbf{A}\,\mathrm{diag}(1./sum(\mathbf{A},1))$ $\eta_A = \mathrm{diag}\{1./sum(\mathbf{A},1)\};\ \eta_S = \mathrm{diag}\{1./sum(\mathbf{S},1)\}$
Euclidean distance with regularization $\sum_{ik}(x_{ik} - [\mathbf{AS}]_{ik})^2 + \alpha_S\|\mathbf{S}\|_1 + \alpha_A\|\mathbf{A}\|_1$	$\mathbf{S} \leftarrow \mathbf{S} .* \left[\mathbf{A}^T\mathbf{X} - \alpha_S\right]_\varepsilon ./ \left[\mathbf{A}^T\mathbf{A}\mathbf{S}\right]_\varepsilon$ $\mathbf{A} \leftarrow \mathbf{A} .* \left[\mathbf{X}\mathbf{S}^T\right] - \alpha_A]_\varepsilon ./ \left[\mathbf{A}\mathbf{S}\mathbf{S}^T\right]_\varepsilon$, $\mathbf{A} \leftarrow \mathbf{A}\,\mathrm{diag}(1./sum(\mathbf{A},1))$ $\mathbf{S} \leftarrow \left[(\mathbf{A}^T\mathbf{A})^+(\mathbf{A}^T\mathbf{X} - \alpha_S)\right]_\varepsilon$,

Table 6.2, continued

Minimization of cost function subject to $a_{ij} \geq 0$ and $s_{ik} \geq 0$	Iterative learning algorithm
	$A \leftarrow [(XS^T - \alpha_A)(SS^T)^+]_\varepsilon$
Beta divergence $$\sum_{ik}\left(x_{ik}\frac{x_{ik}^\beta - [AS]_{ik}^\beta}{\beta(\beta+1)} + [AS]_{ik}^\beta \frac{[AS]_{ik} - y_{ik}}{\beta+1}\right)$$	$A \leftarrow A.*\left((X./(AS+\varepsilon)^{.1-\beta})S^T\right)./\left((AS+\varepsilon)^{.\beta}S^T\right)$
	$A \leftarrow A \operatorname{diag}\{1./sum(A,1)\}, \quad \beta = [-1,1]$
Itakura-Saito distance $$\sum_{ik}\left(-\log\frac{x_{ik}}{[AS]_{ik}} + \frac{x_{ik}}{[AS]_{ik}} - 1\right)$$	$S \leftarrow S.*\left[(A^TP)./(A^TQ+\varepsilon)\right]^{.\omega}$
	$A \leftarrow A \operatorname{diag}(1./sum(A,1)), \quad \omega = [0.5,1]$
	$P \leftarrow X./(AS+\varepsilon)^{.2}, \quad Q \leftarrow 1./(AS+\varepsilon)$

An essential feature of the NMF approach is that it reduces the data set from its full data space to lower dimensional NMF space determined by rank n (typically, $n < (mN)/(m + N)$). For any rank n, the NMF algorithms group the available data into classes or clusters of components. The key open issue is to find whether a given rank n decomposes the data into "meaningful" components. In general, the NMF algorithms may or may not converge to the same meaningful solutions on each run, depending on the random initial conditions and the kind of the algorithm we use. If a clustering into n classes is strong, we would expect that sample assignment to clusters would vary little from run to run. Although NMF is pure algebraic factorization, it was shown that as the rank n increases, the method may uncover some structure or substructures, whose robustness can be evaluated by running the algorithm for gradually increasing n. In fact, NMF may reveal hierarchical structure when it exists, but does not force such structure on the data like SCA or ICA does. Thus, NMF may have some advantages in exposing meaningful components and discover fine substructures.

The utility of NMF for estimating latent (hidden) components and their clusters or classes from EEG data (represented in the frequency or time-frequency domains) stems from its non-negativity constraints, which facilitates the detection of sharp boundaries among classes. These components are typically sparse, localized and relatively independent, which often makes physiologically and neuroanatomically meaningful signal decompositions. Despite its promising features, NMF has limitations due to non-uniqueness of solutions and difficulties to find optimal dimensions of matrices $\mathbf{A}$ and $\mathbf{S}$, as well as interpretation of some components.

6.9.1 Multi-layer NMF

In order to improve performance of the NMF, especially for ill-conditioned and badly scaled data, and also to reduce risk to get stuck in local minima of non-convex minimization, we have developed a simple hierarchical and multi-stage procedure in which we perform sequential decomposition of nonnegative matrices as follows: In the first step, we perform the basic decomposition (factorization) $\mathbf{X} = \mathbf{A}_1\mathbf{S}_1$ using any available NMF algorithm. In the second stage, the results obtained from the first stage are used to perform the similar decomposition: $\mathbf{S}_1 = \mathbf{A}_2\mathbf{S}_2$ using the same or different update rules, and so on. We continue our decomposition taking into account only the last achieved components. The process can be repeated arbitrary many times until some stopping criteria are satisfied. In each step, we usually obtain gradual improvements of the performance. Thus, our model has the form: $\mathbf{X} = \mathbf{A}_1\mathbf{A}_2 \cdots \mathbf{A}_L\mathbf{S}_L$, with the basis nonnegative matrix defined as $\mathbf{A} = \mathbf{A}_1\mathbf{A}_2 \cdots \mathbf{A}_L$. Physically, this means that we build up a system that has many layers or cascade connection of L mixing subsystems. The key point in our novel approach is that the learning (update) process to find parameters of sub-matrices $\mathbf{S}_l$ and $\mathbf{A}_l$ is performed sequentially, i.e. layer by layer. In each step or each layer, we can use the same cost (loss) functions, and consequently, the same learning (minimization) rules, or completely different cost functions and/or corresponding update rules.

In summary, the NMF is a promising technique for extracting, clustering and classifying of latent components. However, the challenge that still remains is to provide a meaningful physiological interpretation for some of NMF discovered hidden components or classes of components when the structures of the true sources are completely unknown.

6.10   DISCUSSION AND CONCLUSIONS

In this chapter, we discussed several extensions and modifications of blind source separation and decomposition algorithms for spatio-temporal decorrelation, independent component analysis, sparse component analysis, and non-negative matrix factorization, where various criteria and constraints are imposed such as linear predictability, smoothness, mutual independence, sparsity, and non-negativity of extracted components. Especially, we described generalization and extension of ICA to MSD-ICA, which relaxes considerably the condition on independence of original sources. Using these concepts in many cases, we are able to reconstruct (recover) the original brain sources and to mixing and separating matrices even if the original sources are not independent and in fact they are strongly correlated. Moreover, we propose a simple method for checking validity and true performance of BSS separation by applying the bank of filters with various frequency characteristics.

Furthermore, we have proposed a simple and efficient BSS approach for blind extraction from raw EEG data-specific components to improve sensitivity and specificity of early detection of Alzheimer's disease. The basic principle is to order and cluster automatically the estimated components and project back to the scalp level only the suitable group of components which are significant electrophysiological markers of Alzheimer disease. The suboptimal selection of indexes and the number of ordered components has been performed by extensive computer simulation and optimization procedure.

References

Amari, S. & Cichocki, A. (1998). Adaptive blind signal processing - neural network approaches. *Proceedings IEEE*, *86*, 1186–1187.

Amari, S., Cichocki, A. & Yang, H. (1996). A new learning algorithm for blind signal separation. In David S. Touretzky, M. C. M. & Hasselmo, M. E. (Eds.), *Advances in Neural Information Processing Systems 1995*, Volume 8 (pp. 757–763). MIT Press: Cambridge, MA.

Amari, S., Hyvärinem, A., Lee, S.-Y., Lee, T.-W. & Sanchez, V. (2002). Blind signal separation and independent component analysis. *Neurocomputing*, *49(12)*, 1–5.

Amari, S. & J.-F.Cardoso (1997). Blind source separation — semiparametric statistical approach. *IEEE Trans. on Signal Processing*, *45(11)*, 2692–2700.

Bach, F. & Jordan, M. (2003). Beyond independent components: trees and clusters. *Journal of Machine Learning Research*, *4*, 1205–1233.

Barros, A. K. & Cichocki, A. (2001). Extraction of specific signals with temporal structure. *Neural Computation*, *13(9)*, 1995–2000.

Bell, A. & Sejnowski, T. (1995). An information maximization approach to blind separation and blind deconvolution. *Neural Computation*, *7, no. 6*, 1129–1159.

Belouchrani, A., Abed-Meraim, K., Cardoso, J.-F. & Moulines, É. (1997). A blind source separation technique using second-order statistics. *IEEE Trans. Signal Processing, 45(2)*, 434–444.

Belouchrani, A. & Amin, M. (1996). A new approach for blind source separation using time-frequency distributions. *Proc. SPIE, 2846*, 193–203.

Belouchrani, A. & Cichocki, A. (2000). Robust whitening procedure in blind source separation context. *Electronics Letters, 36(24)*, 2050–2053.

Bobin, J., Moudden, Y., J.-L., Starck & Elad, M. (2006). Morphological diversity and source separation. *IEEE Signal Processing Letters, 13*, 409–412.

Cardoso, J.-F. & Laheld, B. (1996). Equivariant adaptive source separation. *IEEE Trans. Signal Processing, 44(12)*, 3017–3030.

Chenubhotla, S. C. (2004). *Spectral Methods for Multi-scale Features Extraction and Data Clustering.* Ph.D Thesis, University of Toronto.

Choi, S., Cichocki, A. & Amari, S. (1998). Flexible independent component analysis. In *Proc. of the 1998 IEEE Workshop on NNSP* (pp. 83–92). Cambridge, UK.

Choi, S., Cichocki, A. & Amari, S. (2002a). Equivariant nonstationary source separation. *Neural Networks, 15*, 121–130.

Choi, S., Cichocki, A. & Amari, S. (2002b). Equivariant nonstationary source separation. *Neural Networks, 15(1)*, 121–130.

Choi, S., Cichocki, A. & Belouchrani, A. (2002c). Second order nonstationary source separation. *Journal of VLSI Signal Processing, 32(1–2)*, 93–104.

Cichocki, A. & Amari, S. (2003). *Adaptive Blind Signal And Image Processing (New revised and improved edition).* New York: John Wiley.

Cichocki, A., Amari, S., Zdunek, R., He, Z. & Kompass, R. (2006a). Extended SMART algorithms for non-negative matrix factorization. *LNAI 4029, Springer*, 548–562.

Cichocki, A., Amari, S. M., Siwek, K., Tanaka, T. & et al. (2004a). ICALAB Toolboxes for Signal and Image Processing *www.bsp.brain.riken.go.jp*. JAPAN.

Cichocki, A. & Belouchrani, A. (2001). Sources separation of temporally correlated sources from noisy data using bank of band-pass filters. In *Third International Conference on Independent Component Analysis and Signal Separation (ICA-2001)* (pp. 173–178). San Diego, USA.

Cichocki, A., Bogner, R., Moszczyński, L. & Pope, K. (1997a). Modified Hérault-Jutten algorithms for blind separation of sources. *Digital Signal Processing, 7(2)*, 80 – 93.

Cichocki, A. & Georgiev, P. (2003). Blind source separation algorithms with matrix constraints. *IEICE Transactions on Fundamentals of Electronics, Communications and Computer Sciences, E86-A(1)*, 522–531.

Cichocki, A., Kasprzak, W. & Skarbek, W. (1996). Adaptive learning algorithm for principal component analysis with partial data. In Trappl, R. (Ed.), *Cybernetics and Systems '96. Thirteenth European Meeting on Cybernetics and Systems Research*, Volume 2 (pp. 1014–1019). Austrian Society for Cybernetic Studies, Vienna.

Cichocki, A., Li, Y., Georgiev, P. G. & Amari, S. (2004b). Beyond ICA: Robust sparse signal representations. In *Proceedings of 2004 IEEE International Symposium on Circuits and Systems (ISCAS2004)*, Volume V (pp. 684–687). Vancouver, Canada.

Cichocki, A., Rutkowski, T. M. & Siwek, K. (2002). Blind signal extraction of signals with specified frequency band. In *Neural Networks for Signal Processing XII: Proceedings of the 2002 IEEE Signal Processing Society Workshop* (pp. 515–524). Martigny, Switzerland: IEEE.

Cichocki, A., Shishkin, S., Musha, T., Leonowicz, Z., Asada, T. & Kurachi, T. (2005). EEG filtering based on blind source separation (BSS) for early detection of Alzheimer disease. *Clinical Neurophysiology, 116*, 729–737.

Cichocki, A. & Thawonmas, R. (2000). On-line algorithm for blind signal extraction of arbitrarily distributed, but temporally correlated sources using second order statistics. *Neural Processing Letters, 12(1)*, 91–98.

Cichocki, A., Thawonmas, R. & Amari, S. (1997b). Sequential blind signal extraction in order specified by stochastic properties. *Electronics Letters, 33(1)*, 64–65.

Cichocki, A. & Unbehauen, R. (1993). Robust estimation of principal components in real time. *Electronics Letters, 29(21)*, 1869–1870.

Cichocki, A. & Unbehauen, R. (1994). *Neural Networks for Optimization and Signal Processing (New revised and improved edition)*. New York: John Wiley & Sons.

Cichocki, A. & Unbehauen, R. (1996). Robust neural networks with on-line learning for blind identification and blind separation of sources. *IEEE Trans. Circuits and Systems I : Fundamentals Theory and Applications, 43(11)*, 894–906.

Cichocki, A., Unbehauen, R. & Rummert, E. (1994). Robust learning algorithm for blind separation of signals. *Electronics Letters, 30(17)*, 1386–1387.

Cichocki, A. & Zdunek, R. (2006). NMFLAB Toolboxes for Signal and Image Processing *www.bsp.brain.riken.go.jp*. JAPAN.

Cichocki, A., Zdunek, R. & Amari, S. (2006b). Csiszar's divergences for non-negative matrix factorization: Family of new algorithms. *LNCS, Springer, 3889*, 32–39.

Cichocki, A., Zdunek, R. & Amari, S. (2006c). New algorithms for non-negative matrix factorization in applications to blind source separation. In *Proc. IEEE International Conference on Acoustics, Speech, and Signal Processing, ICASSP-2006*.

Cruces, S., Cichocki, A. & Castedo, L. (2000). An iterative inversion approach to blind source separation. *IEEE Trans. on Neural Networks, 11(6)*, 1423–1437.

Cruces, S. A., Castedo, L. & Cichocki, A. (2002). Robust blind source separation algorithms using cumulants. *Neurocomputing, 49,* 87–118.

Cruces, S. A. & Cichocki, A. (2003). Combining blind source extraction with joint approximate diagonalization: Thin algorithms for ICA. In *Proceedings of 4th International Symposium on Independent Component Analysis and Blind Signal Separation (ICA2003)* (pp. 463–468). Kyoto, Japan: ICA.

Cruces, S. A., Cichocki, A. & Amari, S. (2004). From blind signal extraction to blind instantaneous signal separation: criteria, algorithms and stability. *IEEE Transactions on Neural Networks, Special issue on Information Theoretical Learning, 15,* 859–873.

DeKosky, S. & Marek, K. (2003). Looking backward to move forward: Early detection of neurodegenerative disorders. *Science, 302(5646),* 830–834.

Delorme, A. & Makeig, S. (2004). EEGLAB: an open source toolbox for analysis of single-trial EEG dynamics. *J. Neuroscience Methods, 134:9-21, 2004, 134,* 9 21.

Dhillon, I. & Sra, S. (2005). Generalized nonnegative matrix approximations with Bregman divergences. In *NIPS -Neural Information Proc. Systems, Vancouver Canada.*

Donoho, D. L. & Elad, M. (2004). Representation via l1 minimization. *The Proc. National Academy of Science, 100,* 2197–2202.

Fiori, S. (2003). A fully multiplicative orthoghonal-group ICA neural algorithm. *Electronics Letters, 39(24),* 1737–1738.

Georgiev, P. G. & Cichocki, A. (2004). Sparse component analysis of overcomplete mixtures by improved basis pursuit method. In *Proceedings of 2004 IEEE International Symposium on Circuits and Systems (ISCAS2004),* Volume V (pp. 37–40). Vancouver, Canada.

Gharieb, R. R. & Cichocki, A. (2003). Second-order statistics based blind source separation using a bank of subband filters. *Digital Signal Processing, 13,* 252–274.

He, Z. & Cichocki, A. (2006). K-EVD clustering and its applications to sparse component analysis. In *6th International Conference on Independent Component Analysis and Blind Signal Separation* (pp. 90–97). Springer LNCS 3889.

Himberg, J., Hyvärinen, A. & Esposito, F. (2004). Validating the independent components of neuroimaging time series via clustering and visualization. *NeuroImage, 22(3)*, 1214–1222.

Hyärinen, A. & Oja, E. (2000). Independent component analysis: Algorithms and applications. *Neural Networks, 13*, 411–430.

Hyvärinen, A., Karhunen, J. & Oja, E. (2001). *Independent Component Analysis.* New York: John Wiley.

Jahn, O., Cichocki, A., Ioannides, A. & Amari, S. (1999). Identification and elimination of artifacts from MEG signals using efficient independent components analysis. In *Proc. of th 11th Int. Conference on Biomagentism BIOMAG-98* (pp. 224–227). Sendai, Japan.

Jelic, V., Johansson, S., Almkvist, O., Shigeta, M., Julin, P., Nordberg, A., Winblad, B. & Wahlund, L. (2000). Quantitative electroencephalography in mild cognitive impairment: Longitudinal changes and possible prediction of Alzheimer's disease. *Neurobiological Aging, 21(4)*, 533–540.

Jeong, J. (2004). EEG dynamics in patients with Alzheimer's disease. *Clinical Neurophysiology, 115(7)*, 1490–1505.

Jung, H.-Y. & Lee, S.-Y. (2000). On the temporal decorrelation of feature parameters for noise-robust speech recognition. *IEEE Transactions on Speech and Audio Processing, 8(7)*, 407–416.

Jung, T., Makeig, S., Humphries, C., Lee, T.-W., McKeown, M., Iragui, V. & Sejnowski, T. (2000). Removing electroencephalographic artifacts by blind source separation. *Psychophysiology, 37*, 167–178.

Karhunen, J. & Pajunen, P. (1997). Blind source separation and tracking using nonlinear PCA criterion: A least-squares approach. In *Proc. 1997 Int. Conference on Neural Networks (ICNN'97)*, Volume 4 (pp. 2147–2152). Houston, Texas, USA.

Kompass, R. (2005). A generalized divergence measure for non-negative matrix factorization. Neuroinfomatics Workshop, Torun, Poland.

Kreutz-Delgado, K., Murray, J. F., Rao, B. D., Engan, K., Lee, T.-W. & Sejnowski, T. J. (2003). Dictionary learning algorithms for sparse representation. *Neural Computation, 15(2)*, 349–396.

Lee, D. D. & Seung, H. S. (1999). Learning of the parts of objects by non-negative matrix factorization. *Nature, 401*, 788–791.

Li, Y., Cichocki, A. & Amari, S. (2004). Analysis of sparse representation and blind source separation. *Neural Computation, 16(6)*, 1193–1204.

Li, Y., Cichocki, A. & Amari, S. (2006). Blind estimation of channel parameters and source components for EEG signals: A sparse factorization approach. *IEEE Transactions on Neural Networks, 17*, 419–431.

Li, Y., Cichocki, A., Amari, S., Shishkin, S., Cao, J. & Gu, F. (2003). Sparse representation and its applications in blind source separation. In *Seventeenth Annual Conference on Neural Information Processing Systems (NIPS-2003)*. Vancouver.

Lin, C.-J. (2005). Projected gradient methods for non-negative matrix factorization. Technical report, Department of Computer Science, National Taiwan University.

Mainecke, F., Ziehe, A., Kawanabe, M. & Müller, K.-R. (2002). A resampling approach to estimate the stability of one dimensional or multidimensional independent components. *NeuroImage, 49(13)*, 1514–1525.

Makeig, S., Debener, S., Onton, J. & Delorme, A. (2004a). Mining event-related brain dynamics. *Trends in Cognitive Science, 8*, 204–210.

Makeig, S., Delorme, A., M., M. W., Townsend, J., Courchense, E. & Sejnowski, T. (2004b). Electroencephalographic brain dynamics following visual targets requiring manual responses. *PLOS Biology, 2*, 747–762.

Matsuoka, K., Ohya, M. & Kawamoto, M. (1995). A neural net for blind separation of nonstationary signals. *Neural Networks, 8(3)*, 411–419.

Merritt, M. & Zhang, Y. (2004). An interior-point gradient method for large-scale totally nonnegative least squares problems. Technical report, Department of Computational and Applied Mathematics, Rice University, Houston, Texas, USA.

Minami, M. & Eguchi, S. (2002). Robust blind source separation by beta-divergence. *Neural Computation, 14*, 1859–1886.

Miwakeichi, F., Martinez-Montes, E., Valds-Sosa, P. A., Nishiyama, N., Mizuhara, H. & Yamaguchi, Y. (2004). Decomposing EEG data into space-time-frequency components using Parallel Factor Analysis. *NeuroImage, 22(3)*, 1035–1045.

Molgedey, L. & Schuster, H. (1994). Separation of a mixture of independent signals using time delayed correlations. *Physical Review Letters, 72(23)*, 3634–3637.

Musha, T., Asada, T., Yamashita, F., T., T. K., Chen, Z., Matsuda, H., Uno, M. & Shankle, W. (2002). A new EEG method for estimating cortical neuronal impairment that is sensitive to early stage Alzheimer's disease. *Clinical Neurophysiology, 113(7)*, 1052–1508.

Nishimori, Y. (1999). Learning algorithm for ICA by geodesic flows on orthogonal group. In *Joint Conference on Neural Networks (IJCNN'99)*, Volume 2 (pp. 1625–1647).

Petersen, R. (2003). *Mild Cognitive Impairment: Aging to Alzheimers Disease*. New York: Oxford University Press.

Petersen, R., Stevens, J., Ganguli, M., Tangalos, E., Cummings, J. & DeKosky, S. (2001). Practice parameter: Early detection of dementia: Mild cognitive impairment (an evidence-based review). *Neurology, 56*, 1133–1142.

Rosipal, R., Girolami, M., Trejo, L. J. & Cichocki, A. (2001). Kernel PCA for feature extraction and de-noising in nonlinear regression. *Neural Computing & Applications, 10*, 231–243.

Sajda, P., Du, S. & Parra, L. (2003). Recovery of constituent spectra using non-negative matrix factorization. In *Proceedings of SPIE – Volume 5207* (pp. 321–331.). Wavelets: Applications in Signal and Image Processing.

Stone, J. (2001). Blind source separation using temporal predictability. *Neural Computation, 13(7)*, 1559–1574.

Tanaka, T. & Cichocki, A. (2004). Subband decomposition independent component analysis and new performance criteria. In *Proceedings of International Conference on Acoustics, Speech, and Signal Processing (ICASSP2004)*, Volume V (pp. 541–544). Montreal, Canada.

Theis, F. J., Georgiev, P. G. & Cichocki, A. (2004). Robust overcomplete matrix recovery for sparse sources using a generalized Hough transform. In *Proceedings of 12th European Symposium on Artificial Neural Networks (ESANN2004)* (pp. 223–232). Bruges, Belgium.

Tong, L., Liu, R.-W., Soon, V.-C. & Huang, Y.-F. (1991). Indeterminacy and identifiability of blind identification. *IEEE Trans. on Circuits and Systems, 38(5)*, 499–509.

Vialatte, F., Cichocki, A., Dreyfus, G., Musha, T., Shishkin, S. L. & Gervais, R. (2005). Early diagnosis of Alzheimer's disease by blind source separation, time frequency representation, and bump modeling of EEG signals. In *Artificial Neural Networks: Biological Inspirations ICANN 2005, 15th International Conference Warsaw, Poland, September 11-15, 2005 Proceedings*, Volume LNCS 3696 (pp. 683–692).

Vorobyov, S. & Cichocki, A. (2002). Blind noise reduction for multisensory signals using ICA and subspace filtering, with application to EEG analysis. *Biological Cybernetics, 86(4)*, 293–303.

Wagner, A. (2000). Early detection of Alzheimer's disease: An fMRI marker for people at risk? *Nature Neuroscience, 10(3)*, 973–974.

Wang, Z., Lee, Y., Fiori, S., Leung, C.-S. & Zhu, Y.-S. (2003). An improved sequential method for principal component analysis. *Pattern Recognition Letters, 24*, 1409–1415.

Washizawa, Y. & Cichocki, A. (2005). On line k-plane clustering learning algorithm for sparse component analysis. In *IEEE International Conference on Acoustics, Speech, and Signal Processing,*. ICASSP-2006, Toulouse, France.

Zdunek, R. & Cichocki, A. (2006). Non-negative matrix factorization with quasi-newton optimization. *LNAI 4029, Springer*, 870–879.

Zhang, L., Cichocki, A. & Amari, S. (2004). Multichannel blind deconvolution of nonminimum-phase systems using filter decomposition. *IEEE Transactions on Signal Processing, 52(5)*, 1430–1442.

Zibulevsky, M., Kisilev, P., Zeevi, Y. & Pearlmutter, B. (2002). Blind source separation via multinode sparse representation. In *In Advances in Neural Information Processing Systems, (NIPS2001)* (pp. 185–191). Morgan Kaufmann.

Ziehe, A., Müller, K.-R., Nolte, G., Mackert, B.-M. & Curio, G. (2000). Artifact reduction in biomagnetic recordings based on time-delayed second order correlations. *IEEE Trans. on Biomedical Engineering, 47*, 75–87.

Zou, H., Hastie, T. & Tibshirani, R. (2006). Sparse principal component analysis. *Journal of Computational and Graphical Statistics, 15*, 265–286.

7

Quantifying Scaling Properties of Neurophysiological Time Series

Thomas C. Ferree
University of California, San Francisco

Mark A. Kramer
University of California, Berkeley

David J. McGonigle
Neurosciences Cognitive et Imagerie Cerebrale, UPR 640-LENA

Rudolph C. Hwa
University of Oregon

Among the noninvasive techniques available for human functional neuroimaging, the electroencephalogram (EEG) provides a measure of brain electrical activity with millisecond temporal resolution and centimeter spatial resolution (Nunez, 1981). Modern EEG systems typically feature 128 electrodes positioned over the scalp, giving a global view of brain dynamics that is complementary to anatomical images. A significant challenge is how best to represent the rich dynamical information in these large, complicated data sets. Traditionally, the methods employed by experimental psychology and neuroscience have been motivated by the need to consolidate these data across experimental conditions and subject groups, usually to facilitate hypothesis testing with either the t or F statistic. As we see here, although such averaging allows standard statistical tools to be used, it is employed at the expense of the true complexity of the data.

The EEG measures the time-dependent voltage on the scalp, at a set of measurement electrodes, relative to some reference electrode. Figure 7.1 shows a typical example of spontaneous EEG data collected from a normal human subject resting with eyes closed. The

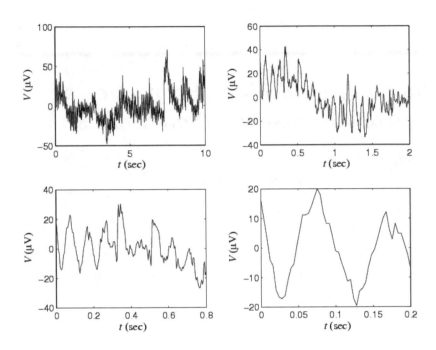

Fig. 7.1: Typical example of spontaneous EEG data collected from a normal human subject, resting with eyes closed. The same data are shown at four different scales of temporal resolution.

time series exhibits fluctuations across the entire range of collected time scales. It is common in neuroscience to describe these fluctuations as oscillations. This implicitly presumes that the data can be linearly decomposed into sinusoidal components, however, which may not be realistic for EEG data. Spectral-temporal analysis, typically based on the moving-window Fourier transform or wavelets, often reveals non-stationarity in the spectral content of the data over time, but it still emphasizes isolated frequencies. Although these spectral approaches are natural if the fluctuations on a certain time scale behave independently of others, their use is motivated more by providence.

Scaling analysis is a complementary way of characterizing fluctuations in a time series, by relating the size of the fluctuations *across* time scales. This approach is natural when the size of the fluctuations on neighboring time scales relate to one another in a particular way. We give a precise definition of *scaling* in the next section. Briefly, given some measure of the fluctuations in a system, which is a function of measurement scale, *scaling* behavior refers to a property of that measure that is independent of scale.

7.1   THEORY

The aim of this section is to explain scaling analysis and place it in the context of the more familiar analysis techniques applied to EEG time series. To this end, we discuss linear analyses of transient responses and spontaneous EEG and nonlinear analyses derived from studying chaotic systems. We describe each of these approaches only briefly, but enough to point out their differing assumptions and interpretations.

7.1.1   Linear Technique: Event-Related Averaging (ERA)

By definition, linear methods assume that a linear dynamical system underlies the data. Linear methods yield simple, interpretable results when applied to a linear system. We discuss two linear analysis methods: event-related averaging (ERA) and Fourier spectral analysis (FSA).

Experiments that involve time-localized events (e.g., due to brief, externally generated stimuli) are assumed in linear response theory to have event-related responses superimposed on a background EEG signal. The most common analysis approach for extracting this response is ERA: averaging short data epochs defined around each event. In EEG, the result is called the event-related potential (ERP). In magnetoencephelography (MEG), the analogous result is called the event-related field (ERF).

In general, the response $V(t)$ of a linear system to an input $S(t)$ has a well-known form:

$$V(t) = \int_{-\infty}^{t} dt' \; k(t - t') \; S(t') + N(t) \qquad (7.1)$$

where $k(t-t')$ is the linear response kernel, $S(t')$ is the input, and $N(t)$ represents noise. The upper limit of integration reflects causality.

If $S(t')$ is an impulse (i.e., very brief compared to the time scales inherent in k), then it may be approximated mathematically by a Dirac delta function $\delta(t')$. With $S(t') = S_0\,\delta(t')$, the integral in Equation 7.1 evaluates to

$$V(t) = S_0\,k(t) + N(t),\qquad(7.2)$$

where $t \geq 0$. In EEG, the input $S(t')$ represents a stimulus (or some other brief event, such as subject response), and $V(t)$ represents the voltage measured at a single electrode on the scalp. The assumption that the noise $N(t)$ adds linearly to the response is central to linear analysis. This assumption is reasonable in certain special cases (e.g., amplifier shot [thermal] noise and ambient [60 Hz] noise in the recording environment), but cannot be expected to hold rigorously when $N(t)$ represents other neural activity not captured in the ERP.

The total number of neurons contributing to the signal in each channel is generally large compared with the number responding to the stimulus (Nunez, 1995). Thus the measured response $k(t)$ to an impulse is usually small compared with the background EEG. It is possible to estimate $k(t)$ in the time domain, however, by repeating the experiment in M trials and averaging the results. Assuming that the response $k(t)$ is identical across trials gives

$$\overline{V}(t) \equiv \frac{1}{M}\sum_{i=1}^{M} V_i(t) = S_0\,k(t) + \frac{1}{M}\sum_{i=1}^{M} N_i(t).\qquad(7.3)$$

In the ideal case that $N(t)$ is drawn from a Gaussian distribution with mean zero and standard deviation σ [i.e., $N_i(t) = \mathrm{GRV}(0,\sigma)$], then averaging over trials gives

$$\overline{V}(t) = S_0\,k(t) + \mathrm{GRV}\left(0, \frac{\sigma}{\sqrt{M}}\right).\qquad(7.4)$$

Here the noise is reduced by a factor $1/\sqrt{M}$. Although this *brain noise*, being defined simply as the contribution of the spontaneous and stimulus-related neural activity that is not captured by the ERP, is unlikely to be Gaussian, it is still expected (or hoped) that averaging reduces the contribution of the noise to the measured response. The averaging prescription in (7.3) implicitly defines brain noise in the context of the ERP.

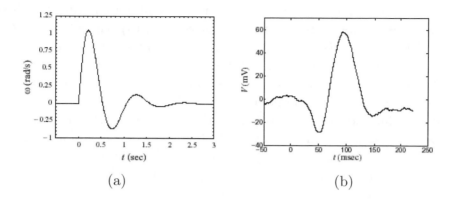

(a)   (b)

Fig. 7.2: The linear impulse response function: (a) mass on a spring, subject to damping; and (b) event-related potential, due to brief auditory tone beep.

Example Linear System: Mass on a Spring

To illustrate the concept of linear impulse response, consider the simplest oscillatory system: a mass on a spring. Certainly this is not a reasonable model of the neural system underlying the scalp EEG, but it does illustrate the basic assumptions implicit in linear analysis. Specifically, consider a mass m connected to a spring with elasticity constant c, subject to velocity-dependent damping with constant b and external forcing function $F(t)$. The equation of motion is

$$m\frac{d^2x}{dt^2} + b\frac{dx}{dt} + cx = F(t). \tag{7.5}$$

The general solution to (7.5) may be expressed as in (7.1). The kernel $k(t)$ has the form

$$k(t) \propto e^{-\beta t}\sin(\omega_1 t - \phi) \tag{7.6}$$

where $\omega_1 \equiv \sqrt{\beta^2 - \omega_0^2}$, $\omega_0 \equiv \sqrt{c/m}$, $\beta \equiv b/2m$, and ϕ is a constant phase shift. If the system were higher dimensional (e.g., multiple masses coupled by springs), then the response kernel would be a sum of damped sinusoids, with the number of unique frequencies and decay constants determined by the dimension and parameters of the entire system.

The response properties of a damped oscillator are intuitive. When we measure the transient brain response to our experiment (i.e., ERP or ERF), it is natural to extend that intuition to an interpretation of the sequence of peaks and troughs present in the evoked waveform. Yet it is unclear whether such a waveform is even qualitatively like a simple mechanical oscillator. Figure 7.2(a) shows the impulse response function $k(t)$ given by Equation 7.6. The height of successive peaks decreases monotonically. The frequency of oscillation and rate of damping are simply related to the underlying system parameters. This situation is satisfying because these measurable quantities can be used to estimate the parameter values in the underlying linear system, for example. However, this kind of detailed interpretation may not extend to nonlinear systems or neurophysiological data.

For comparison, Figure 7.2(b) shows an ERP recorded from a ball electrode located on the cortical surface over auditory areas, in response to a brief tone pulse (R. T. Knight, personal communication). At first glance, the similarity with Figure 7.2(a) is remarkable. One qualitative difference is that the second peak of the ERP is larger than the first peak—an impossible situation for a mass on a spring. Obviously, the mechanisms for generating the transient ERP are fundamentally different from those of a simple oscillator. When a small (e.g., 1 mm^2) patch of cortex is viewed as a neural mass, comprised of excitatory and inhibitory neurons, the EEG oscillations arise from the local cortical circuitry. A mesoscopic view of the system lumps the neural degrees of freedom in each small patch of cortex into a few state variables, coupled by differential equations (Freeman, 1975). The equations have local properties, which might be qualitatively likened to a system of coupled mechanical oscillators, at least insofar as successive peaks and troughs are rebounds of a local state variable. In contrast, the early auditory ERP arising from the brain stem has a series of peaks and troughs, which are in fact transient responses generated along different locations of the auditory nerve (see Cone-Wesson & Wunderlich, 2003, for a review). The nature of the apparent oscillatory activity in the early auditory ERP, therefore, is not even qualitatively like a simple mechanical oscillator. Thus, although one can apply linear analysis techniques to any data set, only if the system being studied is linear can a thorough understanding and relatively unambiguous interpretation be made.

7.1.2   Linear Technique: Fourier Spectral Analysis (FSA)

By far the most common method for analyzing spontaneous EEG data is based on the Fourier transform. Let $\tilde{V}(f)$ represent the Fourier transform of the measured signal $V(t)$. Theoretically, the power spectrum $P(f)$ is defined as

$$P(f) = |\tilde{V}(f)|^2. \tag{7.7}$$

It is straightforward to show that $P(f)$ is equal to the Fourier transform of the temporal autocorrelation of V with itself. In linear response theory, it is normally assumed that (a) the measured signal $V(t)$ may be decomposed linearly into *response* and *noise* terms, as in Equation 7.1; and (b) these terms are not linearly correlated. By the convolution theorem, the Fourier transform of the integral involving k and S in Equation 7.1 is equal to the product of their Fourier transforms. Thus, the power spectrum may be written

$$P(f) = |\tilde{k}(f)\tilde{S}(f)|^2 + |\tilde{N}(f)|^2. \tag{7.8}$$

Here $\tilde{k}(f)$, $\tilde{S}(f)$, and $\tilde{N}(f)$ are the Fourier transforms of $k(t)$, $S(t)$, and $N(t)$, respectively. The first term in Equation 7.8 represents the neural response, and the second term represents the noise contribution. The cross-terms cancel because we have assumed that the response and noise are linearly uncorrelated. If $N(t)$ is Gaussian, then $|\tilde{N}(f)|^2 = N_0^2 = $ constant, and the noise appears in plots of $P(f)$ as a constant *floor*.

Normally, the EEG power spectrum $P(f)$ has large low-frequency content that is often called $1/f$-like, one or more discernible peaks, and a broad-banded component (extending at least to 50 Hz) that is not constant, but falls off gradually with increasing f. When analyzing spontaneous EEG (i.e., without controlling the input to the system), the separation into brain response and brain noise is ambiguous, so we may drop the separate noise term $\tilde{N}(f)$. The structure in $P(f)$ may arise from structure in $\tilde{k}(f)$, $\tilde{S}(f)$, or both. Even if $\tilde{k}(f)$ were independent of frequency, peaks in the baseline input to the cortex, represented now by $\tilde{S}(f)$, would still generate peaks in $P(f)$. Alternatively, if the input to the cortex under resting conditions is viewed as Gaussian white noise (Steyn-Ross, Steyn-Ross, Sleigh &

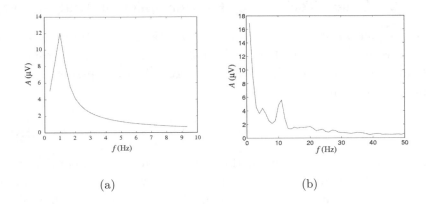

(a)   (b)

Fig. 7.3: Fourier power spectrum of: (a) mass on a spring, subject to white noise input; and (b) spontaneous EEG, normal subject resting with eyes closed. The peak near 10 Hz is the familiar α-rhythm.

Liley, 1999), then peaks in $P(f)$ give information about the linear response function of the underlying cortical system:

$$P(f) = S_0^2 \, |\tilde{k}(f)|^2. \tag{7.9}$$

The complex modulus $|\tilde{k}(f)|$ is called the *gain* of the system.

Figure 7.3(a) shows $|\tilde{k}(f)|$, obtained by computing the Fourier transform of the linear response kernel in Equation 7.6. The existence of a single peak (at the natural frequency: $\omega_1 = 1$ Hz, in this example) reveals the single oscillatory mode of the system. If the system were higher dimensional, $P(f)$ would have multiple peaks at a discrete set of frequencies, corresponding to the *normal modes* of the system. For comparison, Figure 7.3(b) shows the Fourier amplitude spectrum [i.e., $A(f) = \sqrt{P(f)}$] of the time series in Figure 7.1. It has large low-frequency power, a prominent peak in the α-band (8-13 Hz), and a broad-banded contribution that decreases with f, but extends at least to 50 Hz. Our objective in data analysis is to summarize the voltage data illustrated in Figure 7.1. The FSA (shown in Figure 7.3(b)) provides some summary measures (such as the α-band peak), but in general it may be difficult to distinguish peaks from a truly broad-banded component in short segments of EEG data.

Estimating the Fourier power spectrum

The power spectrum shown in Figure 7.3(b) is not the true power spectrum of the EEG data; it is only an estimate. The simplest and most common way of estimating the power spectrum of any discrete time series begins with the fast Fourier transform (FFT). Let t_i be the times at which the voltage is sampled, for $i = 1, ..., N$. The duration of the time series is $T = N\Delta t$, where Δt is the sampling interval. Here we assume that N is even. The Fourier components of V, denoted $\tilde{V}$, are computed at a discrete set of frequencies $f_k = (k - 1)\Delta f$, where $k = 1, 2, ..., N/2 + 1$, and the frequency resolution is $\Delta f = 1/T$. The product $\tilde{V}^*\tilde{V} = |\tilde{V}|^2$, where $\tilde{V}^*$ is the complex conjugate of $\tilde{V}$, generates the *periodogram* estimate of the power spectrum (Press, Tuekolsky, Vetterling & Flannery, 1992).

Because the FFT assumes signal periodicity, which is never valid for real data, the periodogram is contaminated by a well-known artifact. In the time domain, this artifact arises because the aperiodic signal has a discontinuity across the end-points, violating the implicit periodic boundary conditions. In the frequency domain, this artifact arises because the signal has power at frequencies outside the discrete set $\{f_k\}$. This causes significant spillage of power into neighboring frequency bins. Spillage can be minimized by windowing the data (i.e., multiplying it by a *tapering function*) that smoothly reduces the time series to zero at both ends. A popular choice is the Hann window: $w(t) = [1 - \cos(2\pi t/T)]/2$. This restores the periodic boundary condition and reduces the amount of spillage into neighboring bins.

The difficulty with estimating the power spectrum using a single tapering function (such as the Hann window) is that it reduces the contribution of data near the ends of each segment while emphasizing the data in the middle. In this sense, windowing assumes stationarity of the time series. Multitaper methods use a family of tapering functions that weight various parts of the time series separately, such that a linear combination of tapered transforms provides an optimal estimate of the power spectrum (Percival & Walden, 1993). Later in this chapter, we show the results of scaling analysis, based on DFA and FSA for both methods of tapering.

To obtain a good statistical estimate of the power spectrum, one must divide the time series into M segments. Each segment is sep-

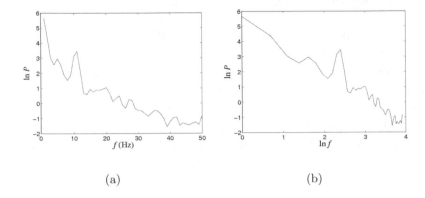

Fig. 7.4: Fourier power spectrum, same as in Figure 7.3(b), plotted two different ways: (a) log-linear, and (b) log-log.

arately windowed, then Fourier transformed, and the squared power values at each frequency are averaged across segments. Dividing the data into M segments reduces the frequency resolution, thereby increasing the minimum observable frequency to $\Delta f = M/T$ and assumes stationarity of the time series.

Visualizing the Fourier Power Spectrum

Because the EEG power spectrum $P(f)$ typically falls off as a function of frequency, plotting $A(f) = \sqrt{P(f)}$ reduces the relative height of large peaks, making small peaks more readily visible. It is also common to plot $P(f)$ on log-linear axes (i.e., $\ln P$ vs. f) so that the small values of $P(f)$ become even more visible. Figure 7.4(a) shows the power spectrum of Figure 7.3(b) plotted this way. Indeed, it is much easier to see the structure at high frequencies, but this does not fundamentally change the way one thinks about the power spectrum. Here one still looks for peaks (as a way of identifying normal modes) or for differences in power between experimental conditions or subject groups. In either case, the emphasis is usually on particular frequency bands.

There is a third way of visualizing the power spectrum, which leads to scaling analysis. It has long been noted that many complex systems produce power spectra with $1/f$-like behavior (Bak, 1996). More generally, the spectra may exhibit power-law behavior: $P(f) \propto 1/f^\beta$, where $\beta > 0$. If this behavior holds over a range of f, then $\ln P \propto -\beta \ln f$, and plotting $P(f)$ in log-log axes reveals the power-law behavior as a straight line with slope $-\beta$. Figure 7.4(b) shows P plotted on log-log axes. Unlike the linear-linear and log-linear plots, the frequency values in log-log plots are distributed unevenly on the f-axis, with the density of points exponentially greater for larger f. The values of $\ln P$ decrease with $\ln f$, but not monotonically. The erratic behavior of the power spectrum, especially at high frequencies, makes it difficult to identify the scaling behavior that may be present. In this figure, the slope of $\ln P$ versus $\ln f$ appears similar on either side of the peak. This is generally not the case in EEG.

7.1.3   Nonlinear Technique: Chaos Analysis

Over the last few decades, the study of nonlinear dynamical systems has provided many new techniques for time-series analysis. The identification of chaotic behavior (characterized by sensitive dependence on initial conditions) in low-dimensional, deterministic systems, came as a surprise. It was thought previously that only high-dimensional, stochastic systems could give rise to such complicated dynamics (Gleick, 1987). Although chaotic dynamics are inherently unpredictable and usually much more complicated than linear dynamics, chaotic attractors provide a structure to the data that is more organized than stochastic noise.

Example: Lorenz System

We first consider a simple model system that exhibits deterministic chaos to illustrate differences in the interpretation of the Fourier power spectrum. The Lorenz system is a set of three ordinary differential equations:

$$\frac{dx}{dt} = a(y - x)$$
$$\frac{dy}{dt} = bx - y - xz \tag{7.10}$$
$$\frac{dz}{dt} = xy - cx,$$

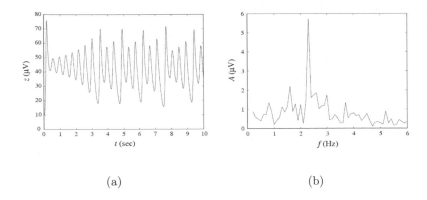

(a)   (b)

Fig. 7.5: Lorenz equations in chaotic parameter regime: (a) time series of the variable $z(t)$, equivalent to the projection of the Lorenz butterfly attractor onto the z-axis; (b) Fourier amplitude spectrum of $z(t)$.

which were devised to model weather dynamics (Lorenz, 1963). There are three independent variables, $x(t)$, $y(t)$, and $z(t)$, and no forcing term. The system is autonomous and generates its own dynamics without external input. Figure 7.5(a) shows the time course of one of the variables $z(t)$ for a common choice of parameters: $a = 10$, $b = 28$, $c = 8/3$. The time series appears nearly periodic, which suggests we apply FSA.

Figure 7.5(b) shows the Fourier amplitude spectrum of $z(t)$. It is broad-banded (i.e., it has nonzero power across a wide range of frequencies). The dominant peak near 2.25 Hz reflects the dominant period that is visible in Figure 7.5(a). The many smaller peaks that are visible in Figure 7.5(b) do not have a simple interpretation; the smaller peaks do not reveal additional normal modes of a higher-dimensional linear system, nor are they due to stochastic noise. Rather, they are attributable to the fundamental aperiodicity of chaotic motion. Thus, it is not sensible to interpret each peak individually (e.g., as a distinct normal mode) even though they may appear in the calculated spectrum. This example shows potential pitfalls of applying intuition from linear systems to interpret the power spectrum of a nonlinear dynamical system undergoing chaotic motion.

The trajectory of the Lorenz system, through its three-dimensional phase space—$(x(t), y(t), z(t))$—forms the famous butterfly attractor (Lorenz, 1963). The butterfly attractor has a fractal structure, meaning that the spatial distribution of points in phase space exhibits fractal self-similarity. This fractal structure may be quantified in terms of the space-filling properties of its points (such as the fractal dimension). The time series $z(t)$ is a projection of the butterfly attractor onto a single, one-dimensional axis. Because the attractor is a chaotic attractor and possesses fractal structure, it is not surprising that the time series shown in Figure 7.5(a) is aperiodic. However, the attractor lends structure to the data; $z(t)$ is not white noise, although its dynamics are unpredictable.

Applications to EEG data

The study of model chaotic dynamical systems has led to techniques for identifying and quantifying chaotic properties of observed time series—for example, the fractal dimension (Grassberger & Procaccia, 1983). Now the field of *observed chaos* is vast and rapidly growing.[1] Its application to EEG time-series data is based on the idea that chaos measures provide informative summary statistics, which may correlate with brain state, function, or pathology (Lehnertz, Arnhold, Grassberger & Elger, 2000).

Given (7.10) one may characterize the fractal properties of the Lorenz system. But for EEG time-series data, the governing dynamical equations (which we assume exist) are unknown. When only a measured time series is available, the *embedding theorem* provides an alternative route to the same quantities (Takens, 1981). The idea is to *embed* the time series in a higher dimensional space by plotting the time series versus lagged versions of itself. If the measured time series is $z(t)$, then the embedded time series is $[z(t), z(t + \tau), z(t + 2\tau), ..., z(t+(D_E-1)\tau)]$, where D_E is called the *embedding dimension*. The delay τ is often chosen so that each new coordinate provides the most new information about the dynamics. Common choices for τ are based on the autocorrelation function and the mutual information (Abarbanel, 1996). The embedding theorem proves that topological

---

[1]See (Abarbanel, 1996) for a summary of methods, and (Schreiber, 1999) for a critical review.

properties of the attractor (e.g., fractal dimension and Lyapunov exponents) are the same in this embedding space as in the phase space of the original system variables. This is the basis for most chaos analysis of EEG time series to date.

This approach has been applied extensively to analyze EEG data (Pritchard & Duke, 1992). For example, in the normal waking state, resting with eyes open, the dimension of the EEG appears to be too large to be analyzed as deterministic chaos; we return to this point later. Closing the eyes produces coherent α-waves (8-13 Hz) over posterior brain areas, and the fractal dimension becomes small enough to measure: 5.6-6.2. As arousal decreases, the fractal dimension also decreases: in deep sleep, 4.5 (Babloyantz, Salazar & Nicolis, 1985); in coma, 3.8 (Babloyantz & Destexhe, 1988); and in petit mal epilepsy, the fractal dimension falls near 2.0 (Babloyantz & Destexhe, 1986).

The difficulty with delay-time embedding scalp EEG data is the competing nature of two assumptions: that the underlying system be low-dimensional and stationary. To quantify the density of points in the embedded space, the system must be allowed to traverse its attractor many times. Intuitively, the higher the dimension of the attractor, the more time that requires. If the system is highly nonstationary, as is generally the case for neurophysiological data, then the topology of the attractor may change before accurate estimates can be obtained. This limits the practicality of applying the embedding theorem to most EEG data sets. In addition, the EEG certainly contains either stochastic components or deterministic components whose dynamics are so high dimensional as to be indistinguishable from stochastic noise. Moreover, the embedding theorem applies only when the time-series data are noise-free. These observations have led to suggestions for new concepts to characterize EEG data (Freeman, 2000).

7.1.4   Nonlinear Technique: Scaling Analysis

We now describe the theoretical framework behind a scaling analysis, which quantifies the temporal fluctuations of a time series in terms of power laws. It is motivated first by the observation that the brain is a highly complex system, and second by the difficulty justifying the assumptions of either linear or chaos analysis. Although our understanding of complex systems in physics is still in its infancy (Bar-Yam, 1997), it has been noted that many complex systems in nature tend to exhibit power-law behaviors (Bak, 1996), and that this provides a handle for beginning to understand otherwise intractable complexity.

Whenever a system property is measured, there is an inherent dependence on scale introduced by the measuring device. For a system to exhibit power-law behavior means that some quantity F, measured on a scale k, depends on k simply as a power law:

$$F \propto k^{\alpha} . \tag{7.11}$$

If this expression holds, then the dimensionless exponent α provides a succinct characterization of F across a range of scales k. This is potentially a major step forward in data reduction. That the power law reflects scale independence of $F(k)$ may be seen as follows. If k is rescaled to ck, then

$$F \to (ck)^{\alpha} \propto k^{\alpha} \tag{7.12}$$

and the dependence on k, including the value of α, is preserved. If F is scale-independent in this way, then F is said to exhibit *power-law scaling* behavior. For mathematical fractals, such behavior can persist without limit, whereas for physical systems it can hold only on finite intervals.

Detrended Fluctuation Analysis (DFA)

In order to quantify the temporal fluctuations of an EEG time series, as a function of time scale τ, we use detrended fluctuation analysis (DFA). DFA was first developed to describe the correlation properties in DNA nucleotides (Peng et al., 1992), and was later extended to heartbeat time series (Peng, Havlin, Stanley & Goldberger, 1995). It has been applied to EEG previously in several forms (Hwa & Ferree, 2002; Linkenkaer-Hansen, Nikouline, Palva & Ilmoniemi, 2001; Watters, 1998). We describe the technique first in its generic form. We then describe its application to EEG by previous groups, and its adaptation by our group to continuous time series like EEG.

Let a time series be denoted by $y(t)$, where t is discrete time ranging from 1 to T. Divide the entire range of t to be investigated into B equal windows, discarding any remainder, so that each window has $k = \text{floor}(T/B)$ time points. Within each window, labeled b ($b = 1, \cdots, B$), perform a least-square fit of $y(t)$ by a straight line, $\overline{y}_b(t)$ (i.e., $\overline{y}_b(t) = \text{Linear-fit}[y(t)]$ for $(b-1)k < t \leq bk$). That is the semi-local trend for the bth window. Define $F_b^2(k)$ to be the variance of the fluctuation $y(t)$ from $\overline{y}_b(t)$ in the bth window, that is,

$$F_b^2(k) = \frac{1}{k} \sum_{t=(b-1)k+1}^{bk} [y(t) - \overline{y}_b(t)]^2. \tag{7.13}$$

This is a measure of the semi-locally detrended fluctuation in window b. The average of $F_b^2(k)$ over all windows is

$$F^2(k) = \frac{1}{B} \sum_{b=1}^{B} F_b^2(k). \tag{7.14}$$

$F(k)$ is then the RMS fluctuation from the semi-local trends in B windows each having k time points. The study of the dependence of $F(k)$ on the window size k is the essence of the scaling analysis in DFA. If it is a power-law behavior

$$F(k) \propto k^{\alpha}, \tag{7.15}$$

then the scaling exponent α is an indicator of the nature of the fluctuations. If $y(t)$ is a random walk (i.e., the partial integral of a zero-mean Gaussian random process), then $\alpha = 1/2$, and deviations from this value reflect the nature of the correlations in the original time series (Heneghan & McDarby, 2000). The scale k may also be expressed in physical units: $\tau = k\Delta t$, where Δt is the sampling interval.

Applications to EEG data

In its original formulation (Peng, Havlin, Stanley & Goldberger, 1995), DFA was applied to a discrete time series: the heart interbeat interval. The fluctuations of the intervals from their long-time average were treated as the steps taken by a random walker, and the partial integral of the steps was used as $y(t)$ in the DFA. In this way, the time series of interbeat intervals could be interpreted in terms of a correlated Gaussian random process. When DFA was first applied to EEG data (Watters, 1998), the EEG time series was integrated by exact analogy with the heartbeat problem. In other words, Watters let $y(t)$ equal the partial integral of the EEG time series $V(t)$. In a later application (Linkenkaer-Hansen, Nikouline, Palva & Ilmoniemi, 2001), the time-dependent Fourier power in the α-band was treated as a Gaussian random process, and its zero-mean integral was used as $y(t)$ in DFA. We argue that the smoothness of the EEG time series makes it more like a random walk than like a Gaussian random process, and there is no need to integrate it. Instead, we apply DFA without integration or Fourier pre-processing directly to the EEG time series to reveal any scaling properties with a minimum of assumptions (Hwa & Ferree, 2002). In other words, we let $y(t) = V(t)$.

Quantifying DFA scaling exponents

In a previous study (Hwa & Ferree, 2002), we applied DFA on time scales τ ranging from 1 sec (longest) to 0.02 sec (shortest). The longest time scale was chosen for the analysis of 10-second data segments to allow averaging over at least 10 segments. The shortest time scale was chosen based on the sampling interval $\Delta t = 1/250$ sec and the desire to have at least five points contribute to F in each window. To better resolve the range of time scales when plotted logarithmically, we used natural logarithm (ln) rather than $\log_{10}$. The choice of natural log does not change the existence (or absence) of power-law behavior or the numerical values of the scaling exponents α.

Figure 7.6 shows the result (thin line) of applying DFA to the 10-second segment of resting EEG time series shown in Figure 7.1. The smoothness of this curve over most of the range, especially compared with the power spectra in Figures 7.3(b) and 7.4, is most striking. The curve has two nearly straight regions, which we call Regions I and II, separated by a bend. To quantify the scaling in these two regions, we performed a linear fit (thick lines) in Region I for $-3.9 < \ln \tau < -3$ and denoted the slope by α_1, and similarly in Region II for $-2 < \ln \tau < 0.22$, denoting the slope by α_2. The exponent α_1 describes the behavior on short time scales and α_2 on long time scales. Visual inspection of log-log plots in a previous study involving 28 subjects, and 128 channels per subject, showed this scaling behavior almost

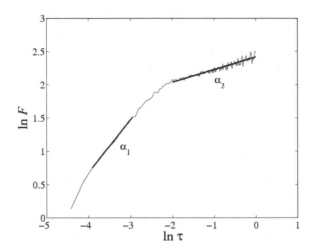

Fig. 7.6: Power-law scaling behavior in the EEG time series of Figure 7.1. The fluctuation measure $F(\tau)$ versus τ (thin line) and best-fit lines determining α_1 and α_2 in Regions I and II (thick lines).

ubiquitously (Hwa & Ferree, 2002).

Interpreting DFA Scaling Exponents

Because our application of DFA differs from that of previous authors, in that we do not integrate the EEG time series, some comments are in order on the theoretical significance of the α values obtained here. We find that usually $\alpha_2 < \alpha_1$. Because the EEG time series is bounded, it is expected that, as $k \to \infty$, $F(k) \to$ constant, and the asymptotic slope $\alpha_\infty \to 0$. One may therefore be tempted to regard the change of slope in Figure 7.6 as the prelude to the asymptotic behavior and dismiss the significance of α_2. There are several arguments against such a view. First, α_2 is generally far from zero, and fluctuates widely across channels. Second, there are a significant number of cases where $\alpha_2 > \alpha_1$, as shown in Figure 7.7(a). Thus, α_2 cannot merely reflect saturation. Third, we have shown that α_2 plays as much role as α_1 in reflecting group differences in stroke patients (Hwa & Ferree, 2004).

We claim that both α_1 and α_2 contain meaningful information

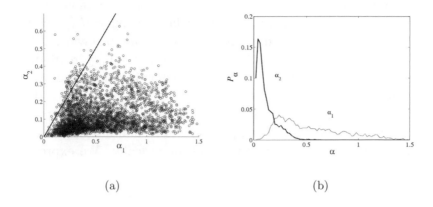

(a)   (b)

Fig. 7.7: Distributions of scaling exponents α_1 and α_2 for all 28 subjects in Hwa and Ferree (2002): (a) scatter plot showing how α_1 and α_2 relate in each channel, and (b) histograms showing the overall occurrence of α_1 and α_2 separately.

about fluctuations in the EEG time series. In support of this point, we now show that the scaling exponents are not (linearly) correlated. Figure 7.7(a) shows a scatter plot of α_1 versus α_2 for the group of 28 subjects in our sample (Hwa & Ferree, 2002), which includes both normal subjects and acute stroke patients. The diagonal line has unit slope. The distribution of points in this space shows that the scaling exponents are not linearly correlated. Some points are found above the line, indicating $\alpha_2 > \alpha_1$, as mentioned previously. Figure 7.7(b) shows the probability distributions of α_1 (thin line) and α_2 (thick line) for the group of 28 subjects. The values of α_2 are sharply peaked, whereas the values of α_1 are much more widely distributed. The maximum value of α_2 is near 0.5, whereas the maximum value of α_1 is near 1.5. Therefore, we retain both exponents in subsequent analyses (e.g., comparisons across conditions or groups).

7.1.5 Relationship between DFA and FSA

Several authors have discussed the relationship between DFA and the Fourier power spectrum (Heneghan & McDarby, 2000; Rangarajan & Ding, 2000). Starting with a stochastic time series having power-law autocorrelations (i.e., $C(\tau) \propto \tau^{\gamma}$), it is possible to show that, (a) the Fourier power spectrum has power-law behavior: $P(f) \propto 1/f^{\beta}$; (b) the DFA fluctuation measure has power-law behavior: $F(\tau) \propto \tau^{\alpha}$, and 3) the FSA and DFA exponents are simply related. All previous authors, however, considered stochastic signals and included integration of the time series as a first step. Because we do not integrate the EEG time series, their results are not directly applicable. We discuss next the relationship between our non-integrated form of DFA and FSA, both analytically and numerically. We express this relationship at three levels of detail.

Heuristic

Figure 7.6 shows a violation of scaling behavior of $F(\tau)$ near $\tau = 0.1$ sec. Scaling behavior implies there is no intrinsic scale to the data, and a violation of scaling implies the existence of a characteristic scale. Looking at the original time series in Figure 7.1, and its power spectrum shown in Figures 7.3(b), 7.4(a), and 7.4(b), the dominant time scale is clearly the ~ 10 Hz α-rhythm. To make intuitive contact between DFA and FSA, therefore, we can associate the time scale τ at which the bend occurs with the frequency f of the dominant frequency in the data

$$\tau \simeq \frac{1}{f}. \tag{7.16}$$

Thus, it appears that the peak in $P(f)$ is related to the bend in $F(\tau)$. This is reminiscent of integrating across a Dirac δ-function to yield a Heaviside step-function. That intuition is not far from correct, as we now show.

Analytic

Starting with a continuous time series $V(t)$, it is possible to derive a formula relating the DFA fluctuation measure $F^2(\tau)$ to the Fourier power spectrum $P(f)$ (Robinson, 2003). It can be shown that

$$F^2(\tau) = \int df\, P(f)\, W(\pi f \tau) \tag{7.17}$$

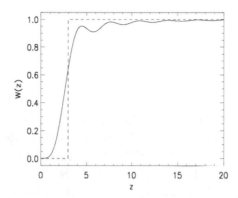

Fig. 7.8: The weighting function $W(z)$ (solid line), and step-function approximation $H(\pi f \tau - 3)$ (dashed line).

where the weighting function $W(z)$ is

$$W(z) = 1 - \left(\frac{\sin(z)}{z} \right)^2 - 3 \left(\frac{\cos(z)}{z} - \frac{\sin(z)}{z^2} \right)^2. \qquad (7.18)$$

Figure 7.8 shows the function $W(z)$ (solid line), and an approximation given by the unit step function $H(\pi f \tau - 3)$ (dashed line). The relation in Equation 7.17 holds only for the form of DFA in which the original time series is *not* integrated (Hwa & Ferree, 2002).

Approximate

When the power spectrum is available, it is possible to evaluate (7.17) and determine an analytic expression for $F(\tau)$. (We find an analytic expression for $F(\tau)$ useful when analyzing model time series, for example, which are constructed to have a particular $P(f)$.) Unfortunately, the integral in Equation 7.17 is difficult to evaluate, and an analytic result often cannot be determined. Here we discuss an approximation to Equation 7.17 that greatly simplifies the integration to provide an approximate analytic result, thereby aiding intuition. The shape of the weight function $W(z)$, shown in Figure 7.8, suggests we approximate $W(z)$ as a unit step function $H(\pi f \tau - 3)$ with step at $f \simeq 1/\tau$. Using this approximation, we replace $W(\pi f \tau)$ in (7.17) with $H(\pi f \tau - 3)$ and find,

$$F^2(\tau) \simeq \int_{1/\tau}^{\bar{f}} df\, P(f). \qquad (7.19)$$

Here we have set $H(0) = 1$. In this approximation, the squared DFA result $F^2(\tau)$ is simply the integral of the power spectrum $P(f)$ between frequencies $1/\tau$ and $\bar{f}$. The lower frequency limit $1/\tau$ is set by the window length τ in the DFA. When the window length is small, the integration limits in Equation 7.19 extend over a limited, high-frequency range. When the window length is large, the integration limits in Equation 7.19 extend over a broad frequency range that includes low frequencies. The upper frequency limit $\bar{f}$ corresponds to the maximum observable frequency (i.e., the Nyquist frequency).

7.2   SCALING PROPERTIES OF MODEL TIME SERIES

The aim of this section is to build intuition for DFA. To do so, we apply DFA analysis to simulated time-series data. Our discussion follows the format in Rangarajan and Ding (2000). For each example, we present both FSA and DFA results side-by-side, and relate the two using Equations 7.17 and 7.19. We conclude this section with a simple example that mimics the DFA results observed in EEG data.

7.2.1   Example: White noise

We first consider the case where the time series $V(t)$ consists of Gaussian random numbers with zero mean and standard deviation of one. In Figure 7.9 we plot the FSA and DFA results for this time series. We show in Figure 7.9(a) that the power spectrum is approximately constant, as expected for Gaussian random numbers. We show in Figure 7.9(b) that the DFA result is also approximately constant, and that the scaling exponent is approximately zero.

We can use Equation 7.19 to confirm the DFA result shown in Figure 7.9(b). Because $P(f) \simeq$ constant, and the integral in Equation 7.19 is simply proportional to the difference of the limits,

$$F^2(\tau) \propto \bar{f} - 1/\tau. \qquad (7.20)$$

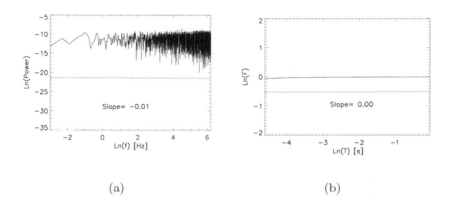

(a)   (b)

Fig. 7.9: Analysis of normally distributed Gaussian random numbers. The sampling rate is $\Delta t = 0.001$. In each figure, the fit to the slope is shown (dotted lines): (a) The power spectrum (solid line) is nearly constant, as expected for data consisting only of noise, and the slope is approximately zero; and (b) the DFA result (solid line). The slope is constant and near zero.

Noting that, for almost all τ, $\bar{f} \gg 1/\tau$, we drop the $1/\tau$ term in Equation 7.20 and find,

$$F(\tau) \propto \bar{f}^{1/2} = \text{constant}. \tag{7.21}$$

This analytic approximation confirms the numerical result shown in Figure 7.9(b): the DFA measure $F(\tau)$ of Gaussian random numbers is constant and exhibits only trivial scaling behavior with $\alpha = 0$.

7.2.2   Example: Long-Range Correlated Process

We now consider a time series for which $P(f) \propto f^{-\beta}$, where $\beta > 0$. To generate a time series with $f^{-\beta}$ behavior in its power spectrum, we follow the procedure discussed in Rangarajan and Ding (2000). We show in Figure 7.10(a) the power spectrum for a time series where we have chosen $\beta = 2$ and note that the fit to the slope of $\ln P$ versus $\ln f$ is approximately -2, as expected. In Figure 7.10(b), we show the corresponding DFA result for the same time series. The scaling behavior is confirmed by the constant slope of 0.51.

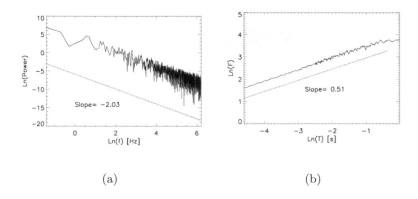

(a)   (b)

Fig. 7.10: Analysis of time-series data possessing a long-range power-law correlation. The sampling rate is $\Delta t = 0.001$. In each figure, the fit to the slope is shown (dotted lines.) (a) The power spectrum (solid line) scales as $1/f^2$; and (b) the DFA result (solid line). The power-law behavior is the same for all τ and the slope is near $1/2$.

We can use the approximation in Equation 7.19 to confirm the numerical results shown in Figure 7.10. Substituting $P(f) = f^{-\beta}$ into Equation 7.19 we find,

$$F^2(\tau) \propto \bar{f}^{-\beta+1} - \frac{1}{\tau}^{-\beta+1}. \tag{7.22}$$

The first term in Equation 7.22 is a constant and not interesting. We drop this term and solve for $F(\tau)$ to find,

$$F(\tau) \propto \frac{1}{\tau}^{(-\beta+1)/2} = \tau^{(\beta-1)/2}. \tag{7.23}$$

Equation (7.23) provides an approximate relationship between the scaling exponent β in FSA, and the scaling exponent α in DFA:

$$\alpha = (\beta - 1)/2. \tag{7.24}$$

Note that this result differs from that discussed in Rangarajan and Ding (2000), where the authors considered rescaled range analysis, not DFA. For the case shown in Figure 7.10, we set $\beta = 2$ in Equation

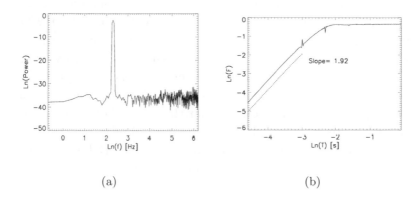

(a)   (b)

Fig. 7.11: Analysis of a sinusoidal time series with frequency $f_0 = 10$ Hz. The sampling rate is $\Delta t - 0.001$. (a) The power spectrum of the sinusoid has a sharp peak at $\ln(f) = 2.3$ or $f \approx 10$ Hz; and (b) the DFA result (solid line). A break in scaling occurs near $\ln(\tau) =\approx -2.3$ or $\tau =\approx 0.1$s. The slope in the scaling region (for small τ) is approximately 1.9.

7.23 and find $F(\tau) \propto \tau^{1/2}$, thus $\alpha = 1/2$. This approximate analytic result agrees with the numerically determined slope of $F(\tau)$, plotted in Figure 7.10(b).

7.2.3   Example: Sinusoid

Next we consider the case where the time series $V(t)$ is a sinusoid of frequency $f_0 = 10$ Hz. The corresponding power spectrum is a Dirac delta function (i.e., $P(f) = \delta(f - f_0)$), and the integral in Equation 7.17 is trivial. We find,

$$F^2(\tau) = W(\pi f_0 \tau). \qquad (7.25)$$

In Figure 7.11(b), we plot the DFA result. The break in scaling of $F(\tau)$ (from a positive slope to a near zero slope) occurs at $\ln \tau_\star \approx -2.3$ or $\tau_\star \approx 0.1$ s, which corresponds to $f_\star \equiv 1/\tau_\star \simeq 10$ Hz $= f_0$. For this example, the break in scaling at $\tau_\star$ allows us to approximate the frequency of the sinusoid f_0.

Using Equation 7.25, we can determine an approximation to the slope of the scaling region (in our example, $-4.5 < \ln \tau < -3.0$). In this region, τ is small and therefore permits a Taylor series expansion of Equation 7.25 about $\tau = 0$. We find to leading order $F(\tau) \propto \tau^2$ or $\ln F \propto 2 \ln \tau$. This analysis suggests that, for the sinusoidal time series $V(t)$, the DFA result will possess a scaling exponent of approximately $\alpha = 2$ for small τ. Fitting the curve in Figure 7.11(b) for $-4.5 < \ln \tau < -3.0$, we find a slope of 1.9 in agreement with the analytic approximation. We note that this result holds in general for any sinusoid. In summary, if $V(t)$ is a sinusoid of frequency f_0, then a break in scaling of $F(\tau)$ occurs at $\tau \simeq 1/f_0$. Before this break, $F(\tau) \propto \tau^\alpha$ for small τ, and the scaling exponent $\alpha \simeq 2$.

7.2.4 Example: Sinusoid + Long-Range Correlated Process

Scaling behavior in the human scalp EEG has been reported previously (Hwa & Ferree, 2002). In this final example, we propose a simulated time series intended to mimic DFA results obtained from experimental EEG data. Namely, we develop a simple example possessing (a) two scaling regions, and (b) scaling exponents in agreement with the numerical ranges of exponents found in scalp EEG data.

To mimic the DFA results from scalp EEG, we construct a simulated time series $V(t)$ that is the sum of two parts. The first part is a sinusoid with frequency $f_0 = 10$ Hz and unit amplitude. The second part is a long-range correlated process with $\beta = 2$ and maximum value of 0.02. The power spectrum $P(f)$ is shown in Figure 7.12(a). Because of the increased power near 10 Hz, this $P(f)$ does not maintain power-law behavior over all frequencies. This break in the scaling is more clearly revealed through the DFA result, plotted in Figure 7.12(b). From the DFA result, the two scaling regions are obvious. We fit each scaling region to determine the slope and found slopes $\alpha_1 = 1.07$ and $\alpha_2 = 0.17$. These results are in general agreement with slopes from experimental scalp EEG results, discussed later.

An analytic approximation for the DFA results shown in Figure 7.12(b) can be determined. We start with Equation 7.17 and set $P(f) = f^{-\beta} + \delta(f - f_0)$. The integral in Equation 7.17 separates into two parts, which can be approximated and evaluated using Equations

7.23 and 7.25. We find

$$F(\tau) \approx \sqrt{\tau^{(\beta-1)/2} + W(\pi f_0 \tau)}. \qquad (7.26)$$

We plot this result with $\beta = 2$ and $f_0 = 10$ Hz in Figure 7.12(c). Fitting the slopes in the two scaling regions, we find $\alpha_1 = 1.2$ and $\alpha_2 = 0.16$, in qualitative agreement with the numerical results shown in Figure 7.12(b).

Of course, we do not purport that scalp EEG signals can be decomposed into sinusoidal and long-range correlated stochastic processes. In the process of interpreting the scaling behaviors seen in real data, however, a reasonable question arises: What is the simplest model time series that has these properties? This example suggests that the scaling in Regions I and II could be explained by a single, long-range correlated process, and the break in scaling could be due only to the familiar α-peak. We cannot rule out the possibility, but it seems unlikely that neurophysiological data would decompose this cleanly. In our analysis of the DFA scaling exponents of scalp EEG time series, we do not assume decompositions of this form.

7.2.5 Comparison of Periodogram and Tapering Methods

We have seen how the power spectrum $P(f)$ behaves quite erratically, such that plots of $\ln P$ versus $\ln f$ do not make scaling behavior visible even if it is present in the data. In contrast, DFA does a much better job of rendering scaling behavior visible. It is reasonable to ask whether the erraticity of $P(f)$ is due to windowing issues. To consider this, we compute $P(f)$ for the simulated data of the previous example in three ways: the unwindowed periodogram, the Hann-windowed periodogram, and the multitaper estimate. We show the results in Figure 7.13(a); note the peak near 10 Hz ($\ln f \simeq 2.3$ Hz) in all three methods. The multitaper result is relatively smooth, but is quite erratic, especially at higher f. Practically speaking, the multitaper method is computationally demanding, at least compared with the periodogram, for which computation times are similar to DFA.

We have discussed how the DFA fluctuation measure F can be computed directly using Equations 7.13 and 7.14 or by integrating

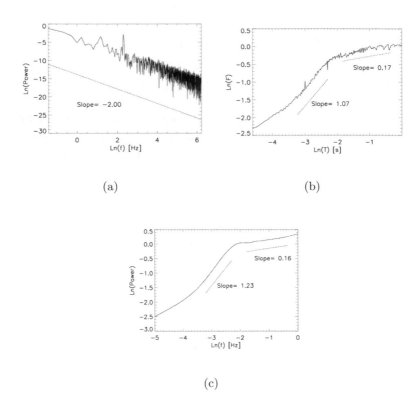

(a)   (b)

(c)

Fig. 7.12: Analysis of a compound time series comprised of a sinusoid with frequency $f_0 = 10$ Hz, and a long-range correlated process with $\beta = 2$ and maximum value of 0.02. The sampling rate is $\Delta t = 0.001$. (a) The power spectrum, although generally maintaining a negative slope, has a sharp peak at $\ln(f) = 2.3$ or $f \approx 10$ Hz; (b) the DFA result (solid line). A break in scaling occurs near $\ln \tau \approx -2.3$ or $\tau \approx 0.1$ sec. There are two scaling regions with slopes near 1.0 for small τ and 0.17 for larger τ; (c) plot of the analytic result from Equation 7.26. There are two scaling regions with slopes near 1.23 for small τ and 0.16 for larger τ.

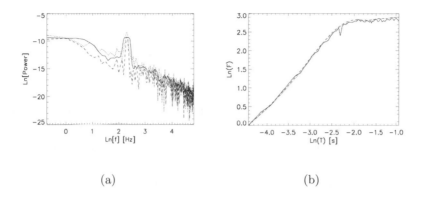

(a)   (b)

Fig. 7.13: Comparison of FSA and DFA results computed various ways. The time series is the same as in Figure 7.12. (a) The power spectrum calculated three ways: the periodogram (dotted line), the Hann-windowed power spectrum (dashed line), and the multitaper method (solid line); and (b) the DFA result calculated three ways: the direct method (solid line), the Robinson method with no windowing of the power spectrum (dotted line), and the Robinson method with a Hann window applied in the power spectrum calculation (dashed line). Each curve is shifted vertically for visualization. All three methods give very similar results.

the power spectrum using Equation 7.17. We have also shown in Figure 7.13(a) how windowing the data affects the power spectrum $P(f)$. One may wonder whether this windowing affects the DFA result calculated using (7.17). To consider this, we use the same time-series data whose power spectra are shown in Figure 7.13(a) (a sinusoid with $f_0 = 10$ Hz and a long range correlated process with $\beta = 2$). In Figure 7.13(b) we plot the DFA result calculated using Equations 7.13 and 7.14 (solid line), using Equation 7.17, where $P(f)$ is the un-windowed periodogram (dotted line) and $P(f)$ is the Hann-windowed power spectrum (dashed line). Here we have shifted the DFA results so that each has a minimum of 0.0 for ease of visual comparison. We find that the results are nearly identical for all three methods. This result supports the assertion that DFA reveals scaling behavior more readily than FSA, as a result of the integral relationship between the two.

7.3 SCALING PROPERTIES OF NEUROPHYSIOLOGICAL TIME-SERIES

The application of DFA to neurophysiological data allows the fluctuations in each EEG time series to be summarized by two scaling exponents: α_1 and α_2. This provides summary statistics for the vast amount of data collected in EEG. The aim of this section is to describe the numerics of these findings globally, considering many sensor channels in many subjects. We compare the scaling exponents between two groups in a stroke study and EEG and MEG scaling behaviors in a sleep study.

7.3.1 Scaling Properties in EEG

We collected scalp EEG data using a 128-channel EEG system (Electrical Geodesics, Inc., Eugene, Oregon). Data were referenced to the vertex. After deleting bad channels, data were re-referenced at each time point to the average potential. This approximates a monopolar recording at the location of each measurement electrode by minimizing the effect of the location of the reference electrode (Nunez, 1981). We selected 10-sec segments that were free of obvious artifacts. The segments were subjected to DFA, and descriptive statistics were computed over electrodes and groups.

Figure 7.7(b) showed the distribution of scaling exponents for the 28 subjects in our study (Hwa & Ferree, 2002). We noted that α_1 was widely distributed on the range [0,1.5]. We contrast this EEG behavior with MEG in the next section. The first two columns of Table 7.1 quantify the overall behaviors of these scaling exponents.

Application: Acute Stroke Detection

The results for 28 subjects, shown in Figure 7.7, fall into two groups (Luu et al., 2001). Ten subjects were acute stroke patients, for whom EEG data were collected within the acute stage (few hours-1.5 days). The remaining 18 subjects were an age-match control group, with clean MRI and no previous history of neurological incident.

Table 7.1: Statistics of EEG scaling exponents

	EEG Both		EEG Control		EEG Stroke	
	α_1	α_2	α_1	α_2	α_1	α_2
Min	0.0156	0.0007	0.0156	0.0007	0.0702	0.0057
Max	1.4829	0.6269	1.4388	0.5812	1.4829	0.6269
Mean	0.5341	0.1148	0.4421	0.0756	0.6984	0.1846
Median	0.4541	0.0839	0.3671	0.0588	0.6674	0.1692

We (Hwa, He & Ferree, 2003; Hwa & Ferree, 2004) computed *within subjects* the mean and normalized variance of α_1 and α_2 over the scalp, and used these quantities to distinguish the two groups. Keeping the focus here on the scaling exponents, we simply concatenated within each group the scaling exponents from all good data channels in all subjects. Figure 7.14 shows the distributions of α_1 and α_2 for (a) the control group, and (b) the stroke group. In the stroke group, both means appear increased, and α_2 is visibly less peaked. The last four columns of Table 7.1 list the statistics of these distributions. Indeed, in the stroke group, the means of both α_1 and α_2 are larger, which is consistent with our findings based on within-subject statistics (Hwa, He & Ferree, 2003). Interestingly, the minimum and maximum values are not very different between the two groups.

The finding of higher mean values of α_1 and α_2 was discussed in detail in Hwa and Ferree (2003). Because the DFA scaling exponents reflect the *relative* size of fluctuations at neighboring time scales, larger α_1 and α_2 reflect relatively larger fluctuations on the longest time scales within each of Regions I and II. This increase in the size of fluctuations on the longest time scales is consistent with the notion of "EEG slowing," which has been noted in stroke since the time of paper chart recordings. It was also shown that the increased within-subject means in stroke patients was not due to a few channels, but instead involved nearly all of the channels (Hwa, He & Ferree, 2003). This argues for a global effect of stroke on the EEG. The

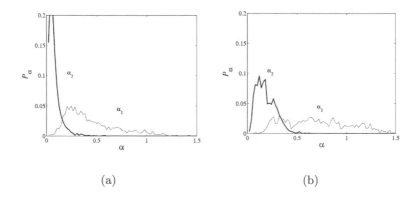

(a)   (b)

Fig. 7.14: Distributions of scaling exponents α_1 and α_2, shown together in Figure 7.7, but separated here into two groups: (a) 18 normal subjects, and (b) 10 stroke patients.

observation of a global effect in stroke via these analysis techniques is consistent with the many reports of diaschesis, i.e., remote effects of lesions. However, a global effect in EEG is quite different from the focal anomalies seen in MRI.

7.3.2   Scaling Properties in MEG

Theoretical Considerations

EEG and MEG have similar, but not identical, neurophysiological origins. In both cases, the fundamental physiological process is neuronal activity, but isolating exactly which aspect of neuronal activity gives rise to the measured fields is rather complicated. In response to the opening and closing of ion channels, caused by changes in transmembrane potential, neurotransmitter binding, and other factors, ionic currents flow in the transmembrane, intracellular, and extracellular spaces. When making noninvasive, electrophysiological recordings in humans, the electric potential (EEG) or magnetic field (MEG) is measured at the scalp. From this remote distance, the current source density is usually represented as a dipole due to the behavior of the multipole expansion under the constraint of current conservation (Nunez, 1981).

This phenomenological source summarizes the net effect of actual ionic currents, as well as secondary sources due to the discontinuity in conductivity at the cell membrane and other tissue boundaries. Because conductivity discontinuities affect electric and magnetic solutions differently, the effective dipoles of EEG and MEG are not identical. Nevertheless, in both cases, the effective dipole is associated with dendritic currents (i.e., not axonal action potentials), thus the effective dipole current flows parallel to the direction of the primary dendritic branch. The quasi-static limit of bioelectromagnetism applies equally to electric and magnetic fields, so that the fields at the scalp are determined at each time point solely by the values of the source currents at the same time point (Plonsey, 1969). Thus, the phenomenological dipoles of EEG and MEG can be considered essentially the same, and the differences between EEG and MEG lie at higher levels.

Assuming that the definitions of dipole in EEG and MEG are perfectly synonymous, EEG and MEG have other differences that arise from more macroscopic considerations. First, the magnetic field (MEG) propagates through the head volume to the detectors, almost unaffected by the shape and conductivity of the different head tissues. This statement is rigorously true for a spherical head and holds approximately for a non-spherical head. In contrast, the electric potential (EEG) propagates from source to sensors in a way that depends sensitively on the shape and conductivity of each of the head tissues. Usually the head is considered to be comprised of four tissues: scalp, skull, CSF, and brain. The large conductivity differences between these tissues are the most important to account for, but to be precise, one should also account for defects in the skull such as eye holes and fontanelles, conductivity differences between gray and white matter, and white matter anisotropy. Because MEG is relatively insensitive to these details, the head is easier to model in computer simulations. For the same reasons, the magnetic field measured by MEG is less distorted by volumetric current flow and gives a higher-resolution view of brain activity.

The different resolutions of EEG and MEG can be conceptualized in terms of half-sensitivity volumes (HSVs, Malmivuo & Plonsey, 1995). The HSV represents the volume of brain that each sensor integrates over, with a certain threshold criterion on sensitivity. Because EEG fields are spread by the skull and other factors, the HSV for EEG is generally larger than MEG. For nearby EEG electrodes, the HSV can be similar to that of MEG, but most EEG electrodes are not nearby, thus the HSV for EEG is generally larger.

Another macroscopic difference between EEG and MEG is the sensitivity to orientation of neuronal current sources. The dipole sources of EEG and MEG (i.e., the apical dendrites of pyramidal cells) are oriented along the local normal to the cortical surface. The cortical surface is folded so that its normal can range from parallel to perpendicular relative to the scalp. Because of the geometry of magnetic fields, it turns out that MEG is nearly blind to radial sources. However, because each MEG sensor integrates over a volume that typically encompasses dipoles of all orientations, each MEG channel is sure to measure some brain activity. There is no reason to think that spontaneous activity on a gyrus, for example, is systematically different from spontaneous activity in the adjacent sulci, thus the orientation issue should not be a major one for relating spontaneous EEG and MEG fluctuations.

Comparison with EEG

Because EEG and MEG measure similar quantities, we expect that DFA applied to MEG will also show scaling behavior. If the bend seen in EEG is related to the α-rhythm, we expect two scaling regions separated by a bend. Because MEG sensors integrate over a smaller brain volume, however, we expect some differences related to this fact.

To test these hypotheses, we recorded EEG and MEG data simultaneously from a normal human volunteer. The MEG data were recorded using a dual 37-channel biomagnetometer device with the dewars positioned bilaterally over the temporal regions (Magnes II; Biomagnetic Technology, San Diego). Simultaneously recorded EEG data were recorded using a Nihon-Kohden digital EEG system, with 11 electrodes positioned roughly according to the standard 10/20 system. The sampling rate for both EEG and MEG was 520.8 Hz, and the data were high-pass filtered at 1 Hz. The duration of the recording session was 40 minutes. The subject was sleep-deprived, and fell asleep almost immediately.

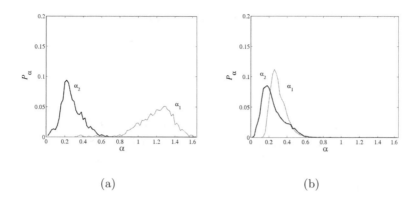

(a)   (b)

Fig. 7.15: Distributions of scaling exponents α_1 and α_2 for (a) EEG, and (b) MEG, recorded simultaneously for a normal subject sleeping.

To perform the scaling analysis, we divided each 40-minute time series into 240 10-sec segments and applied DFA to each segment exactly as before. Specifically, Regions I and II were defined the same as in Figure 7.6. As expected, the DFA results for the MEG appeared qualitatively similar to the DFA results for the EEG. There are two scaling regions separated by a bend. The linearity of the log-log plots within each region was quite impressive, and suggests that the scaling exponents so determined are reasonable summary statistics of the temporal fluctuations in MEG time series.

Figure 7.15 shows the distributions of the scaling exponents for EEG and MEG, plotted as in Figures 7.7 and 7.14. The EEG distributions of α_1 and α_2 are different in detail from those in Figures 7.7 and 7.14, although the distribution of α_2 appears quite similar to that of the stroke group in Figure 7.14(b). The EEG distribution of α_1 is shifted upward, nevertheless, the distribution extends over a similar range. It is not clear whether the shift in the α_1 distribution reflects subject-specific differences or sleep-related physiology, and it is not possible to determine that with these data. Our main purpose is to compare the DFA results for EEG and MEG.

Figure 7.15(b) shows the distributions of α_1 and α_2 for MEG data recorded simultaneously with the EEG in the same subject. Simultaneous recording controls perfectly for subject state (i.e., sleep

Table 7.2: Statistics of MEG scaling exponents.

	EEG Asleep		MEG Asleep	
	α_1	α_2	α_1	α_2
Min	0.3263	0.0238	0.1338	0.0283
Max	1.6518	0.6654	0.8401	0.8816
Mean	1.1933	0.2746	0.3045	0.2434
Median	1.2178	0.2532	0.2881	0.2152

stages), and allows a more meaningful comparison between EEG and MEG results. The α_2 distribution is nearly identical in EEG and MEG. In contrast, the α_1 distribution is shifted dramatically downward. Table 7.2 shows some statistics of the α distributions shown in Figure 7.15. In MEG, the maximum α_1 is only 0.84—nearly half the value seen in all the EEG data analyzed so far. We tentatively conclude, therefore, that this difference is related to the difference in spatial resolution between EEG and MEG.

The substantial difference between the distributions of α_1 in EEG versus MEG can be explained in terms of their differences in half-sensitivity volumes and the concept of *dispersion*. Dispersion refers to a connection between spatial and temporal frequencies. For electromagnetic waves propagating in vacuum, for example, the dispersion relation is $f = c/\lambda$, where f is frequency, c is the speed of light in vacuum, and λ is the wavelength. This relation associates higher spatial frequencies with higher temporal frequencies. This idea has been applied to the study of brain waves, to argue that the coherence of high-frequency temporal oscillations, which is required for signal superposition at the sensors, should be limited to shorter spatial scales (Nunez, 1995). As described previously, MEG reflects brain activity integrated over a volume that is typically much smaller than that in EEG. Therefore, we expect the MEG to signal to better reflect fluctuations on shorter time scales. This would increase $F(\tau)$ for small τ, thereby decreasing α_1. This is precisely what is observed in

Figure 7.15(b).

7.4 SUMMARY

We described scaling analysis of continuous neurophysiological time series, emphasizing a version of detrended fluctuation analysis (DFA) developed by our group (Hwa & Ferree, 2002). The spirit of scaling analysis is on relating the size of fluctuations *across* time scales, rather than on particular scales, and we argue this approach is more justifiable for a complex system such as the brain. As it is applied here, the analysis reduces 10-second segments of resting EEG or MEG data to two dimensionless scaling exponents α_1 and α_2. Practically speaking, this is a major step in data reduction, which facilitates comparisons across experimental conditions and subject groups.

The theoretical section contrasted scaling analysis with linear and nonlinear analysis, especially Fourier spectral analysis. We later described a mathematical relationship between the DFA fluctuation measure $F(\tau)$ and the Fourier power spectrum $P(f)$. Given this relationship, it is reasonable to ask whether there are advantages to DFA, that would warrant its adoption. We argued that, because the fluctuation measure $F(\tau)$ is much smoother than the Fourier power spectrum, DFA is a more direct way to visually identify and quantify scaling behavior.

We applied DFA to model and neurophysiological time series. The model time series were constructed to have particular scaling behaviors and verified the mathematical relationship between $F(\tau)$ and $P(f)$ just described. They also provided intuition on the origin of the bend separating the two scaling regions. The application of DFA to neurophysiological time series showed statistical differences in the scaling exponents between normal and stroke groups, as well as differences between EEG and MEG scaling behaviors. We suggest that the differences between EEG and MEG can be understood in terms of their different spatial resolutions, although further work is required to prove this assertion.

References

Abarbanel, H. D. I. (1996). *Analysis of observed chaotic data.* New York: Springer-Verlag.

Babloyantz, A. & Destexhe, A. (1986). Low-dimensional chaos in an instance of epilepsy. *Proceedings of the National Academy of Sciences of the United States of America, 83,* 3513–3517.

Babloyantz, A. & Destexhe, A. (1988). The creutzfeld-jakob disease in the heirarchy of chaotic attractors. In *From chemical to biological organization* (pp. 307–316). New York: Springer-Verlag.

Babloyantz, A., Salazar, J. M. & Nicolis, C. (1985). Evidence of chaotic activity during the sleep cycle. *Physics Letters A, 11,* 152–156.

Bak, P. (1996). *How Nature Works: The Science of Self-Organized Criticality.* New York: Copernicus.

Bar-Yam, Y. (1997). *Dynamics of complex systems.* Reading, Massachusetts: Perseus Books.

Cone-Wesson, B. & Wunderlich, J. (2003). Auditory evoked potentials from the cortex: audiology applications. *Curr. Opin. Otolaryngol. Head Neck Surg., 11(5),* 372–377.

Freeman, W. J. (1975). *Mass action in the nervous system.* New York: Academic Press.

Freeman, W. J. (2000). A proposed name for quasi-periodic brain activity: Stochastic chaos. *Neural networks, 13,* 11–13.

Gleick, J. (1987). *Chaos: Making a new science.* New York: Penguin Books.

Grassberger, P. & Procaccia, I. (1983). Measuring the strangeness of strange attractors. *Physica D, 9,* 189–208.

Heneghan, C. & McDarby, G. (2000). Establishing the relation between detrended fluctuation analysis and power spectral density for stochastic processes. *Phys. Rev. E, 62(5),* 6103–6110.

Hwa, R. C. & Ferree, T. C. (2002). Scaling properties of fluctuations in the human electroencephalogram. *Phys. Rev. E, 66,* 021901.

Hwa, R. C. & Ferree, T. C. (2004). Stroke detection based on the scaling properties of human EEG. *Physica A, 38,* 246–254.

Hwa, R. C., He, W. & Ferree, T. C. (2003). The global effects of stroke on the human electroencephalogram. *J. Integr. Neurosci., 2(1),* 45–53.

Lehnertz, K., Arnhold, J., Grassberger, P. & Elger, C. E. (Eds.). (2000). *Chaos in the Brain?* Singapore: World Scientific.

Linkenkaer-Hansen, K., Nikouline, V. V., Palva, J. M. & Ilmoniemi, R. J. (2001). Long-range temporal correlations and scaling behavior in human brain oscillations. *Journal of Neuroscience, 21(4),* 1370.

Lorenz, E. (1963). Deterministic nonperiodic flow. *Journal of Atmospheric Sciences, 20,* 130 141.

Luu, P., Tucker, D. M., Englander, R., Lockfeld, A., Lutsep, H. & Oken, B. (2001). Localizing acute stroke related eeg changes: Assessing the effects of spatial undersampling. *J. Clin. Neurophys., 18(4),* 302–317.

Malmivuo, J. & Plonsey, R. (1995). *Bioelectromagnetism.* New York: Oxford University Press.

Nunez, P. L. (1981). *Electric Fields of the Brain.* New York: Oxford University Press.

Nunez, P. L. (1995). *Neocortical Dynamics and Human EEG Rhythms.* New York: Oxford University Press.

Peng, C. K., Buldyrev, S. V., Goldberger, A. L., Havlin, S., Sciortino, F., Simons, M. & Stanley, H. E. (1992). Long-range correlation in nucleotide sequences. *Nature, 356,* 168–170.

Peng, C.-K., Havlin, S., Stanley, H. E. & Goldberger, A. L. (1995). Quantification of scaling exponents and crossover phenomena in nonstationary heartbeat time series. *Chaos, 5,* 82.

Percival, D. B. & Walden, A. T. (1993). *Spectral Analysis for Physical Applications.* New York: Cambridge University Press.

Plonsey, R. (1969). *Bioelectric Phenomena.* New York: McGraw-Hill.

Press, W. H., Tuekolsky, S. A., Vetterling, W. T. & Flannery, B. P. (1992). *Numerical Recipes in C.* New York: Cambridge University Press.

Pritchard, W. S. & Duke, D. W. (1992). Measuring chaos in the brain: A tutorial review of nonlinear dynamical eeg analysis. *International Journal of Neuroscience, 67*, 31–80.

Rangarajan, G. & Ding, M. (2000). Integrated approach to the assessment of long-range correlation in time series data. *Phys. Rev. E, 61*, 4991.

Robinson, P. A. (2003). Interpretation of scaling properties of electroencephalographic fluctuations via spectral analysis and underlying physiology. *Phys. Rev. E, 67*, 032902.

Schreiber, T. (1999). Interdisciplinary application of nonlinear time series methods. *Physics Reports, 308(1)*, 2–64.

Steyn-Ross, M. L., Steyn-Ross, D. A., Sleigh, J. W. & Liley, D. T. J. (1999). Theoretical electroencephalogram stationary spectrum for a white-noise driven cortex: Evidence for a general anesthetic-induced phase transition. *Phys. Rev. E, 60(6)*, 7229–7331.

Takens, F. (1981). Detecting strange attractors in turbulance. *Lect. Notes Math., 898*, 366–381.

Watters (1998). Fractal structure in the electroencephalogram. *Complexity International, 5*, 1–8.

8

Applications of Independent Component Analysis to Electroencephalography

Tzyy-Ping Jung and Te-Won Lee
University of California, San Diego

Independent component analysis (ICA) is a signal processing and data analysis technology that was first introduced in the late 1980s. ICA is a multivariate analytical approach that aims at the retrieval of an ensemble of independent source signals out of an ensemble of linear mixtures. It can achieve signal separation by determining the inverse of the mixing process blindly, without prior knowledge of the original source signals or the mixing process. In the past few years, blind source separation by ICA has received significant interest in biomedical signal processing and interpretation such as the analysis of electroencephalogram (EEG, Makeig, Bell, Jung & Sejnowski, 1996) and functional magnetic resonance imaging (fMRI, McKeown, Makeig, Brown, Jung, Kinderman & Sejnowski, 1998) data.

The EEG is a non-invasive measure of brain electrical activity recorded as changes in potential difference between points on the human scalp. Although these weak signals recorded from the surface of the scalp have been studied for nearly 80 years, their origins (*where*), exact dynamics (*what*) and relationship to brain function has been difficult to assess because signals recorded at the scalp are mixtures of signals from multiple brain generators. Furthermore, the general problem of determining the distribution of brain electrical sources from electromagnetic field patterns recorded on the scalp surface is mathematically underdetermined. Spatial smearing of EEG data by volume conduction does not involve significant time delays, suggesting that Independent Component Analysis is suitable for performing blind source separation on EEG data (Makeig et al., 1996). ICA, applied to multi-channel EEG data, derives independent sources from highly correlated EEG signals statistically and without regard to the physical location or configuration of the source generators. Rather than modeling the EEG as a unitary output of a multidimensional dynamical system, or as "the roar of the crowd" of independent microscopic generators, ICA assumes that the EEG is the output of a number of statistically independent, but spatially fixed, potential-generating systems that may either be spatially restricted or widely distributed (Makeig, Jung, Ghahremani, Bell & Sejnowski, 1997).

In this chapter we outline the assumptions made in standard ICA algorithms, explore its validity for analyzing EEG signals, and review the contributions of this signal-decomposition framework to the EEG community.

8.1   INDEPENDENT COMPONENT ANALYSIS

ICA was originally proposed to solve the blind source separation problem—to recover N source signals, $s = s_{1(t)}, \ldots, s_{N(t)}$, after they are linearly mixed by multiplying by $\mathbf{A}$, an unknown matrix while assuming as little as possible about the natures of $\mathbf{A}$ or the component signals (Cardoso & Laheld, 1996; Cichocki, Unbehauen & Rummert, 1994; Karhunen, Oja, Wang, Vigario & Joutsensalo, 1995; Comon, 1994). The problem can be formulated as follows:

$$\mathbf{x} = \mathbf{A}s + \mathbf{n} \tag{8.1}$$

The observed data is $\mathbf{x}$ and $\mathbf{A}*s$ refers to the mixing of the source signals. $\mathbf{n}$ refers to additive noise such as sensor noise. Due to its generality of describing data generation, there are many physical phenomena that can be described by Equation 8.1. In acoustic environments, $\mathbf{x}$ are recordings from an array of microphones where the acoustic signal sources (s) have been mixed through the environment ($\mathbf{A}$). In cardiac data analysis, $\mathbf{x}$ are recordings from electrodes on the chest providing information about electrical pulse activities in the heart (source signals s); due to simultaneous activations, the electrodes also measure a mixture of heart source signals. Brain activities are also known to be localized in the cortex and sparsely distributed. Electrodes ($\mathbf{x}$) on the scalp measure a combination ($\mathbf{A}$) of simultaneous brain source activities (s).

In general, we are interested in obtaining source signals that are masked by a physical mixing due to the environment. The only information available to us is the observed recording $\mathbf{x}$. In statistics, this problem is also known as a data-generative model with hidden variables s. Specifically, one usually tries to recover a version, $\mathbf{u} = \mathbf{Wx}$, of the original sources, s, identical save for scaling and permutation, by finding a square matrix, $\mathbf{W}$, specifying filters that linearly invert the mixing process.

Although the general form of the mathematical formulation in 8.1 is computationally intractable, there are certain realistic assumptions that can be made leading to practical solutions.

One key assumption in ICA is the statistical independence of source signals. Statistical independence means the joint probability density function (pdf) of the output factorizes:

$$p(s) = \prod_{i=1}^{N} p_i(s_i) \qquad (8.2)$$

while decorrelation, which is common in many other statistical analysis techniques, means only that $< ss^T >$, the covariance matrix of s, is diagonal (here $<>$ means average). Linear mixing of the source signals ($\mathbf{A}*s$) is an important assumption that may or may not be true depending on the physical mixing that occurs. In acoustic environments, the linearity of sound source that get mixed at the microphones is a reasonable assumption that has been verified in many acoustic signal processing applications. There are also several biomedical applications where the linear assumption is approximately correct.

The number of source signals N and the number of sensor signals M is very important in determining the complexity of the solution. In standard ICA algorithms, M is assumed to be greater or equal to N, which means that the matrix $\mathbf{A}$ is invertible (ideally a square matrix) and therefore $\mathbf{W}$ can represent a solution such that the sources can be recovered. In case of M smaller than N, the problem is known as the underdetermined problem. The assumption on the sensor noise $\mathbf{n}$ is usually that it is small and therefore negligible. In most applications, good sensors are available such that electronic noise can be avoided.

The assumptions of independence, linearity, square mixing matrix, and low sensor noise are essential to deriving standard ICA algorithms and can be summarized as follows:

$$p(\mathbf{u}) = \prod_{i=1}^{N} p_i(u_i) \tag{8.3}$$

and

$$\mathbf{u} = \mathbf{W}\mathbf{x} \tag{8.4}$$

The unmixed signals $\mathbf{u} = \mathbf{W}\mathbf{x}$ are estimates of the original sources, s, identical save for scaling and permutation. The recovered signals are found by estimating a square matrix, $\mathbf{W}$, specifying spatial filters that linearly invert the mixing process. The learning algorithm for learning W is commonly accomplished by formulating a cost function and an optimization process. There are many possible cost functions and many more optimization processes. This is one of the main reasons that there are so many different algorithms for solving the blind source separation problem.

There are different viewpoints or cost functions such as information maximization (Nadal & Parga, 1994), maximum likelihood (Pham, 1996; Pearlmutter & Parra, 1996), higher order statistics, or other adaptive filtering techniques that approximate a solution for $\mathbf{W}$. The common factor between those different cost functions are that they are all related to the mutual information cost function (Hyvarinen, Karhunen & Oja, 2002; Lee, Girolami, Bell & Sejnowski, 2000a). Mutual information or Kullback Leibler divergence measures the difference between the joint probability of the estimated source signals and its factorial version (Cover & Thomas, 1991):

$$I(\mathbf{u}) = \int p(\mathbf{u}) \log \frac{p(\mathbf{u})}{\prod_{i=1}^{N} p_i(u_i)} d u \tag{8.5}$$

There are also many optimization methods that can be deployed to estimate W. Gradient ascent or descent techniques are common in information maximization or maximum likelihood approaches (Bell & Sejnowski, 1995b; Lee, Girolami & Sejnowski, 1999), and fixed point optimization such as FastICA (Hyvarinen, Karhunen & Oja, 2002) is also popular due to their simple implementations. Although the assumptions made may be oversimplified or provide only rough approximations of a unknown mixing process, the solutions provided by the standard ICA algorithms are very powerful and wide reaching.

More recently, many new approaches have been proposed to relax some of the ICA assumptions. For example, overcomplete representations (Lewicki & Sejnowski, 2000) can separate more sources from the data than the available number of sensors (Lee, 1998) and Bayesian techniques may be used to estimate the source signals and infer the number of sources (Chan, Lee & Sejnowski, 2002). The simple instantaneous mixing model can be extended to include time delayed and convolved source signals (Lambert, 1996; Lee, 1998; Visser, Otsuka & Lee, 2003; Yellin & Weinstein, 1996). Researchers are also trying to elevate core assumptions such as the linear mixing and independence assumption (Lee, Lewicki & Sejnowski, 2000b).

8.2 THE APPLICATION OF ICA TO EEG DATA

In 1996, Makieg and colleagues (1996) first proposed to apply ICA to multiple-channel EEG activity recorded from the scalp for separating joint problems of source identification and source localization. The method has opened a new window for researchers to study functionally distinct brain sources in response to different cognitive events and/or subject responses by revealing *what* temporally independent activations compose the observed scalp recording, without specifying *where* in the brain these activations arise. In the following sections, we examine the assumptions underlying the application of ICA to EEG and Event-related Potential (ERP) and demonstrate its application to a variety of electrical recordings from the human brain.

8.2.1 Assumptions of ICA Applied to EEG data

The ICA algorithm appears effective (Bell & Sejnowski, 1995a) for performing source separation in domains where (a) summation of different signals at the sensors is linear, (b) propagation delays in the mixing medium are negligible, (c) sources are statistically independent, and (d) the number of independent signal sources is the same as the number of sensors, meaning if we employ N sensors, the ICA algorithm can separate N sources.

In the case of EEG signals, N scalp electrodes pick up correlated signals, and we would like to know what effectively independent components generated these mixtures. Assumptions (a) and (b) are reasonable because source currents carried to the scalp electrodes by volume conduction at EEG frequencies, through cerebrospinal fluid, skull, and scalp, are effectively linear and instantaneous. If we assume that the complexity of EEG dynamics can be modeled, at least in part, as a collection of a modest number of statistically independent brain processes, the EEG source analysis problem satisfies assumption (c). However, assumption (d)—that the EEG is a mixture of exactly N or fewer sources—is questionable, because we do not know the effective number of statistically independent brain signals contributing to the EEG recorded from the scalp. Makieg and colleagues (2002) reported a number of numerical simulations in which 600-point signals recorded from the cortex of a patient during preparation for operation for epilepsy were projected to simulated scalp electrodes through a three-shell spherical head model. They used electrocorticographic (ECoG) data in these simulations as a plausible best approximation to the temporal dynamics of the unknown EEG brain generators. Results confirm that the ICA algorithm could accurately identify the activation waveforms and scalp topographies of relatively large and more temporally-independent ECoG signals from the simulated scalp recordings, even in the presence of multiple low-level and temporally independent sources (synthesized from ECoG data or from uniformly-distributed or Gaussian noise, Makeig et al., 2002).

What are the Independent EEG Components?

For EEG or their counterparts, magenetoencephalographic or event-related flux), the rows of the input matrix, $\mathbf{x}$, are EEG signals recorded at different electrodes, and the columns are measurements recorded at different time points. ICA finds an unmixing matrix, $\mathbf{W}$, that decomposes or linearly unmixes the multi-channel scalp data into a sum of temporally independent and spatially fixed components, $\mathbf{u} = \mathbf{W}\mathbf{x}$. The rows of the output data matrix, $\mathbf{u}$, are time courses of activation of the ICA components. The columns of the inverse matrix, $\mathbf{W}^{-1}$, give the relative projection strengths of the respective components at each of the scalp sensors. These scalp weights give the scalp topography of each component and provide evidence for the components' physiological origins (e.g., eye activity projects mainly to frontal sites). The projection of the ith independent component onto the original data channels is given by the outer product of the ith row of the component activation matrix, $\mathbf{u}$, with the ith column of the inverse unmixing matrix, and is in the original channel locations and units (e.g., μV). Thus, brain activities of interest accounted for by single or multiple components can be obtained by projecting selected ICA component(s) back onto the scalp, $\mathbf{x}_0 = \mathbf{W}^{-1}\mathbf{u}_0$, where $\mathbf{u}_0$ is the matrix of activation waveforms, with rows representing activations of irrelevant component activation(s) set to zero (Jung et al., 1998b).

8.3 CONTRIBUTIONS OF ICA TO EEG/ERP ANALYSIS AND INTERPRETATION

8.3.1 EEG Artifact Removal or Correction

One of the biggest problems in EEG interpretation and analysis is the interference from large and distracting artifacts arising from eye movements, eye blinks, muscle noise, heart signals, and line noise. Asking subjects to fixate a visual target may reduce voluntary eye movements (blinks and saccades) in cooperative subjects during brief EEG sessions, but it does not eliminate involuntary eye movements and cannot be used when the subject is performing a task requiring eye movements. Therefore, data from frontal and temporal electrodes located near the eyes or scalp muscles are often discarded, because these are more heavily contaminated by artifacts than central scalp channels. Another common strategy is to reject all EEG epochs containing artifacts larger than some arbitrarily selected EEG voltage value. However, when limited data are available or when blinks and muscle movements occur too frequently as in children and some patient groups, the amount of data lost to artifact rejection may be unacceptable. For example, Small (1971) reported a visual ERP experiment conducted on autistic children who produced electrooculographic (EOG) artifacts in nearly 100% of the trials. In this case, the presence of large background EEG signals not time- and phase-locked to experimental events may make ERP averages of the few artifact-free trials too unstable to permit useful analysis.

Another approach to reducing contamination from eye movement artifacts is to regress out reference signals collected near the eyes. Regression methods have been proposed using both time-domain (Hill-yard & Galambos, 1970; Verleger, Gasser & Mocks, 1982) and frequency-domain techniques (Whitton, Lue & Moldofsky, 1978; Woestenburg, Verbaten & Slangen, 1983). All regression methods, whether in time or frequency domains, depend on having one or more clean reference channels (e.g., one or more EOG channels), which cannot be further analyzed after regression. However, these methods share an inherent weakness, in that both eye movements and EEG signals propagate to periocular (EOG) sites. Therefore, regression-based artifact removal procedures also eliminate neural activity common to the reference and other frontal electrodes. Because the regression coefficients are deter-mined largely by the typically large EOG signals, regression methods may also introduce neural activity projecting to the reference channel into other sites (Jung et al., 2000a).

In this application, ICA assumes that EEG data recorded at mul-tiple scalp sensors are a linear sum at the scalp electrodes of acti-vations generated by distinct neural and artifactual sources and the time series of neural and artifactual sources are statistically inde-pendent (Jung et al., 1998a, 1998b, 2000a,b; Makeig et al., 1996b; Vigário, 1997). ICA derives spatial filters with fixed scalp distri-butions and maximally independent time courses to decompose the artifact-contaminated EEG data into a sum of temporally independent components. Our confidence in ICA decomposition of EEG sig-nals is strengthened by the fact that topographic projections (scalp maps) of ICA components tend to have few spatial maxima, sug-gesting a few localized brain sources compared with those of most principal components derived by principal component analysis (PCA, Jung et al., 1998a, 1998b, 2000a,b), which have more complex spatial patterns (Silberstein & Cadusch, 1992), probably due to the spatial orthogonality imposed on the component maps by PCA. Although ICA also imposes a strong criterion (temporal statistical indepen-dence) on the components, ICA does not impose any condition on the spatial filters. As a result, spatial filters derived by ICA are not affected by each other and can collect concurrent activity arising from any spatially overlapping source distributions.

Figure 8.1 shows a 3-sec portion of the recorded EEG time series collected from 29 scalp electrodes placed according to the modified In-ternational 10-20 System and from two EOG placements, all referred

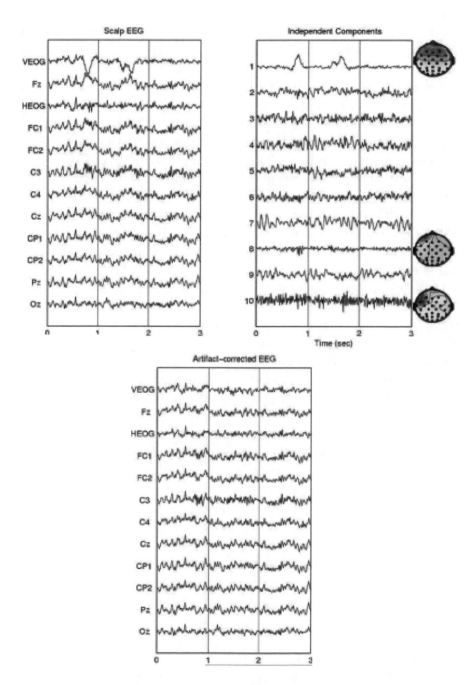

Fig. 8.1: Demonstration of EEG artifact removal by ICA. (A) A 3-sec portion of an EEG time series containing two prominent blinks. (B) Corresponding ICA component activations and scalp maps of ten components accounting for brain activity and artifacts. (C) EEG signals corrected for artifacts by removing the three selected ICA components

to the left mastoid. The sampling rate was 256 Hz. Only twelve of 31 channels are shown in the figure. Figure 8.1B shows the 10 of derived 31 ICA component activations and the scalp topographies for three selected ICA components. The eye blink artifact was isolated to ICA components 1 and 8. Component 10 evidently represented muscle noise from temporal and frontal muscles. The 'corrected' EEG signals obtained by removing the three selected (EOG and muscle noise) components from the data are shown in Figure 8.1C. After eliminating these three artifactual components, by zeroing out the corresponding rows of the activation matrix **u** and projecting the remaining components onto the scalp electrodes, the 'corrected' EEG data (Figure 8.1C) were free of both EOG and muscle artifacts.

ICA-based artifact correction has at least four advantages compared with other artifact removal methods (Jung et al., 2000a,b): (a) ICA simultaneously separates EEG signals including artifacts into independent components based on the characteristics of the data, without relying on the availability of one or more clean reference channels for each type of artifact. This avoids the problem of mutual contamination between regressing and regressed channels. (b) ICA is generally applicable for removal of a wide variety of EEG artifacts. Separate analyses are not required to remove different classes of artifacts. Once the training is complete, artifact-free EEG records in all channels can then be derived by simultaneously eliminating the contributions of various identified artifactual sources in the EEG record. (c) ICA-based artifact removal can preserve all of the recorded trials, a crucial advantage over rejection-based methods when limited data are available, or when blinks and muscle movements occur too frequently, as in some patient groups. (d) Unlike regression methods, ICA-based artifact removal can preserve data at all scalp channels, including frontal and periocular sites.

8.3.2   Decomposition of Functionally Distinct Brain Sources from Unaveraged Single-Trial ERPs

ERPs are the portion of the EEG both time- and phase-locked to experimental events or subject responses. Through time-locked averaging across a set of equivalent experimental events, EEG activity not both time- and phase-locked to event onsets is removed by phase cancellation. What remains is called the event-related potential. Single-trial ERP data are usually averaged prior to analysis to increase their signal/noise relative to non-time and -phase locked electroencephalographic (EEG) activity and non-neural artifacts. However, response averaging ignores the fact that response activity may vary widely between trials in both time course and scalp distribution. This temporal and spatial variability may in fact reflect changes in subject performance or subject state (possibly linked to changes in attention, arousal, task strategy, or other factors). Thus, conventional averaging methods may not be suitable for investigating brain dynamics arising from intermittent changes in subject state and/or from complex interactions between task events (Jung et al., 2001b). Further, response averaging makes possibly unwarranted assumptions about the relationship between ERP features and the dynamics of the ongoing EEG (Jung et al., 2001b).

Analysis of single event-related trial epochs may potentially reveal more information about event-related brain dynamics than simple response averaging, but faces three signal processing challenges: (a) difficulties in identifying and removing artifacts associated with blinks, eye movements, and muscle noise, which are a serious problem for EEG interpretation and analysis; (b) poor signal-to-noise ratio arising from the fact that non-phase-locked EEG activities are often larger than phase-locked response components; and (c) trial-to-trial variability in latencies and amplitudes of both event-related responses and endogenous EEG components (Jung et al., 2001b). Additional interest in analysis of single-trial event-related EEG (or MEG) epochs comes from the realization that filtering out time- and phase-locked activity (by response averaging) isolates only a small subset of the actual event-related brain dynamics of the EEG signals themselves (Makeig & Inlow, 1993; Makeig et al., 2002, 2004).

Figure 8.2 shows the results of the analysis of unaveraged single-trial ERPs. In this example, the EEG/EOG data were collected from a 31 year-old normal subject performing a spatial shift-attention task during which the subject was instructed to attend to one of five squares continuously displayed on a back background 0.8 cm above a centrally located fixation point. The (1.6 x 1.6 cm) squares were positioned horizontally at angles of $0° \pm 2.7°$ and $\pm 5.5°$ in the visual field $2°$ above from the point of fixation. Four squares were outlined in blue while one, marking the attended location, was outlined in green. The location of the attended location was counterbalanced across trial blocks. Stimuli were filled circles and the subject was required to press a right-hand held thumb button as soon as possible following stimuli presented in the attended location. EEG data were collected from 29 scalp electrodes mounted in a standard electrode cap (Electrocap, Inc.) at locations based on a modified International 10-20 System, and from two periocular electrodes placed below the right eye and at the left outer can thus. Data were sampled at 512 Hz within an analog pass band of .01-50 Hz. Although the subject was instructed to fixate the central cross during each 72-sec block, he tended to blink or move his eyes slightly towards target stimuli presented at peripheral locations. Please see Jung et. al. (2001b) for details of the experiments.

To visualize collections of single-trial EEG records, ERP image plots (Jung et al., 1999, 2001b) are useful and often reveal unexpected inter-trial consistencies and variations. Figure 8.2A shows all 652 single-trial ERP epochs recorded from the subject time-locked to onsets of target stimuli (left vertical line). Single-trial event-related EEG epochs recorded at a frontal (Fz), the vertex (Cz), a central parietal (Pz), and an occipital (Oz) site are plotted as color-coded horizontal traces (see color bar) sorted in order of the subject's reaction time latencies (thick black line). The ERP average of these trials is plotted below the ERP image.

ICA, applied to these 652 31-channel concatenated 1-sec EEG records in respond to stimuli presented at the attended locations, separated out: (a) artifact components arising from blinks or eye movements (Figure 8.2B), whose contributions could be removed from the EEG records by subtracting the component projection from the data (Jung et al., 1998b, 2000b, 2001b); (b) EEG components whose activities were either unaffected by experimental events or were affected in ways not revealed by these measures (Figure 8.2C); (c) components showing stimulus time-locked potential fluctuations of consistent polarity many or all trials (Figure 8.2D); (d) components showing response-locked activity covarying in latency with subject response times (Figure 8.2E); (e) components having prominent alpha band (8-12 Hz) activity whose inter-trial coherence (Figure 8.2F, lower middle panel, bottom trace), measuring phase-locking to stimulus onsets, increased significantly after stimulus presentation, even in the absence of any alpha band power increase (middle trace); and (f) mu-rhythm components (Makeig et al., 2000) at approximately 10 Hz that decreased in amplitude when the subject responds (Figure 8.2G). This taxonomy could not have been obtained from signal averaging or other conventional frequency-domain approaches.

Better understanding of trial-to-trial changes in brain responses may allow a better understanding of normal human performance in repetitive tasks and a more detailed study of changes in cognitive dynamics in normal, brain-damaged, diseased, aged, or genetically abnormal individuals. ICA-based analysis allows identification and segregation of spatially-overlapping event-related EEG activities that may show a variety of distinct relationships to task events. ICA also allows investigation of the interaction between phenomena seen in ERP records and its origins in the ongoing EEG. Contrary to the common supposition that ERPs are brief stereotyped responses elicited by some events and independent of ongoing background EEG activity, many ERP features may be generated by ongoing EEG processes (Makeig et al., 2002, 2004). ICA may thus help researchers to take fuller advantage of what until now has been an only partially-realized strength of event-related paradigms—the ability to examine systematic relationships between single trials within subjects (Jung et al., 2001b,a; Makeig et al., 2002, 2004).

8.3.3 Source localization

As mentioned earlier, EEG data collected from any point on the scalp may include activity from multiple processes occurring within a large brain volume. This has made it difficult to localize the sources of the EEG signals. Furthermore, the general problem of determining the distribution of brain electrical sources from electromagnetic field patterns recorded on the scalp surface is mathematically underdetermined. For several decades, ERP and EEG researchers have proposed a number of techniques to localize the sources of brain potentials, either by assuming a known or simple spatial configuration (Scherg & Von Cramon, 1986) or by restricting generator dipoles to lie within and point outward from the cortical surface (Liu, Belliveau & Dale, 1998).

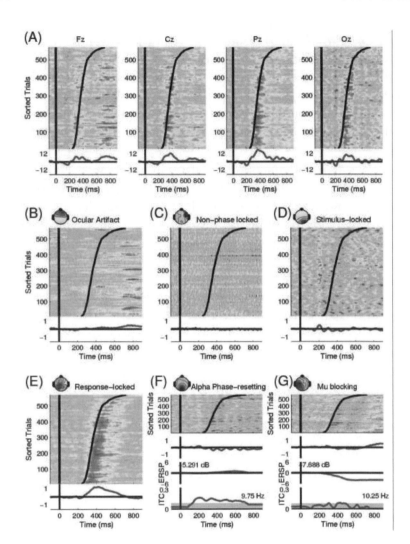

Fig. 8.2: ERP-image plots of correctly responded target response data from a visual selective attention experiment and various independent component categories. (A) Single-trial ERPs recorded at a frontal (Fz), a central (Cz), a parietal (Pz)and an occipital (Oz) electrode from a normal subject and time-locked to onsets of visual target stimuli (left thin vertical line) with superimposed subject response times (RT). (B-G) Single-trial activations of sample independent components accounting for eye blink artifacts, non-phase locked, stimulus-locked and response-locked ERP activities, stimulus phase-reset alpha and response-blocked oscillatory mu activities.

Makeig and colleagues (1996) noted that ICA could be used to separate the problem of EEG (or magneto-encephalography) source identification from the problem of source localization. That is, ICA tells *what* temporally independent activations compose the collected scalp recordings without specifying directly *where* in the brain these activations arise. By separating the contributions of different brain and non-brain sources to the data, however, ICA is also proving to be an efficient preprocessing step prior to source localization (Zhukov, Weinstein & Johnson, 2000). As noted earlier, the columns of the inverse matrix, W^{-1}, give the relative projection strengths of the respective components at each of the scalp sensors. In this model, the ratio of potentials across all the scalp electrodes for each component is fixed, but the real intensity (or potential) is modulated by the corresponding time course of component, the rows of the output data matrix, u. For each component, which should involve one brain or extra-brain network, one can employ inverse solution technique to localize the sources of the activity.

Figure 8.3 shows sample source locations of ICA-preprocessed EEG data. The localization(s) and orientation(s) of equivalent dipole(s) of the ICA components accounting for stimulus-locked and response-locked event-related activities from an autistic subject performing the visual selective attention task as described above were estimated by BESA separately and plotted on the averaged MRI templates. As can be seen, all the scalp topographies of these components can be well fit by a single equivalent dipole (residual variance: 4.65% and 8.05%, respectively), suggesting that its source might be a small patch of unknown size in left medial occipital cortex.

8.4   SUMMARY AND DISCUSSION

ICA of single-trial or averaged ERP data allows blind separation of multichannel complex EEG data into a sum of temporally independent and spatially fixed components. Our results show that ICA can separate artifactual, stimulus-locked, response-locked, and non-event-related background EEG activities into separate components, allowing:

1. Removal of pervasive artifacts of all types from single-trial EEG

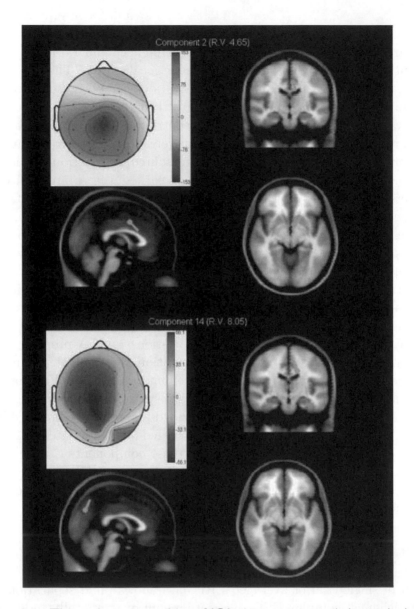

Fig. 8.3: The scalp topographies of ICA components and the equivalent dipole models. The scalp topographies of ICA components accounting for (A) Response-locked and (B) Stimulus-locked activities in unaveraged single-trial ERPs and their equivalent dipoles were obtained by BESA based on a 3-shell spherical head models and overplotted on an MRI template from the MNI database (Montreal Neurological Institute (MNI), Quebec).

records, making possible analysis of highly contaminated EEG records from clinical populations.

2. Identification and segregation of stimulus-, response-locked event-related and event-modulated oscillatory activities in single-trail EEG epochs.

3. Separation of spatially-overlapping EEG activities over the entire scalp and frequency band that may show a variety of distinct relationships to task events, rather than focusing on activity at single frequencies in single scalp channels or channel pairs.

4. Investigation of the interaction between ERPs and ongoing EEG.

5. Better estimation of locations of the sources of EEG signals.

We have also employed component-matching clustering analysis that automatically grouped components from 23 normal controls having similar scalp maps and power spectra. The results show that components accounting for blink, eye movements, temporal muscle activity, event-related activity, and event-modulated mu and alpha activities were similar across subjects (Jung et al., 2001b; Makeig et al., 2004).

Although ICA appears to be generally useful for EEG and fMRI analysis, it also has some inherent limitations. First, ICA can decompose at most N sources from data collected at N scalp electrodes. Usually, the effective number of statistically-independent signals contributing to the scalp EEG is unknown, and it is likely that observed brain activity arises from more physically separable effective sources than the available number of EEG electrodes. Second, the assumption of temporal independence used by ICA cannot be satisfied when the training data set is small or when separate topographically distinguishable phenomena nearly always co-occur in the data. Thus, training data for ICA should always include sufficient information that exhibits distinct reactivities to experimental events or subject responses to allow ICA to extract functionally independent brain signals.

Although results of applying ICA to EEG and ERP data have already shown great promise and given new insights into brain function, the analysis of these results is still in its infancy. They must be validated using other direct or convergent evidence (such as behavior and/or other physiological measurements) before we can interpret their functional significance. Current research on ICA algorithms is focused on incorporating domain-specific constraints into the ICA framework. This would allow information maximization to be applied to the precise form and statistics of biomedical data.

References

Bell, A. J. & Sejnowski, T. J. (1995a). An information-maximization approach to blind separation and blind deconvolution. *Neural Computation*, *7*, 1129–1159.

Bell, A. J. & Sejnowski, T. J. (1995b). Fast blind separation based on information theory. In *Proc. 1995 Intern. Symp. on Nonlinear Theory and Applications (NOLTA)*.

Cardoso, J. F. & Laheld, B. (1996). Equivariant adaptive source separation. *IEEE Trans. on Signal Processing*, *45(2)*, 434–444.

Chan, K.-L., Lee, T.-W. & Sejnowski, T. (2002). Variational learning of clusters of undercomplete nonsymmetric independent components. *Journal of Machine Learning Research*, *3*, 99–114.

Cichocki, A., Unbehauen, R. & Rummert, E. (1994). Robust learning algorithm for blind separation of signals. *Electronics Letters*, *30(17)*, 1386–1387.

Comon, P. (1994). Independent component analysis: A new concept? *Signal Processing*, *36(3)*, 287–314.

Cover, T. M. & Thomas, J. A. (1991). *Elements of Information Theory*. John Wiley.

Hillyard, S. A. & Galambos, R. (1970). Eye-movement artifact in the CNV. *Electroencephalog. Clinical Neurophysiology*, *28(2)*, 173–182.

Hyvarinen, A., Karhunen, J. & Oja, E. (2002). *Independent Component Analysis*. John Wiley and Sons.

Jung, T.-P., Humphries, C., Lee, T., Makeig, S., McKeown, M., Iragui, V. & Sejnowski, T. J. (1998a). Removing electroencephalographic artifacts : Comparison between ICA and PCA. *Neural Networks for Signal Processing, VIII*, 63–72.

Jung, T.-P., Humphries, C., Lee, T., Makeig, S., McKeown, M., Iragui, V. & Sejnowski, T. J. (1998b). Extended ICA removes artifacts from electroencephalographic data. *Advances in Neural Information Processing Systems, 10*, 894–900.

Jung, T.-P., Makeig, S., Humphries, C., Lee, T., McKeown, M. J., Iragui, V. & Sejnowski, T. J. (2000a). Removing electroencephalographic artifacts by blind source separation. *Psychophysiology, 37*, 163–178.

Jung, T. P., Makeig, S., McKeown, M. J., Bell, A. J., Lee, T. W. & Sejnowski, T. J. (2001a). Imaging brain dynamics using independent component analysis. *Proceedings of the IEEE, 89(7)*, 1107–1122.

Jung, T.-P., Makeig, S., Westerfield, M., Townsend, J., Courchesne, E. & Sejnowski, T. J. (2000b). Removal of eye activity artifacts from visual event-related potentials in normal and clinical subjects. *Clinical Neurophysiology, 111*, 1745–1758.

Jung, T. P., Makeig, S., Westerfield, M., Townsend, J., Courchesne, E. & Sejnowski, T. J. (2001b). Analysis and visualization of single-trial event-related potentials. *Human Brain Mapping, 14(3)*, 166–185.

Jung, T.-P., Makeig, S., Westerfield, S., Townsend, J., Courchesne, E. & Sejnowski, T. J. (1999). Analyzing and visualizing single-trial event-related potentials. *Advances in Neural Information Processing Systems, 11*, 118–124.

Karhunen, J., Oja, E., Wang, L., Vigario, R. & Joutsensalo, J. (1995). A class of neural networks for independent component analysis. report a28. Technical report, Helsinki Univ. of Technology.

Lambert, R. (1996). Multichannel blind deconvolution: FIR matrix algebra and separation of multipath mixtures. Master's thesis, University of Southern California.

Lee, T.-W. (1998). *Independent Component Analysis: Theory and Applications*. Kluwer Academic Publishers.

Lee, T. W., Girolami, M., Bell, A. J. & Sejnowski, T. J. (2000a). A unifying information-theoretic framework for independent component analysis. *Computers and Mathematics with Applications, 39*, 1–21.

Lee, T. W., Girolami, M. & Sejnowski, T. J. (1999). Independent component analysis using an extended infomax algorithm for mixed subgaussian and supergaussian sources. *Neural Computation, 11*, 417–441.

Lee, T. W., Lewicki, M. S. & Sejnowski, T. J. (2000b). Unsupervised classification with non-gaussian sources and automatic context switching in blind signal separation. *IEEE Transactions on Pattern Analysis and Machine Intelligence, 22(10)*, 1078–1089.

Lewicki, M. S. & Sejnowski, T. J. (2000). Learning overcomplete representations. *Neural Computation, 12*, 337–365.

Liu, A., Belliveau, J. & Dale, A. (1998). Spatiotemporal imaging of human brain activity using functional mri constrained magnetoencephalography data: Monte carlo simulations. *Proceedings of the National Academy of Sciences U S A, 95*, 8945–8950.

Makeig, S., Bell, A. J., Jung, T.-P. & Sejnowski, T. J. (1996). Independent component analysis if electroencephelographic data. In D. Touretsky, M. Mozer & M. Hasselmo (Eds.), *Advances in Neural Information Processing Systems*, Volume 8 (pp. 145–151). Cambridge, MA: MIT.

Makeig, S., Delorme, A., Westerfield, M., Jung, T. P., Townsend, J., Courchense, E. & Sejnowski, J. (2004). Electroencephalographic brain dynamics following visual targets requiring manual responses. *PLoS Biology, 2(6)*, 747–762.

Makeig, S., Enghoff, S., Jung, T. P. & Sehnowski, T. J. (2000). A natural basis for brain-actuated control. *IEEE Transactions on Rehabilitation Engineering, 8*, 208–211.

Makeig, S. & Inlow, M. (1993). Lapses in alertness: Coherence of fluctuations in performance and EEG spectrum. *Electroencephalogr. Clinical Neurophysiology, 86,* 23–35.

Makeig, S., Jung, T.-P., Ghahremani, D., Bell, A. J. & Sejnowski, T. J. (1997). Blind separation of event-related brain responses into independent components. *Proceedings of the National Academy of Sciences USA, 94,* 10979–10984.

Makeig, S., Jung, T. P., Ghahremani, D. & Sejnowski, T. J. (1996b). Independent component analysis of simulated ERP data. Technical report inc-9606, Institute for Neural Computation, University of California, San Diego, CA.

Makeig, S., Westerfield, M., Jung, T. P., Townsend, J., Courchesne, E. & Sejnowski, T. J. (2002). Electroencephalographic sources of visual evoked responses. *Science, 295,* 690–694.

McKeown, M. J., Makeig, S., Brown, G. G., Jung, T.-P., Kinderman, S. S. & Sejnowski, T. J. (1998). Analysis of fMRI by blind separation into independent spatial components. *Human Brain Mapping, 6(3),* 160–188.

Nadal, J. P. & Parga, N. (1994). Non-linear neurons in the low noise limit: a factorial code maximises information transfer. *Network, 5,* 565–581.

Pearlmutter, B. A. & Parra, L. C. (1996). A context-sensitive generalization of ICA. In *International Conference on Neural Information Processing, Hong Kong* (pp. 151–157).

Pham, D. T. (1996). Blind separation of instantaneous mixture of sources via an independent component analysis. *IEEE Trans. Signal Proc., 44(11),* 2768–2779.

Scherg, M. & Von Cramon, D. (1986). Evoked dipole source potentials of the human auditory cortex. *Electroencephalography Clinical Neurophysiology, 65,* 344–601.

Silberstein, R. B. & Cadusch, P. J. (1992). Measurement processes and spatial principal components analysis. *Brain Topography, 4(4),* 267–276.

Small, J. G. (1971). Sensory evoked responses of autistic children. *Infantile Autism* (pp. 224–239).

Verleger, R., Gasser, T. & Mocks, J. (1982). Correction of EOG artifacts in event-related potentials of EEG: Aspects of reliability and validity. *Psychophysiology, 19(4)*, 472–480.

Vigário, R. N. (1997). Extraction of ocular artifacts from EEG using independent component analysis. *Electroencephalog Clinical Neurophysiology, 103*, 395–404.

Visser, E., Otsuka, M. & Lee, T. W. (2003). A spatio-temporal speech enhancement scheme for robust speech recognition in noisy environments. *Speech Communications, 41(2-3)*, 393–407.

Whitton, J. L., Lue, F. & Moldofsky, H. (1978). A spectral method for removing eye-movement artifacts from the EEG. *Electroencephalog Clinical Neurophysiology, 44*, 735–741.

Woestenburg, J. C., Verbaten, M. N. & Slangen, J. L. (1983). The removal of the eye-movement artifact from the EEG by regression analysis in the frequency domain. *Biological Psychology, 16*, 127–147.

Yellin, D. & Weinstein, E. (1996). Multichannel signal separation: Methods and analysis. *IEEE Trans. Signal Proceedings, 44(1)*, 106–118.

Zhukov, L., Weinstein, D. & Johnson, C. (2000). Independent component analysis for EEG source localization. *IEEE Engineering in Medicine and Biology Magazine, 19*, 87–96.

Author Index

Subject Index

A

Acetylcholine
  and attention, 81–83
  and consolidation of information,
    83–87
  and encoding, 75–77
  and feedback suppression, 77–79
  and long-term potentiation, 79
  and modulation of inhibitory neurons,
    67–70
  and spiking activity, 60–62, 79–81
  and suppression of excitatory feedback,
    62–67
  and theta rhythm, 87
  and volume transmission, 70–74
Advertising, 135–136
Afferent input, 60–62
Aging, cognitive, 1–4
Alzheimer's disease
  BSS/GCA diagnostic methods,
    219–226
  and memory chain model, 141, 144
  neuropsychometric measures of, 4–9
  usefulness of early diagnosis, 218–219
  vs. mild cognitive impairment, 2–4
  vs. vascular dementia, 226–227
Alzheimer's Disease Assessment Scale, 8
Amari's performance index, 251
Amnesia
  difficulty of modeling, 119
  memory chain model, 138–145
  in semantic dementia, 146
  TraceLink model, 126, 136–138
AMUSE algorithm, 215, 222, 224, 235–236
Animal models, 149
Animal studies, relevance of, 19
Apoliprotein E (apoE), 3, 6–7

Artifact removal, 319–322
Attention, 81–83
Auditory spatial attention, 176–178
Auditory Verbal Learning Test, 3
Autobiographical memory, 136

B

Back-propagation networks, 123
Balanced contributions property, 167
Balloon model, 40–41
Bayesian techniques, 317
Behavioral response to neural activation
  max activation model, 47–50
  overview, 42–44
  threshold model, 44–47
Blind source separation (BSS)
  and Alzheimer's disease diagnosis,
    219–226
  basic approaches, 207–210
  and independent component analysis,
    313–314
  and preprocessing of EEG and EMG
    recordings, 211–218
  and spatio-temporal decorrelation,
    234–236
  theoretical foundations, 201–206
  using linear predictability and adaptive
    band pass filters, 236–241
  validity for real-world data, 249–251
  vs. generalized component analysis,
    221
BOLD signal
  linear models, 34–39
  nonlinear models, 39–42
  overview, 33–34

347